Comprehensive Healthcare Simulation

Series Editors

Adam I. Levine
Department of Anesthesiology
Mount Sinai Medical Center
New York, USA

Samuel DeMaria Jr.
Department of Anesthesiology
Mount Sinai Medical Center
New York, USA

More information about this series at http://www.springer.com/series/13029

John T. Paige
Shirley C. Sonesh
Deborah D. Garbee
Laura S. Bonanno
Editors

Comprehensive Healthcare Simulation: InterProfessional Team Training and Simulation

Springer

Editors
John T. Paige
Department of Surgery
Louisiana State University (LSU) Health
New Orleans School of Medicine
New Orleans, LA
USA

Deborah D. Garbee
Associate Dean for Professional Practice
Community Service and Advanced
Nursing Practice
Professor of Clinical Nursing
LSUHSC School of Nursing
New Orleans, LA
USA

Shirley C. Sonesh
Organizational Psychologist
Sonnenschein Consulting, LLC
New Orleans, LA
USA

Laura S. Bonanno
Nurse Anesthesia Program Director
Louisiana State University (LSU) Health
School of Nursing
New Orleans, LA
USA

ISSN 2366-4479 ISSN 2366-4487 (electronic)
Comprehensive Healthcare Simulation
ISBN 978-3-030-28844-0 ISBN 978-3-030-28845-7 (eBook)
https://doi.org/10.1007/978-3-030-28845-7

This Springer imprint is published by the registered company Springer Nature Switzerland AG
The registered company address is: Gewerbestrasse 11, 6330 Cham, Switzerland

To our families, for their support and inspiration, and to all our health professional students. We hope that this work will help foster interprofessional teamwork and collaboration in order to improve the quality of care for all patients.

Foreword I

While many simulation activities started out being addressed to participants from a single discipline, with at most cursory involvement or mention of interprofessional clinical teams, there has been growing realization of the critical importance of simulation-based interprofessional education (IPE) for healthcare workforce development and clinical teamwork. A variety of simulation curricula promote that they address IPE, but actually the term – along with others that are similar in thrust, if not identical (e.g., interdisciplinary, multidisciplinary) – can mean a host of different things. In fact, IPE cuts across a huge swath of the 11 (sometimes 12) "dimensions of simulation" activities that I articulated originally in 2004. Some underlying core principles of IPE may be roughly constant across the dimensions (e.g., experiential learning theory; respect for all participant professions), but others will vary particularly depending on the participant populations' level of experience (e.g., early clinical students/trainees vs. experienced clinicians), clinical professions (e.g., nurses, physicians, allied health professionals, clergy, clerks, technicians), goals of the activity (e.g., team-building, team training, systems probing), and many others. Further, these dimensions will strongly influence exactly how simulation activities will be conducted. There is a saying (now attributed to Yale Class of 1882 student, Benjamin Brewster) "In theory there is no difference between theory and practice, while in practice there is." Surely, the details of a simulation activity – the, as we like to say, "Journalism 101″ view, the "who, what, why, where, when… and how" – will greatly influence what each particular IPE curriculum or session looks like.

Hence, with the great and growing interest in simulation-based IPE, and the substantial variation with the simulation community of what it means and how it is conducted, it is appropriate that a textbook on simulation-based IPE should come out at this time. No book, regardless of how many chapters, and indeed no batch of dozens or hundreds of journal papers or conference presentations, can cover the entire spectrum of issues concerning IPE. This book does a good job of addressing a large number of them. The authors are highly qualified and experienced in the area they address. Of course, the field of IPE is vast, and hearing from a finite number of experts means that there will still be more to learn from others as well.

To use some culinary metaphors – admittedly that I've also used before about some other works because the parallels seem so apt – one could describe this book as a buffet presenting dishes from a variety of skilled chefs. This book is clearly not intended to be read in its entirety, and surely not in one fell swoop. No one can eat a meal consisting of every dish created by dozens of master chefs (holiday dinners notwithstanding), nor is every dish (i.e., chapter) relevant to each person's own taste (i.e., interests). But nearly all readers will find much of interest, usually to agree with, occasionally to disagree with, or to trigger debate. Overall, plenty are useful for improving the extent and quality of simulation-based IPE for the future benefit of clinicians and patients. And that, in the end, is what our simulation community is really all about.

Bon appétit!

David M. Gaba, MD
Professor of Anesthesia, Perioperative, and Pain Medicine
Associate Dean for Immersive and Simulation-based Learning
Founding Editor-in-Chief, Simulation in Healthcare
Stanford University School of Medicine, Stanford, CA, USA

Foreword II

Forty years ago, I entered a Bachelor of Science in Nursing program with the intention of caring for and improving the lives of the patients I would have the privilege to serve. I have since gone on to complete two advanced degrees: one for an Advanced Practice Nursing role (CRNA) and the other in Public Health. Upon reflection, I am struck by the "silo" nature of each of these educational programs as I pursued development of knowledge, skill, and confidence in focused areas of study. I, of course, had the opportunity to interact with many other professional roles through these educational experiences and in my parallel clinical practice, but little attention was devoted toward helping me understand how my role should interface with the other professionals with whom I worked. Perhaps more importantly, my understanding of how to collaborate with other professionals to improve the care of patients had to be learned on the job and through trial and error. More than 25 years ago, I began my simulation career with an initial focus on skill training and anesthesia crisis resource management (ACRM). At the time, we relied on the groundbreaking simulation textbook by Dr. David Gaba and coauthors which described how to manage crisis events which occur in the OR and how to think about the process and organize our efforts as a team. Recognizing the importance of crisis management in the training of anesthesiologists and nurse anesthetists, we created a course that we continue to offer to interprofessional anesthesia trainee teams on an annual basis at WISER. This was my first foray into interprofessional education, and over the intervening years, I have seen interest in the concept of interprofessional education (IPE), and the companion concept of interprofessional collaboration (IPC) grows from an idea germinated in the simulation and patient safety movements to an accepted "next step" in the pursuit of higher-quality patient care.

Professional organizations, educational institutions, healthcare leaders, and hospital systems all now agree that enhancing the function of interprofessional teams is important toward improving the healthcare working environment and the quality of care. This interest and agreement is seen in the United States and across the world. A primary problem that I have encountered in my national and international faculty development work is that educators at the undergraduate, graduate, and practicing professional levels struggle to overcome the challenges associated with planning and organizing interprofessional learning activities. As such, the publication of *Interprofessional Team Training and Simulation* is especially timely and important in today's healthcare environment. Authored by an extraordinary interprofessional team of simulation and safety experts, the textbook includes theory, best practices, planning and implementation strategies, and examples of successful courses. This robust resource has the potential to break down barriers and impact the development of effective and efficient simulation-based IPE courses nationally and internationally.

John M. O'Donnell, DrPH, MSN, RN, CRNA, CHSE, FSSH
Professor and Chair, Department of Nurse Anesthesia
University of Pittsburgh School of Nursing
Program Director, Nurse Anesthesia Program
Senior Associate Director, Winter Institute for Simulation
Education and Research (WISER)
Pittsburgh, PA, USA

Foreword III

Effective interprofessional, collaborative practice is essential to providing high-quality and safe surgical care. Roles and responsibilities of various professionals need to be defined in this context and should form the basis for exemplary teamwork. Such interprofessional, collaborative practice requires individuals from different professions to train together, and simulation can be very helpful in supporting such training. Published research has demonstrated the value of simulation-based interprofessional team training in improving the quality of surgical care and enhancing patient safety.

This book is a major contribution to the field of simulation-based interprofessional team training. It defines the underpinnings and theoretical constructs, describes specific approaches to implementing the training, and provides information on establishing a state-of-the-art simulation center. Team training aimed at learners across the continuum of professional development is then addressed. Finally, implementation of interprofessional training focusing on teamwork in specific settings, including the operating room, labor and delivery rooms, critical care settings, and prehospital care, is covered.

This book addresses a range of important topics in the field of simulation-based interprofessional team training. Surgeons, members of interprofessional teams, surgical trainees, and medical students should all find this book helpful in their work. Faculty at simulation centers should find the book useful in implementing effective simulation-based interprofessional team training programs. Also, the approaches described could be used effectively in surgery residency training and medical student education. I believe this book is a very valuable contribution to the literature on this important subject. Implementation of strategies articulated in this book should help to advance both surgical care and surgical training.

Ajit K. Sachdeva, MD, FACS, FRCSC, FSACME
Director, Division of Education
Chair, ACS Program for Accreditation of Education Institutes
American College of Surgeons
Chicago, IL, USA

Preface

In today's dynamic, complex, and interconnected healthcare system, effective teamwork is essential for safe, quality care. Without it, even the latest, most advanced technologies and newest, streamlined processes cannot compensate. In essence, high reliability in healthcare requires highly reliable teams that are able to adapt quickly and seamlessly to ever-changing conditions in care environments in which decisions can have life or death consequences.

Fortunately, the importance of teams and teamwork in healthcare has grown in prominence over the last half-decade with the acknowledgment of the need for interprofessional education (IPE) to foster team interaction and function. The ability to bring together diverse professions to learn with, from, and about each other during team training is a powerful tool in helping to promote the team orientation, mutual support, communication, and coordination necessary for quality patient care.

Improving team dynamics and teamwork using IPE can take many forms. One of the most effective modalities, however, is with simulation-based training (SBT). Its advantages are well-known and manifold, especially its immersive, experiential qualities that permit the consequences of decisions and actions to unfold without risking harm to a patient. Additionally, SBT provides participants the opportunity to identify and treat rare, high-risk conditions and disease processes again and again in order to optimize care in the clinical environment.

Developing, designing, and implementing beneficial IPE programs employing SBT are often challenging endeavors, especially for individuals approaching such tasks for the first time. In order to assist those fortunate souls charged with this important undertaking, we present this latest edition to the *Comprehensive Healthcare Simulation series: Interprofessional Team Training and Simulation*. Our goal in editing this volume is to provide an approachable resource that combines theory, first principles, and applications in a pragmatic, helpful format that enables widespread adoption of IPE using SBT.

To this end, we have brought together a wide range of experts from a variety of professions in healthcare and beyond as contributors to *Interprofessional Team Training and Simulation*, dividing the work into four major parts: (1) Theories and Concepts, (2) Nuts and Bolts, (3) Perspectives of IPE, and (4) Application of Simulation-Based IPE in Clinical Practice. Such a division allows readers to access information related to key aspects of IPE incorporating SBT quickly and efficiently.

In addition, it expands the potential audience by providing important information related to IPE and SBT in general.

Part I of *Interprofessional Team Training and Simulation* provides a theoretical and conceptual framework with which to understand and approach IPE with SBT. In Chap. 1, Zajac, Woods, Dunkin, and Salas address the importance of effective simulation in improving patient care. Chap. 2, by Gregory, then discusses key components of interprofessional education and training. In Chap. 3, Hughes reviews theoretical concepts related to human factors in healthcare and its role in SBT for IPE. Chapter 4 follows in which Feitosa and Fonseca tackle theories related to teamwork and optimizing its training in healthcare. Part I closes with a discussion by Keebler on the essentials of debriefing and its importance to effective training.

With this foundation of key concepts and theories completed, Part II of *Interprofessional Team Training and Simulation* addresses the nitty-gritty details necessary for successful implementation of IPE making use of SBT. Benishek, Lazzara, and Sonesh begin this part with Chap. 6, in which they address challenges and solutions unique to conducting interprofessional, simulation-based training. Chapter 7, by Black, then provides insight in successfully building a simulation-based IPE program. Gardner, DeSandro, Pillow, and Ahmed lend insight into how to optimize in situ simulation-based interprofessional sessions in Chap. 8. Following this discussion, Webster, Tan, Unger, and Lazzara provide advice related to assessment and evaluation related to simulation-based IPE in Chap. 9. Logistics is the next topic in Chap. 10, in which Charles and Koehn tackle this vexing problem in the interprofessional setting. Part II finishes with Chap. 11 in which Rege provides valuable guidance in developing a state-of-the art simulation-based center that can be used for IPE and SBT.

Part III of *Interprofessional Team Training and Simulation* pivots from theory and fundamentals to application. In it, four sets of distinguished authors present viewpoints on conducting IPE with SBT for a variety of learner levels. Chapter 12 begins the part in which Luk, Sander, Young, Jones, and Brown present macro-, meso-, and microlevels of preparation for prelicensure learners considering logistics, roles of champions and stakeholders, outcomes, curriculum development, and preparation of faculty. Chapter 13, by Lee-Jayaram, Steinemann, and Berg, then discusses training postgraduate learners, touching on such topics as the Accreditation Council for Graduate Medical Education (ACGME) requirements and how combining simulation with just-in-time training can result in sustained effects. In addition, the chapter focuses on latent safety concerns, challenges to simulation, and resources to assist with simulation. In Chap. 14, Robertson, Klainer, Bradley, Yule, and Smink outline the experience of operating room team training at Brigham and Women's Hospital in Boston as an example of IPE using SBT for practicing clinicians. They detail key planning topics such as logistics, design and objectives, scenarios, specialty adjustments, and faculty training. Part III closes with Watkins describing the use of simulation for undergraduate and graduate medical education, continuing medical education, maintenance of certification (MOC), and remediation in Chap. 15.

Part IV of *Interprofessional Team Training and Simulation* expands on application by focusing on four examples of interprofessional SBT currently employed in clinical practice. It begins with Ozawa and Mahboobi's review of employing SBT to improve teamwork in the operating room in Chap. 16. Lee, Goffman, Berstein, Feldman, and Bajaj then discuss applying SBT in the labor and delivery setting and its use in implementing change, such as incorporating checklists into care. Chapter 18, by Paige, Bonanno, and Garbee, address applications of SBT to prepare healthcare providers to address critically ill patients and mass casualty situations, touching on interprofessional competencies, obstacles to implementation in the acute care setting, and solutions to overcoming them. The part, and book, then concludes with Chap. 19, in which McCarthy, Patel, and Spain explain applications of IPE and SBT in the prehospital setting, giving examples of its use for emergency medical services (EMS) personnel.

We sincerely hope that, with *Interprofessional Team Training and Simulation*, we have provided a practical, worthwhile, and informative resource for those individuals, both experienced and novice, tasked with the important responsibility of improving teamwork and team interaction using IPE and SBT in order to improve the safety and quality of patient care. If this volume makes such an endeavor easier for them, then we will have succeeded. Enjoy!

New Orleans, LA, USA

John T. Paige
Shirley C. Sonesh
Deborah D. Garbee
Laura S. Bonanno

Success isn't something that just happens – success is learned, success is practiced and then it is shared – Sparky Anderson, Major League Baseball Manager for the World Series Champions Cincinnati Reds (1975, 1976) and Detroit Tigers (1984).

Alone we can do so little; together we can do so much. – Helen Keller, first deaf-blind person to earn a Bachelor of Arts degree.

Acknowledgments

The editors would like to thank the senior editor of the *Comprehensive Healthcare Simulation* series, Dr. Adam I. Levine, who spearheaded the editing of the original *Comprehensive Textbook of Healthcare Simulation* and who invited us to contribute to this worthwhile endeavor with this current volume. In addition, we like to thank Springer Publishing, especially Maureen Alexander, the Developmental Editor for this project, for their support, guidance, patience, and encouragement. Finally, we would like to acknowledge the hard work of Kathryn Kerdolff, Associate Professor and Research Librarian at LSU Health New Orleans Health Sciences Center, for helping to keep us on task and organized.

Contents

Editors and Contributors

About the Editors

John T. Paige, MD, FACS is a Professor of Clinical Surgery with appointments in Anesthesiology and Radiology at the Louisiana State University (LSU) Health New Orleans School of Medicine. He currently serves as the Director of the American College of Surgeons' accredited Learning Center. At LSU Health New Orleans, he worked with Drs. Garbee and Bonanno to introduce and expand simulation-based interprofessional team training at the Health Sciences Center.

Nationally, Dr. Paige is the Co-Chair of the ACS Accredited Education Institutes (AEI) Faculty Development Committee and Chair of the Continuing Education Committee at the Society of American Gastrointestinal and Endoscopic Surgeons (SAGES) and serves on the ACS Surgical Education and Self-Assessment Program (SESAP) Advisory Committee. He has served as Chair of the Association for Surgical Education (ASE) Simulation and Development Committees and as Chair of the Society for Simulation in Healthcare (SSH) Surgical and Perioperative Simulation Interest Groups. In October 2018, he was inducted as an inaugural Associate in the ACS Academy of Mastery Surgical Educators. He has dedicated his career to surgical education and training. His areas of interest include simulation-based skills training, interprofessional education, team training, human factors, patient safety, and debriefing, topics on which he has published and spoken extensively.

Shirley C. Sonesh, PhD is an Organizational Psychologist specializing in the role of teamwork in healthcare and patient safety. She is the Founder of Sonnenschein Consulting, LLC, where she collaborates with universities and healthcare facilities to provide both research and consulting services in the fields of simulation-based training, team training, interprofessional education (IPE), telemedicine, and human automation systems. After earning her PhD in Organizational Behavior from Tulane University's A.B. Freeman School of Business, she worked as a Research Scientist at the University of Central Florida's Institute for Simulation and Training (IST) and then as an Adjunct Professor at Tulane University. At IST, she led the patient safety research unit. Previous consulting engagements have been conducted in the topics of simulation training, IPE, rapid response teams, team decision-making, prehospital care, executive coaching, human automation systems, intelligent adaptive training for the DOD, tele-health, performance measurement systems, selection, and organizational change initiatives, among others.

Dr. Sonesh has published over 16 academic articles, has authored 4 book chapters, engaged in over 35 speaking engagements at national and international conferences, and has recently served as Chair of the Human Factors and Ergonomics in Healthcare (HFES Healthcare) conference.

Deborah D. Garbee, PhD, APRN, ACNS-BC, FCNS is a Professor of Clinical Nursing at LSU Health New Orleans School of Nursing and serves as Associate Dean for Professional Practice, Community Service, and Advanced Practice Nursing. She is Program Director of the Adult Gerontology Clinical Nurse Specialist concentration in the Doctor of Nursing Practice program. She worked with Drs. Paige and Bonanno to develop, implement, and evaluate interprofessional high-fidelity human patient simulation scenarios to train teams of health profession students in team-based competencies.

Dr. Garbee has over 20 years' experience in the operating room and 17 years as an Adult Health Clinical Nurse Specialist. She was honored in March of 2019 at the inaugural induction as a Fellow by the Clinical Nurse Specialist Institute. She is the Nomination Committee Chair for the Southern Regional Education Board Council on Collegiate Education for Nursing. She previously served on the Research Committee of the National Association of Clinical Nurse Specialists. Her research interests include simulation-based education, interprofessional education, communication, and teamwork.

Laura S. Bonanno, PhD, DNP, CRNA is an Associate Professor of Clinical Nursing at the LSU Health New Orleans School of Nursing and the Director of the Nurse Anesthesia Program. Along with Drs. Paige and Garbee, she has promoted and facilitated the use of high-fidelity simulation to train interprofessional students on team-based competencies and has also published and presented on this topic. She has been a practicing Certified Registered Nurse Anesthetist for 24 years and has been in nurse anesthesia education for 20 years. In addition to interprofessional education and simulation, her research interests include clinical education and evaluation of clinical performance.

Dr. Bonanno holds state and national leadership positions. She is an appointed Board Member to the Louisiana State Board of Nursing where she served a 2-year term as President and currently serves as President. On the national level, she serves on the Council on Accreditation of Nurse Anesthesia Educational Programs as President and previously served two years as Vice-President.

Contributors

Rami Ahmed, DO, MHPE Department of Emergency Medicine, Summa Health System, Akron, OH, USA

Komal Bajaj, MD, MS-HPEd Department of Obstetrics & Gynecology and Women's Health, Albert Einstein College of Medicine/Montefiore Medical Center, Bronx, NY, USA

Department of Obstetrics and Gynecology, Jacobi Medical Center, NYC Health + Hospitals, Bronx, NY, USA

Lauren E. Benishek, PhD Johns Hopkins University School of Medicine, Armstrong Institute for Patient Safety and Quality, Baltimore, MD, USA

Benjamin W. Berg, MD SimTiki Simulation Center, John A Burns School of Medicine, University of Hawaii at Manoa, Honolulu, HI, USA

Peter S. Bernstein, MD, MPH Department of Obstetrics & Gynecology and Women's Health, Albert Einstein College of Medicine/Montefiore Medical Center, Bronx, NY, USA

Erik W. Black, PhD, MPH UF Health Shands Children's Hospital, Department of Pediatrics, Gainesville, FL, USA

Laura S. Bonanno, PhD, DNP, CRNA Nurse Anesthesia Program Director, Louisiana State University (LSU) Health School of Nursing, New Orleans, LA, USA

Dorothy M. Bradley, RN, MSN Center for Nursing Excellence, Brigham and Women's Hospital, Boston, MA, USA

Kimberly M. Brown, MD, FACS Dell Medical School, The University of Texas at Austin, Austin, TX, USA

Department of Surgery and Perioperative Care, Austin, TX, USA

Stephen Charles, MS, MA BMH, PHD, CHSE Office of Medical Education, Brody School of Medicine, East Carolina University, Greenville, NC, USA

Heather A. Davidson, PhD Vanderbilt University Medical Center, Center for Patient and Professional Advocacy, Nashville, TN, USA

Stephanie DeSandro, MS, PA-C School of Health Professions, Baylor College of Medicine, Houston, TX, USA

Brian Dunkin, MD Department of Surgery, Houston Methodist Hospital, MITIE—The Houston Methodist Institute for Technology, Innovation & Education, Houston, TX, USA

Jennifer Feitosa, PhD Claremont McKenna College, Claremont, CA, USA

David L. Feldman, MD, MBA, CPE, FAAPL, FACS Healthcare Risk Advisors, The Doctors Company, New York, NY, USA

Adrian Fonseca, MA McKinsey & Company, San Jose, Costa Rica

Deborah D. Garbee, PhD, APRN, ACNS-BC, FCNS Associate Dean for Professional Practice, Community Service and Advanced Nursing Practice, Professor of Clinical Nursing, LSUHSC School of Nursing, New Orleans, LA, USA

Aimee Gardner, PhD School of Health Professions, Baylor College of Medicine, Houston, TX, USA

Department of Surgery, Baylor College of Medicine, Houston, TX, USA

Dena Goffman, MD Department of Quality and Patient Safety, New York-Presbyterian Hospital, New York, NY, USA

Department of Obstetrics and Gynecology, Columbia University Medical Center, New York, NY, USA

Megan E. Gregory, PhD Department of Biomedical Informatics, The Ohio State University College of Medicine, Columbus, OH, USA

The Center for the Advancement of Team Science, Analytics, and Systems Thinking in Health Services and Implementation Science Research (CATALYST), The Ohio State University College of Medicine, Columbus, OH, USA

Ashley M. Hughes, PhD, MS University of Illinois at Chicago, Chicago, IL, USA

Barbara L. Jones, PhD, MSW School of Social Work, The University of Texas at Austin, Austin, TX, USA

Joseph R. Keebler Embry-Riddle Aeronautical University, Daytona Beach, FL, USA

Suzanne B. Klainer, MD Brigham and Women's Hospital, Department of Anesthesia, Harvard Medical School, Boston, MA, USA

Mary L. Koehn, PhD, APRN, CHSE University of Kansas School of Medicine-Wichita, Wichita, KS, USA

Elizabeth H. Lazzara, PhD Department of Human Factors and Behavioral Neurobiology, Embry-Riddle Aeronautical University, Daytona Beach, FL, USA

Colleen A. Lee, MS, RN Weill Cornell Medicine, Physician Organization-Quality and Patient Safety, New York, NY, USA

Jannet Lee-Jayaram, MD SimTiki Simulation Center, John A Burns School of Medicine, University of Hawaii at Manoa, Honolulu, HI, USA

John C. Luk, MD Dell Medical School, The University of Texas at Austin, Austin, TX, USA

Sohail K. Mahboobi, MD, FASA Tufts University School of Medicine, Lahey Hospital & Medical Center, Department of Anesthesiology, Burlington, MA, USA

Jennifer McCarthy, MAS, BS Seton Hall University, School of Health and Medical Sciences, Nutley, NJ, USA

Edwin Tomoya Ozawa, MD, PhD Tufts University School of Medicine, Lahey Hospital & Medical Center, Department of Anesthesiology, Burlington, MA, USA

John T. Paige, MD, FACS Department of Surgery, Louisiana State University (LSU) Health New Orleans School of Medicine, New Orleans, LA, USA

Nicole M. Paradise Black, MD, MEd UF Health Shands Children's Hospital, Department of Pediatrics, Gainesville, FL, USA

Amar Pravin Patel, DHSc, MS CAE Healthcare, Sarasota, FL, USA

M. Tyson Pillow, MD, Med Department of Emergency Medicine, Baylor College of Medicine, Houston, TX, USA

Robert V. Rege, MD Distinguished Teaching Professor of Surgery, Associate Dean for Undergraduate Medical Education, University of Texas Southwestern Medical Center, Dallas, TX, USA

Jamie M. Robertson, PhD, MPH STRATUS Center for Medical Simulation, Brigham and Women's Hospital, Boston, MA, USA

Department of Emergency Medicine, Harvard Medical School, Boston, MA, USA

Department of Surgery, Harvard Medical School, Boston, MA, USA

Eduardo Salas, PhD Department of Psychology Sciences, Rice University, Houston, TX, USA

M. Kathryn Sanders, DNP, MSN School of Nursing, The University of Texas at Austin, Austin, TX, USA

Douglas S. Smink, MD, MPH Department of Surgery, Harvard Medical School, Boston, MA, USA

Center for Surgery and Public Health, Brigham and Women's Hospital, Boston, MA, USA

Shirley C. Sonesh, PhD Organizational Psychologist Sonnenschein Consulting, LLC, New Orleans, LA, USA

Andrew E. Spain, MA Society for Simulation in Healthcare, Washington, MO, USA

Susan Steinemann, MD Department of Surgery, John A Burns School of Medicine, University of Hawaii at Manoa, Honolulu, HI, USA

Amanda C. Tan, BS Fuqua Center for Late-Life Depression, Emory University, Atlanta, GA, USA

Nicholas Unger, BS, MS Department of Research & Synthesis, BlackHägen Design, Dunedin, FL, USA

Scott C. Watkins, MD Vanderbilt University Medical Center, Department of Anesthesiology, Nashville, TN, USA

Kristen L. W. Webster, PhD Johns Hopkins Hospital, Department of Anesthesiology and Critical Care Medicine and Department of Surgery, Baltimore, MD, USA

Johns Hopkins Hospital, Department of Surgery, Parkville, MD, USA

Amanda L. Woods, BS, MA Department of Psychology Sciences, Rice University, Houston, TX, USA

Veronica Young, PharmD, MPH College of Pharmacy, The University of Texas at Austin, Austin, TX, USA

Steven Yule, MA, MSc, PhD Brigham & Women's Hospital/Harvard Medical School, STRATUS Center for Medical Simulation, Boston, MA, USA

Stephanie Zajac, MS, PhD Department of Surgery, Houston Methodist Hospital, MITIE—The Houston Methodist Institute for Technology, Innovation & Education, Houston, TX, USA

Part I

Theories and Concepts

Improving Patient Care: The Role of Effective Simulation

1

Stephanie Zajac, Amanda L. Woods, Brian Dunkin, and Eduardo Salas

Introduction

Simulation has a critical role in creating long-lasting and transformative change in medical education and healthcare systems [1]. In clinical practice, the use of simulated environments across a variety of sectors has been steadily adopted and endorsed [2–4], and there has been record growth in the number of simulation centers across the globe [5]. The state of the science has also developed significantly; while the literature on interprofessional education (IPE) and simulation was once done mostly in silos [6], there is now a drive to understand *how* and *when* simulation-based training improves individual expertise as well as the ability of experts to work together effectively in interprofessional teams.

This opening chapter seeks to set the stage for the remainder of the book by presenting a brief overview of the rise of simulation and its many applications across the healthcare industry. The authors then delineate the potential benefits of simulation over traditional educational models and address best practices for maximizing the efficacy of simulation-based training (SBT). Where applicable, we highlight emerging evidence specifically within the domain of IPE. A number of practical resources are offered throughout the chapter to provide guidance to those who design and develop simulations. Lastly, in recognizing there is still much to learn, we conclude with directions to guide future research and practice.

S. Zajac (✉) · B. Dunkin
Department of Surgery, Houston Methodist Hospital, MITIE—The Houston Methodist Institute for Technology, Innovation & Education, Houston, TX, USA

A. L. Woods · E. Salas
Department of Psychology Sciences, Rice University, Houston, TX, USA

J. T. Paige et al. (eds.), *Comprehensive Healthcare Simulation: InterProfessional Team Training and Simulation*, Comprehensive Healthcare Simulation,
https://doi.org/10.1007/978-3-030-28845-7_1

The Rise of Simulation

The growing prevalence of simulation in healthcare can be traced to several factors, perhaps the most compelling of which is a concern with medical error and the severe consequences that can follow. While the advent of simulation-based training occurred as early as the 1970s [7, 8], more recent reports of medical error causing unnecessary harm to patients have greatly spurred interest in simulation as a structured training technique [9, 10]. Importantly, these reports make clear that the root cause of preventable errors lies not only in individual deficits in knowledge, skill, or judgment (e.g., clinician assessment, history taking), but in the failure to engage in effective interprofessional teamwork (e.g., communication) [11, 12].

Indeed, the ultimate goal of simulation is to enhance patient safety and patient-centered care from a multi-level perspective (e.g., individual, team, organizational) [13, 14]. To achieve this goal, the healthcare field turned to proven strategies from other high-hazard industries similar in complexity. Specifically, the successful implementation of simulation-based methods in high-reliability domains such as aviation, nuclear power, and the military has been an important impetus behind the adoption of simulation in healthcare [15]. Burke and Hutchins [16] offer practical guidance in translating the lessons learned from these communities. For example, the authors note that a team of experts does not make an expert team; investing time and effort into training is required. Furthermore, training must be designed with tools (e.g., simulation) that allow for systematic practice opportunities coupled with developmental feedback to maximize learning. Decker and colleagues [17] leverage existing best practices to put forth a comprehensive set of standards specifically for simulation-based IPE.

Simulation bridges the gap between the classroom and the clinical environment. Changes to the educational paradigm in medicine limit the time available for formal instruction. For example, the Common Program Requirements that mandate no more than an 80 hour work week have recently been upheld [18]. Additionally, advances in medical knowledge, a growing body of research, and technological innovation require that medical professionals be life-long learners. Finally, medical students traditionally educated in separate systems need to learn from and with each other, and to be prepared for an increasingly team-based clinical environment [19]. Simulation provides a flexible method for self-directed and continuous learning that can take place outside of the classroom and across professions [20].

Applications of Simulation

Training and Education

Simulation holds great potential across a variety of applications (*see* Table 1.1). Likely the most widespread use [21], simulation-based training (SBT) is a method for safely bridging the gap between novice and highly competent healthcare professionals across all fields and levels of education [22]. SBT often targets individual

Table 1.1 Applications of Simulation [15, 21]

Application	Description
Training and Education	Improvement of procedural, teamwork, and interprofessional teamwork skills through introduction of conceptual knowledge and skills, as well as deliberate part and whole task practice.
Evaluation and Assessment	Use in high stakes examinations, certification, and establishment of proficiency.
Performance Support	Facilitation of transfer to the workplace environment.
Innovation and Exploration	Adoption of new organizational practices (e.g., patient care protocols) and research such as investigating human factors that affect performance, and testing the usability of clinical equipment.
Culture Change	Use as a "bottom up" tool for creating a safety-oriented culture.

knowledge and procedural skills. However, while individual capability is considered fundamental, the importance of teamwork to ensure patient safety is now widely recognized [15]. In fact, as predicted nearly two decades ago [23], simulation-based training aimed at the principles of teamwork is now routine practice in many healthcare settings. Furthermore, well-validated healthcare team training tools (e.g., TeamSTEPPS) have proven effective at improving attitudes and behavior specifically in interprofessional teams [24]. SBT has now begun to move beyond technical and teamwork competencies to target unit-level (e.g., work-flow processes) [25] and organizational-level (e.g., senior leadership) [26] factors that can directly and indirectly effect patient outcomes [1].

Evaluation and Assessment

Simulation exercises can be used to assess the competency or proficiency of medical students and practicing clinicians, ensuring standards for safe patient care have been met. For example, proficiency-based progression training is a relatively new approach to simulation [27]. Using this paradigm, performance evaluation can be used to establish a benchmark or level of proficiency that constitutes effective and safe performance. Benchmarks represent different stages of skill or knowledge acquisition [28], and trainees are held accountable to reaching established criteria before moving forward or completing the training. Additionally, the use of standardized simulations for high stakes testing has now become an essential piece of medical education (e.g., certification and licensure of internationally trained clinicians) [29]. These simulations have been shown to be reliable, valid, and fair assessments of clinical competence across a variety of domains [30].

Performance Support

Just-in-time training or rehearsal can be viewed as in-situ performance support; clinicians or operative teams can practice previously trained tasks or a specific, unique, or challenging procedure tailored to a single patient immediately before performance [15]. Pre-procedure warm ups for more routine tasks (e.g., essential laparoscopic skills) have proven to be effective at improving technical performance even for experienced clinicians [31]. Furthermore, the advent of innovative technology, such as 3D printing of advanced anatomical models, allows for simulation tailored to specific patient characteristics and for streamlining of an interprofessional team's patient management strategies (e.g., context specific handoffs) [32]. Sarris and Polimenakos [32] argue this type of in-situ simulation facilitates a step-by-step understanding of an individual case for team members across all professions.

Innovation and Exploration

The medical field represents a rapidly changing industry characterized by innovation and exploration across multiple sectors, including organizational policies and practices (e.g., patient care protocols, safety initiatives), medical devices and equipment, and diagnostic and therapeutic interventions [15]. Simulations can be used to determine a clinician's ability to adapt to changing best practices in patient care (e.g., advanced cardiac life support protocol) [33]. Additionally, simulated environments can be used to safely develop and test the effectiveness of new instruments [34], which can then lead the way for revolutions in the state of medical fields (e.g., the shift from open to laparoscopic surgical interventions) [35].

Culture Change

All of the above applications have at the core an increased focus on patient safety and the quality of patient care. Therefore, an overarching purpose of simulation is to impact the culture of a team, department, or healthcare organization to ultimately improve patient outcomes. For example, team training has been conducted with the overall goal of increasing the awareness and knowledge of patient safety activities as well as personal investment and attitudes toward the safety culture [36]. Simulation-based interventions as a strategy for changing safety culture have been met with some success; simulated exercises can lead to improved attitudes and perceptions [37]. Simulation may also aid in breaking down the "silo mentality" that continues to persist as a result of a culture characterized by interprofessional tension and strict hierarchies [38]. Paige and colleagues [38] assert this culture persists in part because of inadequate interprofessional education opportunities; the authors find that early IPE simulation-based interventions can positively influence teamwork related attitudes and behaviors. However, primary empirical studies investigating culture are limited and findings are somewhat inconsistent, indicating the need for future research using methodologies that can address the complexity of the environment (e.g., mixed method approaches) and designs that allow for evaluation of the effects of training across several levels [39].

The Benefits of Simulation

According to Ziv and colleagues [40], balancing the needs of those completing medical education with the obligation to provide the best treatment possible and ensure patient safety is indeed a source of tension. Simulation offers a potential solution by allowing for exposure and practice in a way that is ethical and protects patients from unnecessary risk. Simulation also allows for healthcare professionals at all levels, including undergraduate and graduate medical education as well as practicing clinicians, to learn or maintain skills in a safe environment. When coupled with methods that require proficiency or demonstrated competence before moving to the next level of training or real cases, simulation represents a critical element of much needed educational reform [41]. However, simply exposing healthcare professionals to simulated environments will not ensure learning.

Experience alone has a weak relationship with observed performance; but, engaging in deliberate practice is strongly linked to the development of expertise [42]. Anders Ericsson [42] delineates characteristics that define deliberate practice, including a focus on skill acquisition and not performance, immediate feedback, time to engage in problem-solving and reflection, and repeated opportunities for performance. For obvious reasons (e.g., patient safety, time constraints), deliberate practice in a real healthcare environment is neither feasible nor desirable, and simulation helps fill this gap. Importantly, deliberate practice allows for effective implementation of competency-based education; all trainees are given the opportunity to reach a level of safe performance, although total time spent training or number of specific practice events can vary by trainee [43, 44]. Finally, simulated practice allows for error-management training (i.e., learning from mistakes to deepen understanding and help control consequences) [45], an effective instructional strategy for adapting to the difficult, complex, and dynamic tasks often found in healthcare.

Simulation allows individuals and teams to train on low frequency, high risk events in which there are significant consequences for error [14]. For example, hospital-related events that require the use of advanced cardiac life support (ACLS) are infrequent [46], but failure to effectively manage them holds severe consequences for patients' safety. Wayne and colleagues [44] stress that it is unrealistic to expect even well-trained individuals and teams to manage events for which they have not practiced or prepared for adequately. Therefore, another benefit of simulation is the maintenance of skills needed for low frequency occurrences and for establishing proficiency for required healthcare certifications (e.g., ACLS). Simulation not only benefits the patient, but the healthcare organization's bottom line.

Although the cost of medical simulators can vary widely and are certainly significant, cost efficiency over in-person training is often still great. Real environments require extensive use of highly valued resources such as hours of instructor and faculty time and medical supplies, and can result in extended length of procedures and increased complications [34]. In fact, complications that arise from unsafe or incorrectly executed procedures represent a significant expense; for example, it is estimated that healthcare-associated infections (HAIs) alone can cost U.S. hospitals up to $45 billion annually [47]. One of the most common HAIs, central-line associated bloodstream infections, can be associated with up to $46,000 in cost to the hospital per infection [48]. Simulation-based interventions (e.g., procedure and prevention techniques) have proven to reduce HAIs, and cost-analysis has shown that the cost of infection far outweighs the investment in training [49, 50].

Specifically in the context of IPE, simulation may help address some of the challenges in integrating interprofessional teamwork into existing programs. For example, simulation can be structured to be relevant to learners from all professions, and the details of scenarios adjusted to accommodate new IPE content [51]. Palaganas and colleagues [51] also note that debriefing, which is a core component of simulation, allows for reflection that can shed light on mental models and assumptions around important IPE social issues (e.g., hierarchy, diversity). Simulation allows for hands-on practice of newly learned interpersonal skills, an essential component to skill acquisition that is missing from other common forms of IPE education (e.g., group discussion, case-based learning) [52].

As a final benefit, simulation has proven to be a valuable tool across all four levels of Kirkpatrick's evaluation framework (i.e., reaction, learning, behavior, results) [53]. Qualitative analysis revealed that, after completion of a human patient simulation program, clinicians found that it was a useful tool for hands-on practice, learning, or remediation without risk. Furthermore, the experience motivated trainees to learn more; the most commonly cited program limitation was insufficient time spent engaged in the simulation [54]. A recent meta-analysis on the efficacy of SBT with opportunity for deliberate practice found that, when compared to traditional clinical education, SBT results in greater achievement of specific skill acquisition goals (i.e., learning) [55]. Simulation is also effective for improving cognitively-based learning outcomes (e.g., knowledge of the AHA recommended algorithms for ACLS) [44] and attitudes (e.g., toward patient safety) [36].

To truly demonstrate the utility of simulation, however, evaluation must link an initiative (e.g., education, evaluation, organizational practices) directly to improved on-the-job behavior (i.e., transfer) and patient-related outcomes [56]. Toward this end, training using simulated experiences or patients has proven to be an effective tool for improving technical performance of both individuals and teams in the field (e.g., improved performance in the OR) [33]. Reflecting a movement toward patient centered research, more recent systematic evaluations of the links between simulation performance and patient - and system-level outcomes indicate small to moderate positive relationships across several domains (e.g., surgical, diagnostic, team, procedure-specific) [57, 58]. For example, a multi-site investigation of the efficacy of a simulation program for patient handoff-improvement was associated with a 23% reduction of all medical error and a 30% reduction in preventable adverse events [59].

In sum, simulation has multiple benefits (*see* Table 1.2) that span across a range of applications, and it is therefore not surprising that simulation is taking a larger role in research and clinical practice. In line with the purpose of this book, the remainder of the chapter will be used to focus more specifically on education and

Table 1.2 Benefits of Simulation

Benefit	Example Cites
Solution for competing goals of education and patient safety	Ziv et al. (2003) [40]
Opportunity for repeated and deliberate practice	Wayne et al. (2006) [44]
Exposure to low frequency/high risk events	Aggarwal et al. (2010) [14]
Reduced cost incurred to organization	Kunkler (2006) [34]
Overcomes challenges to effectively integrating IPE	Palaganas et al. (2014) [51]
Efficacy over traditional approaches	McGaghie et al. (2010) [56]

training. Importantly, simulation is defined as "a technique, not a technology, to replace or amplify real experiences with guided experiences, often immersive in nature, that evoke or replicate substantial aspects of the real world in a fully interactive fashion" [15, p. i2]. A key point of this definition stressed by Gaba [15] is that simulation is not the technology or device utilized; indeed, the extent to which SBT is designed and delivered using evidence-based best practices is far more important than the specific technology itself [60].

Best Practices for Simulation Development

The below guidelines are based on the science of learning and training [61, 62], as well as evidence from healthcare and other high-reliability organizations [54, 63, 64]. It is stressed that training should be designed as a continuous process, not a one-time event [61], and that careful preparation is needed well in advance of implementation. While there are numerous factors to consider in the design and development of SBT, the five considerations outlined below represent the building blocks of effective simulation: identification of learning objectives, scenario design and implementation, robust observation protocols, feedback and reflection, and a system-level approach. Importantly, following these guidelines will optimize training outcomes regardless of the specific content to be learned.

Clear and Precise Learning Objectives

Learning objectives can be viewed as the backbone or foundation of simulation programs. These objectives inform the design and delivery of training, as well as criterion development and the subsequent measurement tools [65]. In fact, best practice requires a clear linkage between measurement tools and the learning objectives; this allows for the assessment of change in the desired knowledge, skills, and abilities (KSAs) that should occur as a result of training, and therefore whether the goals of training have been met [63]. Finally, objectives shape the structure of post-simulation feedback and reflection. They can be delivered by a facilitator during the pre-brief to ensure the learners know what is expected of them and to provide a sense of direction, and used to guide discussion during the debrief [66–69].

Developing learning objectives and the associated scenarios is itself an interprofessional initiative, it requires a close partnership between subject matter experts (SMEs) (e.g. surgeons, nurses) and learning experts (e.g., instructional designers) [60, 70]. SMEs are able to provide detailed information on the task (e.g., deconstructed steps of a procedure or event into component parts) [71] as well as the required knowledge and skill for successful task completion. Ultimately, SMEs can inform well-written learning objectives that describe what the learner should *know* or *be able to do* after successfully completing each piece of the program. This information can then be used to inform the five critical elements of a learning objective; specifically, "who will do how much (or how well) of what by when" [72, p. 29].

Carefully Crafted and Implemented Scenario Designs

The importance of collaborating with SMEs extends beyond establishing learning objectives; the domain-specific knowledge and on-the-job experience that these experts possess can enhance "buy-in" on behalf of trainees and yield more realistic and relevant scenarios [60]. Furthermore, this collaboration allows for the creation of simulation with high *psychological* fidelity, arguably the most important dimension of fidelity for teamwork skills training [73]. Psychological fidelity is defined as the extent to which training elicits the underlying psychological constructs (e.g., individual differences in cognitive ability and goal orientation, performance monitoring, and self-efficacy) and processes (e.g., resource allocation, attention) relevant to learning, performance, and generalization in a real-world setting [74]. Kozlowski and Deshon [74] argue that this type of fidelity is responsible for transfer and adaptability of individuals and teams. Finally, it is argued that to successfully develop and implement scenarios, both SMEs and learning experts must together act as champions within the department or organization, supporting the value of the effort as well as providing feedback and guidance throughout implementation [75].

Carefully designed scenarios provide the opportunity to display targeted technical skills or teamwork competencies through the use of "trigger events" (e.g., a change in patient parameters) based on critical incident data [60, 76, 77]. The behavioral responses elicited from trigger events can then facilitate a structured approach to measuring performance in highly dynamic and often times complex scenarios. This structured approach to scenario development is a sophisticated, multi-stage process; fortunately, there are a number of readily available scenario development tools that can be leveraged (e.g., TEACH Sim) [78].

Robust Observation Protocols

Measures that capture behaviorally manifested technical and teamwork competencies are critical to accurately assessing performance [63, 75]. Many reliable and validated measurement tools that involve an observational approach are currently used in healthcare (e.g., Objective Structured Assessment of Technical Skills, TeamSTEPPS™ Team Performance Observation Tool, Mayo High Performance Teamwork Scale) [75, 79, 80]. However, Rosen and colleagues [63] warn that, while these measures can be successfully transported to new contexts, careful consideration of whether they capture the desired competencies and the purpose of training is first needed.

There are at least three common methods utilized for observational protocols: behavioral observation scales (BOSs) [81], event-based assessment tools (e.g., EBAT) [82], and behaviorally anchored rating scales (BARS) [83]. All of these methods focus on observable behaviors, and therefore reduce the opportunity for bias or error and increase the ability to provide developmental feedback [63]. However, each has its own strengths; for example, EBATs focus raters' attention and reduce the amount of judgment needed, BARS are easily modified and provide concrete examples of behavior, and BOSs more readily capture typical behavior [63, 84]. Before implementing any protocol, however, rater training is a necessary first step. Toward this end, Feldman and colleagues [85] offer a number of strategies (e.g., rater error, performance dimension training, and frame-of-reference training) that can increase rater accuracy and enhance the validity of performance assessments.

Robust observation protocols are not only used to observe and describe behavior, but to evaluate against a pre-determined standard and diagnose performance [86]. In competency-based medical education, evaluation should occur against a desired level of proficiency or performance often set by experts or standards for safety [87]. Performance diagnosis, which determines the cause of effective or ineffective behavior [88], can then be used for guided practice and the delivery of specific and targeted feedback on performance.

Providing Diagnostic and Developmental Feedback and Reflection

When delivered correctly, feedback can be a powerful learning tool. After-action reviews (AARs) or debriefs, a technique originally borrowed from the military community, are a means of delivering systematic, structured feedback that allows for active reflection and discussion in a non-punitive environment [89, 90]. A recent meta-analysis uncovered that debriefs can improve both individual and team effectiveness by as much as 25% [90]. Furthermore, the efficacy of debriefs holds across both real and simulated environments as well as non-medical and medical trainees. The design and delivery of a debrief can greatly influence its effectiveness; fortunately, the literature offers several evidence-based strategies [91], and tools to measure the quality of debriefings in a consistent and reliable manner are available (e.g., Objective Structured Assessment of Debriefing) [92].

To maximize the potential for learning, observations of performance should be quickly translated into feedback (i.e., immediately following the simulation) [63]. Discussion should focus on the behavioral processes that led to individual or team outcomes and not on the outcomes alone. The reason for this is twofold: (1) outcomes can be effected by a host of other factors not related to performance (e.g., patient condition), and (2) focusing on outcomes does not allow for discussion of specific effective or ineffective behaviors or *why* certain outcomes occurred [93]. Indeed, while it is essential to discuss strengths or what individuals or teams are doing well, feedback must also target errors and areas that need development in order to create positive behavioral change.

The importance of a supportive and psychologically safe environment cannot be overstated; trainees must feel comfortable admitting mistakes and openly talking about errors. Discussion should take a non-threatening approach, with the facilitator working closely with the trainees to understand the sense-making process (i.e., process by which trainees interpret and make meaning of information) [94] and uncover the cognitive frames or mental models, assumptions, and beliefs behind actions [95]. Rudolph and colleagues [95] provide advice to the facilitator, and outline a method for debriefing that emphasizes reflection, curiosity and respect, clear evaluative judgments, and a dialogue characterized by advocacy and inquiry. Finally, feedback should be actionable; expectations and goals for future performance should be coupled with clear means for improvement [96].

Systems Level Approach to Training

Designing an effective SBT program goes well beyond a single training event; in fact, factors both within and outside the learning activity, as well as before, during, and after formal training can all facilitate or hinder the use of learned behavior on the job [21, 61]. The sciences of training and learning have identified several of these universal factors along with guidelines that can be applied to any SBT program. First, it has been well-established that a training needs analysis (TNA) should occur before any investment in training [97]. However, TNAs that are most likely to lead to improvements in the quality of patient care and improved service have the following features: (1) clearly defined aims tailored to a specific organization, (2) inclusion of stakeholders' opinions and more than one method of data collection, and (3) explicit expression of the outcomes and how they relate to the needs of the organization [98]. Conditions that support the transfer of training should be put in place months in advance of any event. These conditions include a supportive learning environment in which expectations for the behaviors trainees will be expected to exhibit are clearly communicated and a system for rewards and sanctions [16, 99]. Perceived utility as well as commitment to the training should also be cultivated early on by creating specific job and career goals, and clearly linking these to the content of training [16].

During training, delivery methods should be aligned with the content to be trained. For example, behavioral modeling training (BMT) is a highly effective method for the acquisition of procedural and interpersonal skills. BMT is most effective when it includes a well-defined set of behaviors to be learned, positive and negative models of behavior, and opportunities for repeated practice [99]. Principles of learning should be incorporated throughout, such as the use of a realistic work environment and tasks [100, 101], encouragement of errors and how they can be managed to mitigate negative consequences [102], and opportunities for practice followed by developmental feedback [103]. The importance of practice cannot be overstated; conditions (i.e., spacing, whole or part task, overlearning) should be carefully considered with respect to individual characteristics (e.g., ability) and task features (e.g., complexity) [104]. An additional team development aid, peer coaching, can extend the learning experience and is especially beneficial for IPE because it can occur in the actual practice setting, facilitates individualized learning, and fosters collaboration between team members [105, 106].

The conclusion of the formal training event should be followed by the creation of an environment that facilitates transfer and a rigorous evaluation of the program. While there are numerous organizational factors that set the stage for transfer, work environment support has proven to be a consistent and powerful predictor of the use of open skills (i.e., skills in which there is no one right way to act) [107] in the workplace [108]. Support from the organization and supervisors serve as situational cues for training [109], and can take the form of opportunities to perform trained tasks clear expectations and provide post-training follow-up and resource availability (e.g., time, funding, equipment) [16, 110, 111]. Executive leadership and other administrative and clinical leaders should establish training as a priority and facilitate its implementation [112]. The organization should also show commitment through the establishment of supportive policies (e.g., reward structure) and change the infrastructure of existing programs to incorporate IPE [108].

Support from peers (e.g., encouragement, guidance or assistance for the use of trained behaviors) can be equally important for the continued use of trained skills, especially in self-directed teams where members are likely to hold great influence over peer behaviors [113, 114]. Finally, implementing simulation into an existing program for *any* purpose should be preceded by careful consideration of how it will be evaluated [55]. Training evaluation should include data on both affective and utility reactions, learning across multiple levels, transfer of learned KSAs on the job, and system-level outcomes (e.g., cost savings to the organization, patient-related outcomes) [70].

Future Research

Evidence of the efficacy of simulation-based training for learning-based outcomes is robust; SBT is associated with consistent, positive effects on learning across multiple domains [55, 58]. However, Schmidt and colleagues [115] point out that evidence for higher levels of Kirkpatrick's evaluation framework [53] is inconsistent; solid conclusions about the efficacy of SBT for transfer of trained skills to the field and patient-related outcomes cannot yet be drawn. This need for future research may be even more salient for simulation-based IPE, as use of trained skills in the field and patient health outcomes are understudied, and reliability and validity of measurement tools are often not reported [116]. Furthermore, Cook and colleagues [58] conclude that we know little about *how* to use simulation in order to optimize the benefits of SBT. The authors assert that theory-based investigations into the efficacy of different instructional design features (e.g., practice schedule, duration) are needed.

On a broader scale, there is a continued need for methodologically rigorous studies that clearly specify targeted outcomes across multiple levels, as well as systematic reporting of simulation details [15]. In order to achieve this, simulation-based research may benefit from a clearer taxonomy of patient- and system-level outcomes. Systematic evaluation of return on investment as an important system-level outcome is also needed; demonstrating the cost-efficiency of simulation in IPE education may lead to increased accessibility of SBT [117]. In the context of IPE, Abu-Rish and colleagues [52] offer a tool (i.e., the Replicability of Interprofessional Education; RIPE) for structured reporting of study details.

Future IPE research should also investigate multi-team system simulations within healthcare, or simulations that encompass the entire patient care pathway (e.g., sub-specialties, pre-hospital and discharge teams) [118]. Aurora and colleagues [118] suggest these macro-simulations are critical for developing leadership and communication in cross-department or cross-site patient care. Finally, beyond initial transfer of learned skills to the workplace, we know little about sustainability of training over time. This may be an especially salient issue for low frequency, high consequence events, and many questions (e.g., how often should refreshers occur?) remain to be answered [1].

Conclusion

Simulation is a useful tool across a variety of applications in healthcare, including training and education, evaluation and assessment, performance support, innovation and exploration, and cultural change. SBT, the most prevalent use of simulation, fills several gaps related to educational reform, including: (1) the ability to engage in deliberate practice without harm to patients, (2) exposure to low frequency events, and (3) opportunity for self-directed learning. Moreover, it has proven cost-efficient and effective for the acquisition of procedural and interprofessional teamwork skills, use of trained skills in the field, and ultimately in improving patient-related outcomes over and above traditional educational models.

This chapter has laid out the five cornerstones of developing effective simulation-based training. First, clear and precise learning objectives are the foundation of simulation curriculum, and are used to inform subsequent scenarios, metric development, and evaluation. Realistic and relevant simulation scenarios must have a high degree of psychological fidelity and be designed with "trigger events" that elicit targeted competencies. These simulation scenarios must be assessed by robust, behaviorally-based observation protocols that are used not only to describe, but to evaluate and diagnose performance. Diagnostic and developmental feedback should be delivered immediately after performance diagnosis. Importantly, feedback should focus on both effective and ineffective behaviors in a psychologically safe environment where trainees feel comfortable discussing errors. Finally, it is necessary to consider factors that will facilitate the transfer of training well beyond the formal training event (e.g., perceived utility, organizational climate). The importance of collaboration between healthcare professionals and experts in training and learning is emphasized throughout; indeed, creating effective simulations requires an interprofessional effort.

References

1. Salas E, Paige JT, Rosen MA. Creating new realities in healthcare: the status of simulation-based training as a patient safety improvement strategy. BMJ Qual Saf. 2013;22(6):449–52.
2. American College of Surgeons (ACS). ACS/ASE medical student simulation-based surgical skills curriculum [Internet]. Chicago, IL: American College of Surgeons; year unknown [cited 2017 Apr 20]. Available from: https://www.facs.org/education/program/simulation-based.
3. Agency for Healthcare Research and Quality (AHRQ). Improving patient safety through simulation research [Internet]. Rockville, MD: Agency for Healthcare and Research Quality; 2012 [Updated 2016 Apr; cited 2017 Apr 20]. Available from: https://www.ahrq.gov/research/findings/factsheets/errors-safety/simulproj11/index.html.
4. National League for Nursing (NLN). A vision for teaching with simulation [Internet]. Washington, DC: National League for Nursing; 2015 Apr [cited 2017 May 2]. Available from: http://www.nln.org/docs/default-source/about/nln-vision-series-(position-statements)/vision-statement-a-vision-for-teaching-with-simulation.pdf?sfvrsn=2.
5. Society for Simulation in Healthcare. SSH hits record growth [Internet]. Washington, DC: Society for Simulation in Healthcare; 2017. [cited 2017 May 2]. Available from: http://www.ssih.org/News/articleType/ArticleView/articleId/2053/SSH-Hits-Record-Growth.
6. Robertson J, Bandali K. Bridging the gap: Enhancing interprofessional education using simulation. J Interprof Care. 2008;22(5):499–508.
7. Gordon MS. Cardiology patient simulator: development of an animated manikin to teach cardiovascular disease. Am J Cardiol. 1974;34(3):350–5.
8. Sajid AW, Gordon MS, Mayer JW, et al. Symposium: a multi-institutional research study on the use of simulation for teaching and evaluating patient examination skills. Annu Conf Res Med Educ. 1980;19:349–58.
9. Donaldson MS, Corrigan JM, Kohn LT, editors. To err is human: building a safer health system. Washington, DC: National Academies Press; 2000.
10. Makary MA, Daniel M. Medical error-the third leading cause of death in the US. BMJ. 2016;3:353–i2139.
11. Schiff GD, Hasan O, Kim S, Abrams R, Cosby K, Lambert BL, Elstein AS, Hasler S, Kabongo ML, Krosnjar N, Odwazny R. Diagnostic error in medicine: analysis of 583 physician-reported errors. Arch Intern Med. 2009;169(20):1881–7.
12. World Health Organization. Framework for action on interprofessional education and collaborative practice. Geneva: WHO; 2010.
13. Barry MJ, Edgman-Levitan S. Shared decision making—the pinnacle of patient-centered care. N Engl J Med. 2012;366(9):780–1.
14. Aggarwal R, Mytton OT, Derbrew M, Hananel D, Heydenburg M, Issenberg B, MacAulay C, Mancini ME, Morimoto T, Soper N, Ziv A. Training and simulation for patient safety. Qual Saf Health Care. 2010;19(Suppl 2):i34–43.
15. Gaba DM. The future vision of simulation in health care. Qual Safety Health Care. 2004;13(suppl 1):i2–10.
16. Burke LA, Hutchins HM. A study of best practices in training transfer and proposed model of transfer. Hum Resour Dev Q. 2008;19(2):107–28.
17. Decker SI, Anderson M, Boese T, Epps C, McCarthy J, Motola I, Palaganas J, Perry C, Puga F, Scolaro K. Standards of best practice: Simulation standard VIII: Simulation-enhanced interprofessional education (sim-IPE). Clin Simul Nurs. 2015;11(6):293–7.

18. American Council for Graduate Medical Education. Common Program Requirements. Chicago, IL: American Council for graduate Medical Education; 2007 Feb 11 [cited 2017 Apr 22]. Available from http://www.acgme.org/Portals/0/PFAssets/ProgramRequirements/CPRs_07012016.pdf.
19. Bandali K, Niblett B, Yeung TP, Gamble P. Beyond curriculum: embedding interprofessional collaboration into academic culture. J Interprof Care. 2011;25(1):75–6.
20. Issenberg SB, McGaghie WC, Hart IR, Mayer JW, Felner JM, Petrusa ER, Waugh RA, Brown DD, Safford RR, Gessner IH, Gordon DL. Simulation technology for health care professional skills training and assessment. JAMA. 1999;282(9):861–6.
21. Rosen MA, Salas E, Tannenbaum SI, Provonost P, King HB. Simulation-based training for teams in health care: designing scenarios, measuring performance, and providing feedback. In: Carayon P, editor. Handbook of HFE in health care and patient safety. 2nd ed. Boca Raton: FLCRC Press; 2011. p. 571–92.
22. Galloway SJ. Simulation techniques to bridge the gap between novice and competent healthcare professionals. Online J Issues Nurs. 2009;14(2)
23. Gaba DM, Howard SK, Fish KJ, Smith BE, Sowb YA. Simulation-based training in anesthesia crisis resource management (ACRM): a decade of experience. Simul Gaming. 2001;32(2):175–93.
24. Brock D, Abu-Rish E, Chiu CR, Hammer D, Wilson S, Vorvick L, Blondon K, Schaad D, Liner D, Zierler B. Interprofessional education in team communication: working together to improve patient safety. BMJ Qual Saf. 2013;22(5):414–23.
25. Neri PM, Redden L, Poole S, Pozner CN, Horsky J, Raja AS, Poon E, Schiff G, Landman A. Emergency medicine resident physicians' perceptions of electronic documentation and workflow: a mixed methods study. Appl Clin Inform. 2015;6(1):27–41.
26. Mohr JJ, Abelson HT, Barach P. Creating effective leadership for improving patient safety. Qual Management Healthcare. 2002;11(1):69–78.
27. Gallagher AG, O'Sullivan GC. Proficiency-based progression simulation training: a to-do list for medicine. Fundamentals of Surgical Simulation. London: Springer-Verlag London Limited; 2011. p. 325–353.
28. Gallagher AG. Metric-based simulation training to proficiency in medical education:-what it is and how to do it. Ulster Med J. 2012;81(3):107–13.
29. Whelan GP, Boulet JR, McKinley DW, Norcini JJ, Van Zanten M, Hambleton RK, Burdick WP, Peitzman SJ. Scoring standardized patient examinations: lessons learned from the development and administration of the ECFMG Clinical Skills Assessment (CSA®). Med Teach. 2005;27(3):200–6.
30. Fried GM, Feldman LS, Vassiliou MC, Fraser SA, Stanbridge D, Ghitulescu G, Andrew CG. Proving the value of simulation in laparoscopic surgery. Ann Surg. 2004;240(3):518–28.
31. Calatayud D, Arora S, Aggarwal R, Kruglikova I, Schulze S, Funch-Jensen P, Grantcharov T. Warm-up in a virtual reality environment improves performance in the operating room. Ann Surg. 2010;251(6):1181–5.
32. Sarris GE, Polimenakos AC. Three-dimensional modeling in congenital and structural heart perioperative care and education: a path in evolution. Pediatr Cardiol. 2017;29:1–3.
33. Okuda Y, Bryson EO, DeMaria S, Jacobson L, Quinones J, Shen B, Levine AI. The utility of simulation in medical education: what is the evidence? Mt Sinai J Med. 2009;76(4):330–43.
34. Kunkler K. The role of medical simulation: an overview. Int J Med Robot Comput Assisted Surg. 2006;2(3):203–10.
35. Ruurda JP, Van Vroonhoven TJ, Broeders IA. Robot-assisted surgical systems: a new era in laparoscopic surgery. Ann R Coll Surg Engl. 2002;84(4):223.
36. Patterson MD, Geis GL, LeMaster T, Wears RL. Impact of multidisciplinary simulation-based training on patient safety in a paediatric emergency department. BMJ Qual Saf. 2013;22:383–93.
37. Wolf FA, Way LW, Stewart L. The efficacy of medical team training: improved team performance and decreased operating room delays: a detailed analysis of 4863 cases. Ann Surg. 2010;252(3):477–85.

38. Paige JT, Garbee DD, Kozmenko V, Yu Q, Kozmenko L, Yang T, Bonanno L, Swartz W. Getting a head start: high-fidelity, simulation-based operating room team training of interprofessional students. J Am Coll Surg. 2014;218(1):140–9.
39. Morello RT, Lowthian JA, Barker AL, McGinnes R, Dunt D, Brand C. Strategies for improving patient safety culture in hospitals: a systematic review. BMJ Quality & Safety. 2013;22(1):11–8.
40. Ziv A, Wolpe PR, Small SD, Glick S. Simulation-based medical education: an ethical imperative. Acad Med. 2003;78(8):783–8.
41. Cooke M, Irby DM, Sullivan W, Ludmerer KM. American medical education 100 years after the Flexner report. N Engl J Med. 2006;355(13):1339–44.
42. Anders EK. Deliberate practice and acquisition of expert performance: a general overview. Acad Emerg Med. 2008;15(11):988–94.
43. McGaghie WC, Miller GE, Sajid A, Telder TV. Competency-Based Curriculum Development in Medical Education. Public Health Paper No. 68. Geneva: World Health Organization; 1978.
44. Wayne DB, Butter J, Siddall VJ, Fudala MJ, Wade LD, Feinglass J, McGaghie WC. Mastery learning of advanced cardiac life support skills by internal medicine residents using simulation technology and deliberate practice. J Gen Intern Med. 2006;21(3):251–6.
45. Bell BS, Kozlowski SW. Active learning: effects of core training design elements on self-regulatory processes, learning, and adaptability. J Appl Psychol. 2008;93(2):296.
46. Peberdy MA, Kaye W, Ornato JP, Larkin GL, Nadkarni V, Mancini ME, Berg RA, Nichol G, Lane-Trultt T, NRCPR Investigators. Cardiopulmonary resuscitation of adults in the hospital: a report of 14 720 cardiac arrests from the National Registry of Cardiopulmonary Resuscitation. Resuscitation. 2003;58(3):297–308.
47. Scott RD. The Direct Medical Costs of Healthcare-Associated Infections in U.S. Hospitals and the Benefits of Prevention. Atlanta, GA: Centers for Disease Control and Prevention; 2009 [cited 2017 May2]. Available from: http://www.cdc.gov/hai/pdfs/hai/scott_costpaper.pdf.
48. Zimlichman E, Henderson D, Tamir O, Franz C, Song P, Yamin CK, Keohane C, Denham CR, Bates DW. Health care–associated infections: a meta-analysis of costs and financial impact on the US health care system. JAMA Intern Med. 2013;173(22):2039–46.
49. Burden AR, Torjman MC, Dy GE, Jaffe JD, Littman JJ, Nawar F, Rajaram SS, Schorr C, Staman GW, Reboli AC. Prevention of central venous catheter-related bloodstream infections: is it time to add simulation training to the prevention bundle? J Clin Anesth. 2012;24(7):555–60.
50. Cohen ER, Feinglass J, Barsuk JH, Barnard C, O'donnell A, McGaghie WC, Wayne DB. Cost savings from reduced catheter-related bloodstream infection after simulation-based education for residents in a medical intensive care unit. Simul Healthc. 2010;5(2):98–102.
51. Palaganas JC, Epps C, Raemer DB. A history of simulation-enhanced interprofessional education. J Interprof Care. 2014;28(2):110–5.
52. Abu-Rish E, Kim S, Choe L, Varpio L, Malik E, White AA, Craddick K, Blondon K, Robins L, Nagasawa P, Thigpen A. Current trends in interprofessional education of health sciences students: a literature review. J Interprof Care. 2012;26(6):444–51.
53. Kirkpatrick DL. Evaluating training programs. Columbus: Tata McGraw-Hill Education; 1975.
54. Bremner MN, Aduddell K, Bennett DN, VanGeest JB. The use of human patient simulators: best practices with novice nursing students. Nurse Educ. 2006;31(4):170–4.
55. McGaghie WC, Issenberg SB, Cohen ME, Barsuk JH, Wayne DB. Does simulation-based medical education with deliberate practice yield better results than traditional clinical education? A meta-analytic comparative review of the evidence. Acad Med. 2011;86(6):706.
56. McGaghie WC, Issenberg SB, Petrusa ER, Scalese RJ. A critical review of simulation-based medical education research: 2003–2009. Med Educ. 2010;44(1):50–63.
57. Brydges R, Hatala R, Zendejas B, Erwin PJ, Cook DA. Linking simulation-based educational assessments and patient-related outcomes: a systematic review and meta-analysis. Acad Med. 2015;90(2):246–56.

58. Cook DA, Hatala R, Brydges R, Zendejas B, Szostek JH, Wang AT, Erwin PJ, Hamstra SJ. Technology-enhanced simulation for health professions education: a systematic review and meta-analysis. JAMA. 2011;306(9):978–88.
59. Starmer AJ, Spector ND, Srivastava R, West DC, Rosenbluth G, Allen AD, Noble EL, Tse LL, Dalal AK, Keohane CA, Lipsitz SR. Changes in medical errors after implementation of a handoff program. N Engl J Med. 2014;371(19):1803–12.
60. Salas E, Wilson KA, Burke CS, Priest HA. Using simulation-based training to improve patient safety: what does it take? Jt Comm J Qual Patient Saf. 2005;31(7):363–71.
61. Salas E, Tannenbaum SI, Kraiger K, Smith-Jentsch KA. The science of training and development in organizations: What matters in practice. Psychol Sci Public Interest. 2012;13(2):74–101.
62. Weaver SJ, Rosen MA, Salas E, Baum KD, King HB. Integrating the science of team training: guidelines for continuing education. J Contin Educ Health Prof. 2010;30(4):208–20.
63. Rosen MA, Salas E, Wilson KA, King HB, Salisbury M, Augenstein JS, Robinson DW, Birnbach DJ. Measuring team performance in simulation-based training: adopting best practices for healthcare. Simul Healthc. 2008;3(1):33–41.
64. Hill RW Jr, Belanich J, Lane HC, Core M, Dixon M, Forbell E, Kim J, Hart J. Pedagogically structured game-based training: development of the ELECT BiLAT simulation: University of Souther California Marina Del Ray Ca, Ins for Creative Technologies; 2006.
65. Salas E, Cannon-Bowers JA. The science of training: a decade of progress. Annu Rev Psychol. 2001;52(1):471–99.
66. Dreifuerst KT. The essentials of debriefing in simulation learning: a concept analysis. Nurs Educ Perspect. 2009;30(2):109–14.
67. Fanning RM, Gaba DM. The role of debriefing in simulation-based learning. Simul Healthc. 2007;2(2):115–25.
68. Jeffries PR. Simulation in nursing education: from conceptualization to evaluation. National League for Nursing; 2007.
69. Reilly DE, Oermann MH. Behavioral Objectives-evaluation in nursing. Lincoln, NE: to Excel Press; 1999.
70. Salas E, Wilson KA, Burke CS, Wightman DC, Howse WR. A checklist for crew resource management training. Ergon Des. 2006;14(2):6–15.
71. Zevin B, Levy JS, Satava RM, Grantcharov TP. A consensus-based framework for design, validation, and implementation of simulation-based training curricula in surgery. J Am Coll Surg. 2012;215(4):580–6.
72. Kern DE. Curriculum development for medical education: a six-step approach. Baltimore: JHU Press; 1998.
73. Beaubien JM, Baker DP. The use of simulation for training teamwork skills in health care: how low can you go? Qual Saf Health Care. 2004;13(suppl 1):i51–6.
74. Kozlowski SW, DeShon RP. A psychological fidelity approach to simulation-based training: theory, research and principles. In: Salas E, Elliot LR, Schflett SG, Coovert MD, editors. Scaled worlds: development, validation, and applications. Burlington: Ashgate Publishing; 2004. p. 75–99.
75. King HB, Battles J, Baker DP, et al. TeamSTEPPS: team strategies and tools to enhance performance and patient safety. In: Henriksen K, Battles JB, Keyes MA, Grady ML, editors. Advances in patient safety: new directions and alternative approaches (vol 3: performance and tools). Rockville: Agency for Healthcare Research and Quality (US); 2008.
76. Rosen MA, Salas E, Silvestri S, Wu TS, Lazzara EH. A measurement tool for simulation-based training in emergency medicine: the simulation module for assessment of resident targeted event responses (SMARTER) approach. Simul Healthc. 2008;3(3):170–9.
77. Tobias S, Fletcher JD, editors. Training & retraining: a handbook for business, industry, government, and the military. New York: Macmillan Library Reference; 2000.
78. Benishek LE, Lazzara EH, Gaught WL, Arcaro LL, Okuda Y, Salas E. The template of events for applied and critical healthcare simulation (TEACH Sim): a tool for systematic simulation scenario design. Simul Healthc. 2015;10(1):21–30.

79. Malec JF, Torsher LC, Dunn WF, Wiegmann DA, Arnold JJ, Brown DA, Phatak V. The mayo high performance teamwork scale: reliability and validity for evaluating key crew resource management skills. Simul Healthc. 2007;2(1):4–10.
80. Martin JA, Regehr G, Reznick R, Macrae H, Murnaghan J, Hutchison C, Brown M. Objective structured assessment of technical skill (OSATS) for surgical residents. Br J Surg. 1997;84(2):273–8.
81. Salas E, Burke CS, Fowlkes JE, Priest HA. On measuring teamwork skills. Comprehensive Handbook of Psychological Assessment. 2004;4:427–442.
82. Fowlkes J, Dwyer DJ, Oser RL, Salas E. Event-based approach to training (EBAT). Int J Aviat Psychol. 1998;8(3):209–21.
83. Devcich DA, Weller J, Mitchell SJ, McLaughlin S, Barker L, Rudolph JW, Raemer DB, Zammert M, Singer SJ, Torrie J, Frampton CM. A behaviourally anchored rating scale for evaluating the use of the WHO surgical safety checklist: development and initial evaluation of the WHOBARS. BMJ Qual Saf. 2016;25(10):778–86.
84. Tziner A, Joanis C, Murphy KR. A comparison of three methods of performance appraisal with regard to goal properties, goal perception, and ratee satisfaction. Group Org Manag. 2000;25(2):175–90.
85. Feldman M, Lazzara EH, Vanderbilt AA, DiazGranados D. Rater training to support high-stakes simulation-based assessments. J Contin Educ Heal Prof. 2012;32(4):279.
86. Salas E, Rosen MA, Held JD, Weissmuller JJ. Performance measurement in simulation-based training a review and best practices. Simul Gaming. 2009;40(3):328–76.
87. Searle J. Defining competency–the role of standard setting. Med Educ. 2000;34(5):363–6.
88. Cannon-Bowers J, Salas E. Team performance measurement in training: a conceptual approach to dynamic assessment. In: Brannick MT, Salas E, Prince CW, editors. Assessment and measurement of team performance: theory, research, and application. New York: Psychology Press; 1997.
89. Villado AJ, Arthur W Jr. The comparative effect of subjective and objective after-action reviews on team performance on a complex task. J Appl Psychol. 2013;98(3):514.
90. Tannenbaum SI, Cerasoli CP. Do team and individual debriefs enhance performance? A meta-analysis. Hum Factors. 2013;55(1):231–45.
91. Sawyer T, Eppich W, Brett-Fleegler M, Grant V, Cheng A. More than one way to debrief: a critical review of healthcare simulation debriefing methods. Simul Healthc. 2016;11(3):209–17.
92. Arora S, Ahmed M, Paige J, Nestel D, Runnacles J, Hull L, Darzi A, Sevdalis N. Objective structured assessment of debriefing: bringing science to the art of debriefing in surgery. Ann Surg. 2012;256(6):982–8.
93. Lyons R, Lazzara EH, Benishek LE, Zajac S, Gregory M, Sonesh SC, Salas E. Enhancing the effectiveness of team debriefings in medical simulation: more best practices. Jt Comm J Qual Patient Saf. 2015;41(3):115–25.
94. Weick KE. Sense making in organizations. Thousand Oaks: Sage; 1995.
95. Rudolph JW, Simon R, Dufresne RL, Raemer DB. There's no such thing as "nonjudgmental" debriefing: a theory and method for debriefing with good judgment. Simul Healthc. 2006;1(1):49–55.
96. Kluger AN, DeNisi A. The effects of feedback interventions on performance: a historical review, a meta-analysis, and a preliminary feedback intervention theory. Psychol Bull. 1996;119(2):254–84.
97. Denby S. The importance of training needs analysis. Ind Commer Train. 2010;42(3):147–50.
98. Gould D, Kelly D, White I, Chidgey J. Training needs analysis. A literature review and reappraisal. Int J Nurs Stud. 2004;41(5):471–86.
99. Taylor PJ, Russ-Eft DF, Chan DW. A meta-analytic review of behavior modeling training. J Appl Psychol. 2005;90(4):692–709.
100. Grossman R, Salas E. The transfer of training: what really matters. Int J Train Dev. 2011;15(2):103–20.
101. Hays RT, Singer MJ. Simulation fidelity in training system design: bridging the gap between reality and training. New York: Springer Science & Business Media; 2012.

102. Helmreich RL, Merritt AC, Wilhelm JA. The evolution of crew resource management training in commercial aviation. Int J Aviat Psychol. 1999;9(1):19–32.
103. Issenberg S, Mcgaghie WC, Petrusa ER, Lee Gordon D, Scalese RJ. Features and uses of high-fidelity medical simulations that lead to effective learning: a BEME systematic review. Med Teach. 2005;27(1):10–28.
104. Baldwin TT, Ford JK. Transfer of training: a review and directions for future research. Pers Psychol. 1988;41(1):63–105.
105. Salas E, Lacerenza C. Team Training for Team Science: Improving Interdisciplinary Collaboration. In: Workshop on Science Team Dynamics and Effectiveness 2013; p. 1.
106. Steinert Y. Learning together to teach together: Interprofessional education and faculty development. J Interprofession Care. 2005;19(sup1):60–75.
107. Yelon SL, Ford JK. Pursuing a multidimensional view of transfer. Perform Improv Q. 1999;12(3):58–78.
108. Blume BD, Ford JK, Baldwin TT, Huang JL. Transfer of training: A meta-analytic review. J Manag. 2010;36(4):1065–105.
109. Rouiller JZ, Goldstein IL. The relationship between organizational transfer climate and positive transfer of training. Hum Resour Dev Q. 1993;4(4):377–90.
110. Cromwell SE, Kolb JA. An examination of work-environment support factors affecting transfer of supervisory skills training to the workplace. Hum Resour Dev Q. 2004;15(4):449–71.
111. Quinones MA, Ford JK, Sego DJ, Smith EM. The effects of individual and transfer environment characteristics on the opportunity to perform trained tasks. Training Res J. 1995;1(1):29–49.
112. Nelson WA, Donnellan JJ, Elwyn G. Implementing shared decision making: an organizational imperative. In: Elwyn G, Edwards A, Thompson R, editors. Shared decision making in health care: achieving evidence-based patient choice. Oxford, UK: Oxford University Press; 2016.
113. Van der Klink M, Gielen E, Nauta C. Supervisory support as a major condition to enhance transfer. Int J Train Dev. 2001;5(1):52–63.
114. Russ-Eft D. A typology of training design and work environment factors affecting workplace learning and transfer. Hum Resour Dev Rev. 2002;1(1):45–65.
115. Schmidt EM, Goldhaber-Fiebert SN, Ho LA, McDonald KM, Shekelle PG, Wachter RM, Pronovost PJ. Use of simulation exercises in patient safety efforts. Making healthcare safer II: an updated critical analysis of the evidence for patient safety practices. Comparative effectiveness review no. 211. Rockville: Agency for Healthcare Research and Quality; 2013. p. 472–9.
116. Zhang C, Thompson S, Miller C. A review of simulation-based interprofessional education. Clin Simul Nurs. 2011;7(4):e117–26.
117. Fung L, Boet S, Bould MD, Qosa H, Perrier L, Tricco A, Tavares W, Reeves S. Impact of crisis resource management simulation-based training for interprofessional and interdisciplinary teams: a systematic review. J Interprof Care. 2015;29(5):433–44.
118. Arora S, Cox C, Davies S, Kassab E, Mahoney P, Sharma E, Darzi A, Vincent C, Sevdalis N. Towards the next frontier for simulation-based training: full-hospital simulation across the entire patient pathway. Ann Surg. 2014;260(2):252–8.

The Impact of Interprofessional Education on Healthcare Team Performance: A Theoretical Model and Recommendations

2

Megan E. Gregory

The work reported here was supported in part by the U.S. Department of Veterans Affairs, Veterans Health Administration, Health Services Research and Development Service, Office of Academic Affiliations, Health Professions Education Evaluation and Research Advanced Fellowship and in part by Center for Innovations in Quality, Effectiveness and Safety (CIN 13-413), Michael E. DeBakey VA Medical Center, Houston, TX. This work is supported in part the Houston VA HSR&D Center for Innovations in Quality, Effectiveness and Safety (CIN 13-413).

The views expressed in this article are those of the author and do not necessarily reflect the position or policy of the U.S. Department of Veterans Affairs or the United States government.

Introduction

Recent estimates suggest that more than 400,000 deaths annually are due to preventable medical errors [1], with an economic impact of up to $1 trillion annually [2]. Among the top contributors to medical errors and patient harm are failures in teamwork processes, such as ineffective communication and leadership issues [3]. However, while ineffective team performance can lead to patient harm, teamwork is a requirement of modern-day healthcare, as medical care can no longer be provided in silo. Rather, the increasing complexity of today's care requires numerous professionals to manage a patient with as many as 63 healthcare professionals needed for a

M. E. Gregory (✉)
Department of Biomedical Informatics, The Ohio State University College of Medicine, Columbus, OH, USA

The Center for the Advancement of Team Science, Analytics, and Systems Thinking in Health Services and Implementation Science Research (CATALYST), The Ohio State University College of Medicine, Columbus, OH, USA
e-mail: megan.gregory@osumc.edu

J. T. Paige et al. (eds.), *Comprehensive Healthcare Simulation: InterProfessional Team Training and Simulation*, Comprehensive Healthcare Simulation,
https://doi.org/10.1007/978-3-030-28845-7_2

single surgical patient [4]. In today's complex healthcare environment, therefore, it is essential that professionals are prepared to work effectively on teams with members of other professions. However, effective teamwork and collaboration is not simply a result of highly-skilled interprofessional members working together. Rather, effective interprofessional teamwork and collaboration in healthcare requires imparting a requisite set of attitudes, behaviors, and cognitions onto healthcare professionals. That is, it is necessary to educate members of various health professions about the value of each interprofessional team member, the role of each profession in regards to patient care, and how to work together to co-manage a patient.

The term *interprofessional education and training (IPE)* has become a buzzword within the healthcare industry and academia alike. For example, a Google search of the term "interprofessional education" yields no less than 425,000 results. But, what is IPE? How does IPE improve healthcare team effectiveness? In this chapter, I will answer these questions by first defining the term *interprofessional education and training* and distinguishing it from similar terms. I will then describe its theoretical underpinnings to explain how IPE can be a driver for effective team performance, and will propose a theoretical model to this end. Subsequently, I will briefly describe factors to consider when developing an IPE intervention.

What Is IPE?

A review of the literature suggests that there is often conflicting terminology in terms of IPE. Terms such as "multiprofessional," "interdisciplinary," and "multidisciplinary" are often used in place of the term "interprofessional." Formally defined, *interprofessional education and training (IPE)* is when students or members of two or more professions learn with, from, and about each other to enhance collaboration, quality of care, and other health outcomes [5, 6]. I distinguish this from *interdisciplinary education,* defined as learners from various specialties within a discipline (e.g., in medicine: pediatrics, anesthesia, etc.). I also distinguish it from *multiprofessional education* (i.e., when learners from two or more professions learn alongside, but not with, from, and about one another) [7]; and *multidisciplinary education* (when learners from two or more disciplines learn alongside, but not with, from, and about one another). To further clarify, IPE may also be interdisciplinary (e.g., comprised of nurses and physicians from obstetrics and cardiology) or intradisciplinary (e.g., comprised of nurse anesthetists and anesthesiologists).

IPE is a form of collaborative learning; that is, it is an instructional method wherein learners work together to achieve a common goal [8]. Learners in IPE may be students, practicing clinicians, or a mix of both, with meta-analytic evidence suggesting it is effective for all of these groups [9].

While IPE can be formal (i.e., IPE is explicitly planned) or informal (i.e., IPE is not explicitly planned but occurs in the process of another activity or due to informal professional interactions), the focus of this chapter is on formal IPE. In a broader sense, IPE is not simply placing various professionals in a room and lecturing them in parallel as a group; rather, learners must actively learn with, from, or about one another to be engaged in IPE.

Evidence for IPE Effectiveness

As previously stated, the healthcare system is plagued by human error, and a major cause of this error is teamwork factors such as miscommunication [3]. One potential way to combat this is by using IPE. As such, a number of studies have been conducted to determine the extent to which IPE leads to improved outcomes.

Results show that when designed and delivered in alignment with the needs of learners, IPE is effective in that in leads to improved outcomes. More specifically, a review of IPE interventions found support for positive learner reactions, increased knowledge, transfer of behaviors to the job, and improved organizational and patient outcomes [10]. This includes, as examples, improved practice around cardiovascular disease [11], reduced morbidity of pre-term infants [12], and fewer medical errors [13]. Altogether, this evidence suggests that IPE produces attitudinal, behavioral, and cognitive learning that transfers to the work environment. This transferred knowledge, in turn, leads to more effective performance on the job, which subsequently leads to improved patient outcomes. In the next section, I will explore in more depth *how* this process occurs.

Theoretical Underpinnings of IPE

The goal of IPE is to induce learning and, ultimately, transfer learned knowledge, attitudes, and skills to a work setting. Learning is defined as "a relatively permanent change in knowledge or skill produced by experience [14]. While there are various types of learning (e.g., conceptual, motor skills, verbal, etc.), those most relevant for IPE are attitude learning and problem solving. That is, IPE is most valuable for improving attitudes towards other professionals, and working with other professionals to solve problems, as opposed to learning advanced profession-specific concepts, principles, and motor skills relevant to only a subset of learners (e.g., the physiology behind cardiac arrest may be relevant to physicians and nurses, but not to psychologists; similarly, the specific techniques employed in cognitive-behavioral therapy are important for psychologists to learn, but may be more information than a pharmacist needs). That is, the awareness of the expertise that other professions have, as well as the roles each team member plays in managing specific patient care issues, is essential to effective teamwork and should be covered in IPE. However, the advanced theory, specific skills, and nuanced concepts behind these profession-specific domains is more optimally taught in silo.

As previously stated, IPE is a form of collaborative learning, wherein learners must work together to achieve a goal. Thus, IPE enhances individual cognitive learning processes by causing one to process additional perspectives, disagreements, and explanations. This can result in a wider knowledge-base and better understanding of a problem, process, or person. Furthermore, collaborative learning can reduce individuals' cognitive labor by improving a team's transactive memory system—defined as a shared awareness of "who knows what" on a team [15]—which thereby allows for deeper specialized learning, as will be further described below.

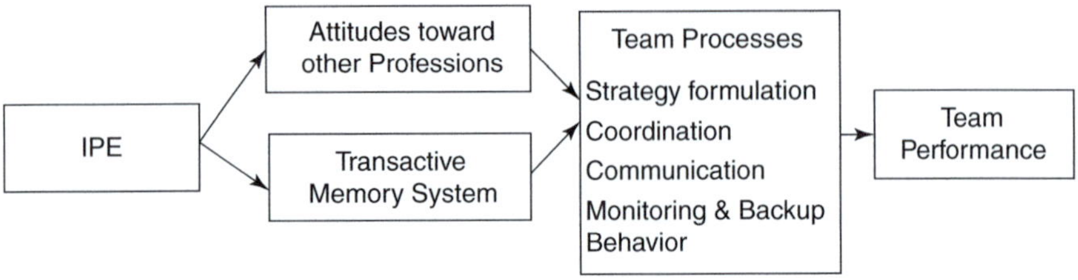

Fig. 2.1 Theoretical model of the relationship between IPE and performance

Moreover, the logic behind IPE is that learning about, with, and from members of other professions will improve individuals' (a) attitudes towards other professionals, (b) knowledge of other professionals' expertise and roles (i.e., the transactive memory system) and (c) team processes (e.g., strategy formulation, coordination, communication, monitoring and backup behavior). More succinctly, IPE improves how members feel about other professions as well as what they know about other professions, and these two outcomes in turn improve how members work together with other professions. Together, these processes should theoretically lead to improved team performance (see Fig. 2.1).

More specifically, the rationale for the need for IPE relies in part on diversity theories from social psychology that explain how individuals classify themselves and others. These include social identity theory [16] and self-categorization theories [17], which posit that individuals derive their identity from the groups or social categories (e.g., professions) in which they are a part of, leading them to prefer their group (profession) over others. For example, individuals tend to rate their ingroup (i.e., the group [e.g., profession] to which they belong) more positively than outgroups [18].

However, as posited by intergroup contact theory [19, 20], and confirmed by empirical evidence [21], simple exposure to groups different than one's own leads to higher tolerance and more positive attitudes towards the group. Thus, engaging in IPE should theoretically improve attitudes towards members of other professions. Empirical evidence has supported this assertion. For instance, one study found that students from five professions had more positive attitudes towards other professions after interprofessional education, as compared to a control group [22]. Similar results were found in other studies, with improvements on attitudes towards other professions improving from pre- to post-IPE [23]. In sum, theory and evidence suggests that individuals from different professions are likely to have improved attitudes towards other professions after engaging in IPE. More formally, I propose the following:

Proposition 1 Interprofessional education leads to more positive attitudes towards other professions.

Further, the categorization-elaboration model (CEM) [24] suggests that teams with members from various social categories or groups can have positive outcomes when members speak up and elaborate on task-relevant information [24]. In a related vein, when members from diverse social categories engage in this type of task-related communication, a team's *transactive memory system* (TMS) is enhanced [25, 26]. Conceptually, TMS is widely considered to be comprised of three dimensions [25]: (1) specialization (the extent to which each team member has differentiated knowledge and expertise), (2) coordination (the effectiveness with which information within a team is used), and (3) credibility (the extent to which members trust others' information). A team with an effective TMS has members with specialized knowledge (thereby allowing each member to develop a deep, rather than broad, level of expertise in an area), high credibility (i.e., members trust one another), and effective coordination (i.e., members know who has what information, and are able to obtain and use it as needed) [25]. Along these lines, engaging in IPE should theoretically increase all three of the dimensions of TMS by increasing task-relevant communication between professional boundaries. As such, I propose the following:

Proposition 2 Interprofessional education leads to a higher-quality transactive memory system.

Improved attitudes towards other professions should facilitate more beneficial interactions, or *team processes*. For example, having a positive and respectful attitude towards a colleague from another profession likely facilitates strategy formulation, insofar that the team is more likely to actively seek input from interprofessional colleagues when creating a plan [27]. Further, interprofessional teams in healthcare often have a hierarchy, with some professions having a higher perceived status then others [28]. Social identity theory would posit that in order to preserve this hierarchy, members of the team are likely to tend to engage behaviors that favor the higher-status professions [29]. Thus, members who feel their profession is perceived as inferior to other professions tend to devalue their contribution to the team [30] and are less likely to speak up as a result [31, 32]. However, this can be counteracted when all members have positive attitudes toward interprofessional team members, as these positive attitudes should lead to increased psychological safety (defined as the extent to which a team member feels safe to take interpersonal risks [e.g., speaking up] in a team setting [33]. Psychological safety has been empirically demonstrated to lead to improved team processes. For instance, research has shown that teams with a high level of psychological safety have more open and effective communication [34], as well as increased participation by interprofessional team members [35]. Thus, I assert:

Proposition 3 The attainment of more positive attitudes towards other professions leads to more effective team processes.

Improved TMS has been found to be related to better performance [36], by way of improved team processes [25, 36–40]. More specifically, TMS facilitates processes such as *strategy formulation* (developing courses of action for goal attainment) [41], *coordination* ("orchestrating the sequencing and timing of interdependent actions") [41], *communication* ("a reciprocal process of team members' sending and receiving information that forms and re-forms a team's attitudes, behaviors, and cognitions") [42], and *team monitoring & backup behavior* (coaching and/or assisting team members with task performance) [41]. As such, I posit:

Proposition 4 Higher-quality transactive memory systems lead to better team processes.

Team processes, in turn, enhance *team performance*, defined as "an emergent phenomenon resulting from the goal-directed process whereby members draw from their individual and shared resources to display taskwork processes, teamwork processes, and integrated team-level processes to generate products and provide services" [43]. Team processes have been empirically demonstrated to improve team performance. For example, research has found that planning processes (such as strategy formulation) leads to team performance [44–46]. Further, communication, coordination, and back-up behavior have also been linked to improved team performance [47–49]. Therefore, I propose:

Proposition 5 Having improved team processes leads to better team performance.

In summary, the proposed model suggests that IPE leads to enhanced team performance by way of improved attitudes and improved TMS, which in turn facilitate more effective team processes and, ultimately, team performance. However, in order to achieve these improved team performance outcomes, it is essential that IPE be developed in alignment with best practices. The next section will discuss this in further depth.

Development of IPE

Moving from the theoretical aspects of IPE, I now will briefly touch on considerations for the development of an IPE effort. As with any type of education and training, the design of IPE should be driven by pre-defined learning objectives (i.e., actionable statements that delineate the learning outcomes that trainees should come away from an educational intervention with [50]; see Fig. 2.2). To

After this training, learners should be able to...
Appreciate the value of each profession's contribution to the healthcare team
Explain the role of different professions in patient care
Demonstrate effective communication when handing over a patient to a member of another profession
Recognize an opportunity to refer a patient to an interprofessional colleague

Fig. 2.2 Examples of learning objectives for IPE

generate additional ideas for IPE learning objectives, see Thistlethwaite and Moran (2010) [51].

As with any training program, it is beneficial to engage in a formal needs analysis before beginning an IPE program [52]. Needs analyses help to more concretely define the learning objectives, or what it is that the organization hopes learners gain from engaging in IPE. This in turn will drive the structure, content, and type of leaners to be included in an IPE program. Along these lines, this section will briefly describe factors to consider when developing an IPE program (see Table 2.1). I will expand on each of these considerations in the following subsections.

Learners in IPE

Physicians and nurses often immediately come to mind when considering learners in IPE; however, in today's complex care environment, it is valuable to include a wider range of health professionals, such as psychologists, social workers, pharmacists, and other allied health personnel. Learners may span one discipline (e.g., labor and delivery), or may cross multiple disciplines (e.g., labor and delivery and surgery). Discipline-specific IPE issues are discussed later in this book.

Furthermore, introducing multiple professions into an IPE effort can be logistically challenging. It is necessary to review the schedules and availability of members of each professional group to find a mutually agreeable time to engage in IPE. Schedules may need to be rearranged and time blocked in order to accommodate all professions. In addition, different professions often have profession-specific

Table 2.1 Considerations for Development of IPE

IPE Development Components	Examples	Considerations
Learners	Physicians Nurses Psychologists Physical therapists Social workers	Which professions will be included? Can you work around each profession's schedule? Will learners be from one or > 1 disciplines?
Content	*Technical* Diabetes management Medication reconciliation *Non-technical* Communication Quality improvement	Is content tied to learning objectives? Is content relevant to all learners? Do you have instructors with appropriate expertise?
Structure	One hour lecture One simulation-based training session Year-long course	Do you have adequate staffing? Can you block time, if necessary? Do you have necessary facilities?
Instructional Methods	Information Demonstration Practice (e.g., simulation)	Do you have necessary resources?

terminology and jargon. This should be taken into consideration when delivering content to learners, such that language that may be unknown or mean something else to one or more of the professions that are engaged in IPE should be explicitly defined.

Content of IPE

At a broad level, IPE can be categorized into technical and non-technical content. In healthcare, technical content often includes clinical topics such as the management of particular diseases. Non-technical content includes "soft-skills" topics such as teamwork, communication, and leadership. The content should be driven by the learning objectives, which should be defined during development of an IPE program. It is also essential to determine who will teach the topic(s) in the IPE program. Do teachers/faculty have the necessary expertise for the topic(s)? If not, can it be acquired or outsourced (e.g., obtaining a guest speaker)?

Importantly, when developing an IPE program and the content therein, it is imperative to explicitly consider the extent to which content is relevant to learners from each profession (and discipline, if applicable). Explicating the role of each profession in regards to the topic at hand will lead to better learning outcomes.

Structure of IPE

IPE can be structured in various ways, ranging from a singular didactic lecture to a multi-semester course. The decision of how to structure an IPE effort should be driven largely by the pre-defined learning objectives. Specifically, the learning objectives specify how much (and what) content should be covered, which drives the amount of time required and the format of the IPE effort. On a more practical level, it is also necessary to consider the resources (e.g., facilities, staffing, protected time) available for IPE. If your learning objectives outpace your resources, it is wise to consider prioritizing and refining your objectives. While there are no hard and fast rules regarding number of learning objectives, you should expect on average to be able to achieve approximately 1–2 learning objectives per hour of training. More specifically, you should also define the particular knowledge, skills, and attitudes (KSAs) that learners should display that will demonstrate attainment of these learning objectives [53]. At least one KSA should be tied to each learning objective [53].

Instructional Methods for IPE

There are various theories that inform the best practices for instructional methods to employ in IPE. Methods should be guided by adult learning theory [54], which posits that for training to be effective, it should be aligned with principles that underlie adult learning. According to Knowles (1973) [54], these principles are: (1) adults must be involved in the learning; (2) adults must be able to see connections between what they are learning and their prior experiences; (3) adults come to a learning experience with a specific goal in mind – they know what they want to obtain from the training; (4) learning should be problem-focused, such that learners can find a solution to a problem; and (5) adults must be internally motivated in order to learn. In accordance with these principles, it is important to use instructional methods that will increase learners' motivation, allow them to be active participants in their learning, and employ content that can relate to their prior experiences.

As such, there are various learning modalities that can be employed for IPE. These include information- (e.g., lectures, discussions, debates), demonstration- (e.g., videos, observations), and practice-based methods (e.g., case-based learning, problem-based learning, role play, simulation). Oftentimes, more than one method is utilized, and research supports that this is most effective [55]. However, the choice of learning modality(ies) for IPE again depends upon learning objectives and resources.

As previously stated, simulation is one form of practice – and is largely the focus of this book. While more detail on the usage of simulation for IPE is provided in subsequent chapters of this book, it is important to consider at this point the unique challenges of simulation-based training for IPE. Simulation-based IPE has been used to train a wide variety of both clinical and non-clinical topics, from disaster management [56], to developing an interprofessional care plan for HIV/AIDS patients [57], to improving attitudes towards other professions [58]. As with any type of simulation-based training, IPE simulation content should be driven and the scenarios should be developed to align with pre-determined learning objectives and KSAs [59]. However, integrating multiple professions and IPE goals adds an additional layer of complexity, wherein content needs to be relevant for all learners, and objectives specified for each professional group. Simulation developers from the various professions targeted in the simulation-based IPE should be involved to ensure relevance and important contextual details for their profession will occur in the scenario.

Conclusion

IPE, as defined in this chapter, entails an active, intentional process where learners from various professions (e.g., physicians, nurses, physical therapists, etc.) learn with, from, and about each other to improve performance outcomes. IPE leads to improved team processes (and subsequent performance) by way of improved attitudes toward other professions, and improved TMS. However, to get the most benefit from IPE, learning objectives should be pre-defined, and organizations should explicitly consider factors such as the learners, content, structure, and methods.

References

1. James JT. A new, evidence-based estimate of patient harms associated with hospital care. J Patient Saf. 2013;9(3):122–8.
2. Andel C, Davidow SL, Hollander M, Moreno DA. The economics of health care quality and medical errors. J Health Care Finance. 2012;39(1):39–50.

3. Joint Commission. Sentinel event statistics released for 2014. Joint Commission; 2015; Available from: http://www.jointcommission.org/assets/1/23/jconline_April_29_15.pdf.
4. Gawande A. Big med [Internet]. New York: The New Yorker; 2012. Available from: http://www.newyorker.com/magazine/2012/08/13/big-med.
5. The Centre for the Advancement of Interprofessional Education (CAIPE). Statement of purpose [Internet]. CAIPE; 2002. Available from: http://www.caipe.org.
6. World Health Organization. Framework for action on interprofessional education & collaborative practice [Internet]. Geneva: WHO. 2010. Available from: http://www.who.int/hrh/nursing_midwifery/en/.
7. Freeth D, Hammick M, Reeves S, Koppel I, Barr H. Effective interprofessional education: development, delivery & evaluation. Oxford, UK: Blackwell; 2005.
8. Gokhale AA. Collaborative learning enhances critical thinking. J Technol Educ. 1995;7(1)
9. Hughes AM, Gregory ME, Joseph DL, Sonesh SC, Marlow SL, Lacerenza CN, et al. Saving lives: a meta-analysis of team training in healthcare. J Appl Psychol. 2016;101:1266–304.
10. Hammick M, Freeth D, Koppel I, Reeves S, Barr H. A best evidence systematic review of interprofessional education. Med Teach. 2007;29:735–51.
11. Ketola E, Sipila R, Makela M, Klockars M. Quality improvement programme for cardiovascular disease risk factor recording in primary care. Qual Saf Health Care. 2000;9:175–80.
12. Horbar JD, Rogowski J, Plsek PE, Delmore P, Edwards WH, Hocker J, et al. Collaborative quality improvement for neonatal intensive care. Pediatr. 2001;107:14–22.
13. Morey JC, Simon R, Jay GD, Wears RL, Salisbury M, Dukes KA, et al. Error reduction and performance improvement in the emergency department through formal teamwork training: evaluation results of the MedTeams project. Healt Serv Res. 2002;37:1553–81.
14. Weiss HM. Learning theory and industrial and organizational psychology. In: Dunnette MD, Hough LM, editors. Handbook of industrial and organizational psychology. 2nd ed. Palo Alto: Consulting Psychologists Press; 1990. p. 171–221.
15. Liang DW, Moreland R, Argote L. Group versus individual training and group performance: the mediating role of transactive memory. Personal Soc Psychol Rev. 1995;21:384–93.
16. Tajfel H, Turner JC. An integrative theory of intergroup conflict. In: Austin WG, Worchel S, editors. The social psychology of intergroup relations. Monterey: Brooks/Cole; 1979. p. 33–47.
17. Turner JC. Towards a cognitive redefinition of the social group. In: Tajfel H, editor. Social identity and intergroup relations. Cambridge: Cambridge University Press; 1982. p. 15–40.
18. Stathi S, Crisp RJ. Imagining intergroup contact promotes projection to outgroups. J Exp Soc Psychol. 2008;44(4):943–57.
19. Allport FH. The structuring of events: outline of a general theory with applications to psychology. Psychol Rev. 1954;61(5):281–303.
20. Pettigrew TF. Intergroup contact theory. Annu Rev Psychol. 1998;49(1):65–85.
21. Green DP, Wong JS. Tolerance and the contact hypothesis: a field experiment. In: Borgida E, Federico CM, Sullivan JL, editors. The political psychology of democratic citizenship. Oxford, UK: Oxford University Press; 2009. p. 228–46.
22. Lindqvist S, Duncan A, Shepstone L, Watts F, Pearce S. Case-based learning in cross-professional groups- the development of a pre-registration interprofessional learning programme. J Interprof Care. 2005;19(5):509–20.
23. Jacobsen F, Lindqvist S. A two-week stay in an interprofessional training unit changes students' attitudes to health professionals. J Interprof Care. 2009;23(3):242–50.
24. Van Knippenberg D, De Dreu CK, Homan AC. Work group diversity and group performance: an integrative model and research agenda. J Appl Psychol. 2004;89:1008–22.
25. Lewis K. Measuring transactive memory systems in the field: scale development and validation. J Appl Psychol. 2003;88:587–604.
26. Kanawattanachai P, Yoo Y. The impact of knowledge coordination on virtual team performance over time. MIS Q. 2007;31(4):783–808.
27. Lie DA, Forest CP, Walsh A, Banzali Y, Lohenry K. What and how do students learn in an interprofessional student-run clinic? An educational framework for team-based care. Med Educ Online. 2016;21:1–10.

28. Currie G, Finn R, Martin G. Accounting for the 'dark side' of new organizational forms: the case of healthcare professionals. Hum Relat. 2008;61(4):539–64.
29. Tajfel H, Turner JC. The social identity theory of intergroup behavior. In: Worchel S, Austin WG, editors. Psychology of intergroup relations. Chicago: Nelson-Hall; 1986. p. 7–24.
30. Berger J, Fisck H, Norman RZ, Zelditch M. The formation of reward expectations in status situations. In: Berger J, Zelditch M, editors. Status, rewards, and influence. San Francisco: Jossey-Bass; 1985. p. 121–54.
31. Kirchler E, Davis JH. The influence of member status differences and task type on group consensus and member position change. J Pers Soc Psychol. 1986;51:83–91.
32. Weisband SP, Schneider SK, Connolly T. Computer-mediated communication and social information: status salience and status differences. Acad Manag J. 1995;38:1124–51.
33. Edmondson A. Psychological safety and learning behavior in work teams. Adm Sci Q. 1999;44:350–83.
34. Siemsen E, Roth AV, Balasubramanian S, Anand G. The influence of psychological safety and confidence in knowledge on employee knowledge sharing. Manuf Serv Oper Manag. 2008;11(3):429–47.
35. Nembhard IM, Edmondson AC. Making it safe: the effects of leader inclusiveness and professional status on psychological safety and improvement efforts in health care teams. J Organiz Behav. 2006;27:941–66.
36. DeChurch LA, Mesmer-Magnus JR. The cognitive underpinnings of effective teamwork: a meta-analysis. J Appl Psychol. 2010;95:32–53.
37. He J, Butler BS, King WR. Team cognition: development and evolution in software project teams. J Manag Inform Syst. 2007;24:261–92.
38. Prichard JS, Ashleigh MJ. The effects of team-skills training on transactive memory and performance. Small Group Res. 2007;38:696–726.
39. Schmutz J, Manser T. Do team processes really have an effect on clinical performance? A systematic literature review. B J Anaesth. 2013;110:529–44.
40. Yoo Y, Kanawattanachai P. Developments of transactive memory systems and collective mind in virtual teams. Int J Organ Anal. 2001;9:187–208.
41. Marks MA, Mathieu JE, Zaccaro SJ. A temporally based framework and taxonomy of team processes. Acad Manag Rev. 2001;26:356–76.
42. Salas E, Shuffler ML, Thayer AL, Bedwell WL, Lazzara EH. Understanding and improving teamwork in organizations: a scientifically based practical guide. Hum Resour Manag. 2015;54:599–622.
43. Salas E, DiazGranados D, Klein C, Burke CS, Stagl KC, Goodwin GF, et al. Does team training improve team performance? A meta-analysis. Hum Factors. 2008;50:903–33.
44. Hiller NJ, Day DV, Vance RJ. Collective enactment of leadership roles and team effectiveness: a field study. Leadersh Q. 2006;17:387–97.
45. Janicik GA, Bartel CA. Talking about time: effects of temporal planning and time awareness norms on group coordination and performance. Group Dyn. 2003;7:122–34.
46. Mathieu JE, Schulze W. The influence of team knowledge and formal plans on episodic team process-performance relationships. Acad Manag J. 2006;49:605–19.
47. LePine JA, Piccolo RF, Jackson CL, Mathieu JE, Saul JR. A meta-analysis of teamwork processes: tests of a multidimensional model and relationships with team effectiveness criteria. Pers Psychol. 2008;61:273–307.
48. Porter COLH. Goal orientation: effects on backing up behavior, performance, efficacy, and commitment in teams. J Appl Psychol. 2005;90:811–8.
49. Tesluk PE, Mathieu JE. Overcoming roadblocks to effectiveness: incorporating management of performance barriers into models of work group effectiveness. J Appl Psychol. 1999;84:200–17.
50. Goldstein I. Training in work organizations. In: Dunnette MD, Hough LM, editors. Handbook of industrial and organizational psychology. 2nd ed. Palo Alto: Consulting Psychologists Press; 1991. p. 507–619.
51. Thistlethwaite J, Moran M. on behalf of the World Health Organization study group on interprofessional education and collaborative practice. Learning outcomes for interprofessional education (IPE): literature review and synthesis. J Interprof Care. 2010;24:503–513.

52. Salas E, Cannon-Bowers JA. The science of training: a decade of progress. Annu Rev Psychol. 2001;52:471–99.
53. Benishek LE, Lazzara EH, Gaught WL, Arcaro LL, Okuda Y, Salas E. The template of events for applied and critical healthcare simulation (TEACH Sim): a tool for systematic simulation scenario design. Simul Healthc. 2015;10(1):21–30.
54. Knowles M. The adult learner: a neglected species. Houston: Gulf Publishing Company; 1973.
55. Salas E, Tannenbaum SI, Kraiger K, Smith-Jentsch KA. The science of training and development in organizations: what matters in practice. Psychol Sci Public Interest. 2012;13(2):74–101.
56. Atack L, Parker K, Rocchi M, Maher J, Dryden T. The impact of an online interprofessional course in disaster management competency and attitude towards interprofessional learning. J Interprof Care. 2009;23(6):586–98.
57. Curran VR, Mugford JG, Law RM, MacDonald S. Influence of an interprofessional HIV/AIDS education program on role perception, attitudes and teamwork skills of undergraduate health sciences students. Educ Health. 2005;18(1):32–44.
58. Joyal KM, Katz C, Harder N, Dean H. Interprofessional education using simulation of an overnight inpatient ward shift. J Interprof Care. 2015;29(3):268–70.
59. Rosen MA, Salas E, Silvestri S, Wu TS, Lazzara EH. A measurement tool for simulation-based training in emergency medicine: the simulation module for assessment of resident targeted event responses (SMARTER) approach. Simul Healthc. 2008;3(3):170–9.

Human Factors in Healthcare: Theoretical Underpinnings for Simulation in Interprofessional Education

3

Ashley M. Hughes

Introduction

One hundred thousand lives are lost each year due to medical error alone [1]; while estimates vary in terms of how much impact is made due to medical error, recent evidence suggests that these numbers have not since improved [2]. Miscommunication, among other teamwork factors is attributed to appear in 70% of all adverse events [3], making poor teamwork a major source of preventable medical error. Within the past 30 years, interventions have targeted improvement of team-related knowledge, skills, and attitudes (KSAs) to mitigate the impact of medical error. One method employed in approximately 75% of medical education institutions is to provide a type of interdisciplinary or interprofessional "team-based" training for students, in the attempt to better prepare them for the workforce [4]. These attempts to enhance teamwork skills have been met with some success; yet, the evidence on interprofessional education (IPE) and learning suggest that not all training programs are created equal. In fact, evidence on teamwork training (i.e., learning activities which directly target the acquisition of teamwork related KSAs) is encouraging in that it is effective at enhancing patient care in a variety of ways (e.g., reduced mortality) [5]. Yet, the literature on IPE is mixed. In fact, studies suggest that while IPE is well-received, it may not be sufficient for enhancing attitudes necessary for cooperative teamwork in applied settings [6]. Systematic reviews on IPE have reported little to no published literature examining the effectiveness of IPE [7] using randomized controlled trials. However, interprofessionality (defined as professionals coming together from different health care disciplines, organizations or professions who contribute unique conceptualizations of the patient, patient needs and response in

A. M. Hughes (✉)
University of Illinois at Chicago, Chicago, IL, USA
e-mail: amhughes@uic.edu

J. T. Paige et al. (eds.), *Comprehensive Healthcare Simulation: InterProfessional Team Training and Simulation*, Comprehensive Healthcare Simulation,
https://doi.org/10.1007/978-3-030-28845-7_3

complex health care situations), [8] is gaining momentum in the medical community, necessitating deeper examination of the drivers to effective IPE [9]. Nonetheless, implementation of Institute of Medicine (IOM) and other evidence-based recommendations require guidance from the science of learning and human performance to direct the future of clinical education across the career continuum and in a multitude of patient care settings (e.g., physical therapy, outpatient clinics, surgery) [10].

What are the human factors that may enable practitioners to develop effective and engaging IPE? Human factors has been defined as "... the scientific discipline concerned with the understanding of interactions among humans and other elements of a system, and the profession that applies theory, principles, data and methods to design in order to optimize human well-being and overall system performance and as a result, provides several solutions within medical education and job design" [11, **para1**]. Following the IOM's 2015 [8] report on the state and need for IPE, more contextualized evidence is needed; in specific, alignment of IPE approaches and methodologies need to be robust and to target enhancing collaboration in context. Recent evidence on health care effectiveness, in particular for understanding interacting components (e.g., sociotechnical issues in organizational policy and electronic health record [EHR] use) of the health care system, points us to a literature base known as human factors. Human factors as a discipline combines perspectives from psychology to industrial and mechanical engineering to optimize humans and their interaction with technical systems, such as person to environment in leveraging health information technologies (HIT). Given the field's practical focus on system solutions and multidisciplinary nature of examining efficiency in large and complex sociotechnical systems, the field of human factors is ripe for informing the future of IPE in the health care setting.

Interprofessional simulation-based education is poised to tackle errors stemming from human factors sources. The Joint Commission for Quality and Safety labels human factors related errors as a leading cause of adverse events, including unsafe use of health information technology (HIT) [3]. Similarly, the National Coordinating Counsel for Medication Error Reporting and Prevention encourages use of a systems-based approach to understanding specific forms of medical error such as medication error [12]. Use of a systems-based approach can be largely understood by leveraging principles of human factors [13]. Sonesh and colleagues [14] leveraged the human factors accident classification system (HFACs) to identify a number of human factors related errors occurring in emergency medical services (EMS) to find that medication labeling, medication placement, medication shortages, and teamwork-related problems (e.g., lack of communication regarding a medication error event or near miss) contribute to the occurrence of medication error. Based on their findings, Sonesh and colleagues [14] recommend leveraging a team-based approach to education as well as systems-wide implementation of standardized medication labeling procedures. Taking this into account, the field of human factors offers several practical principles derived from human factors, theory which are poised to shape the understanding of medical error in context as well as develop successful countermeasures to enhance safety.

Human factors theories and frameworks have a history of influencing positive change in the medical community [15]. The application of human factors to health information technology (HIT) within the context of IPE simulation ensures safe, and satisfactory use by the clinician or user group [16]. Previous research has identified specific human factors frameworks that have proven useful to transforming health care and improving patient safety, such as the Systems Engineering for Improved Patient Safety (SEIPS) model [17, 18]. This includes a focus on a systems-based approach (e.g., multi-level work environment considerations) and the consideration of both environment and human factors to optimize their fit. Using these approaches to guide contextual design may help reduce workload, improve workflow, and minimize the occurrence of errors in real-world persons interacting with technical systems.

While human factors literature is diverse, this literature base enables closer examination of work performed within health care and the ways in which workflow can be optimized. Therefore, a number of theories available from the human factors literature at large are poised to inform the development of effective IPE. This chapter is organized to first cover the theoretical underpinnings of human factors as it pertains to simulation education in IPE. The second portion of this chapter will discuss practical implications and strategies for bolstering IPE effectiveness to ensure cooperation amongst team members from various disciplines. It will conclude with practical recommendations.

Why Is Theory Important? Bridging the Gap from Theory to Practice

The science of effective simulation-based education stems from the science of learning. Human factors theory informs the path forward to designing and implementing effective learning opportunities, such as those inherent in simulation-based IPE programs. In particular, elements of human factors (e.g., systems-based approach, sociotechnical features, human computer interaction principles) inform development of successful learning content, selection of appropriate simulation equipment and components of the IPE program's evaluation(s). The literature on training and education guides development of successful education programs [19, 20]; yet, the guidance provided in this chapter is contextualized to create IPE programs which leverage simulation-based practice opportunities.

Practical frameworks provide guidance for IPE program development throughout the program's temporal lifecycle. In other words, education programs are an iterative process understood in relation to the implementation of the IPE program. These temporal phases of an IPE program are best understood before IPE is implemented (i.e., the IPE development phase), a period during which the IPE program is implemented (i.e., the time from which IPE is piloted or implemented in a widespread fashion), and the period which occurs after learners have completed their IPE opportunity [21, 22]. However, the education program should also be examined for updates and improvements in practice. Recent and ongoing research informs the basis of effective educational practices [23, 24]; yet, a century of research on learning and training has paved a way forward to enable closer examination of specific components of training to enable long-term sustainable benefits. These practices are rooted in key principles tied to human factors learning theories [19–23]. I present human factors guiding principles nested within the applicable portion of the training and education lifecycle. Specifically, I do this to emphasize the importance of human factors and the iterative process of learning (e.g., skill retention; competencies are updated on an as needed basis).

Interprofessional Education Program Design

Problem Identification and Content Development

IPE activities should be crafted with the clinician group in mind. To address a need, IPE activities must align with pre-identified clinical priorities. These priorities stem from needs of the health care group at large, recommendations for improving practice in care (e.g., meeting the American College of Obstetrics and Gynecology's 20 minute from decision to incision for emergent Cesarean sections) [25], or specific needs of a particular unit. The stem cause of the problem should arise from human factors or interprofessional related issues. For instance, if a unit is experiencing difficulty in medication administration for patients (e.g., too much or too little of a given medication is dispensed), and the problem is attributed to poor interprofessional communication, learning goals should center on the interprofessional communication used to verify patient medications and dosage amounts. To thoroughly contextualize and identify competency needs, multiple perspectives must be garnered to provide input into the development of the IPE program. Specifically, key stakeholders within each discipline/profession undergoing IPE should have the opportunity to provide input to the learning content; members of unit or hospital leadership should also be involved early. This assists in creating a meaningful and effective learning program in two ways: (1) The educator/education team gains multiple perspectives on the trainees' needs to develop robust content, and (2) The trainees will be engaged in the program's anticipated outcomes. There is evidence to suggest how well designed simulation scenarios enhance IPE's effectiveness, Smith-Jentsch et al. [26] found that learners who underwent negative experiences which were related to the education content (e.g., poor teamwork experienced on-the-job prior to entry into a course teaching teamwork) experienced greater gains in the learning activity than learners who could not relate to the examples within the education content. Leveraging multiple perspectives and gaining buy-in from key stakeholders early within the education lifecycle ultimately enhances participation, motivation, and learning from IPE.

Learners should be selected purposively to attend the IPE opportunity. This concept applies based on learners' educational experiences, discipline, or profession [27]; framing of the importance of learning in terms of an opportunity rather than a mandate can enhance the motivation of learners to attend [28, 29]. Reviewing the emergent results of the needs analysis can better direct learner identification process. Particularly, emphasizing the anticipated benefits of engaging in the interprofessional learning opportunity can enhance learner acquisition and retention of the content embedded within the IPE [30, 31].

Practice and Simulation Development

Learning occurs when education programs engage learners in meaningful opportunities to practice [20]. Specifically, leveraging IPE related content while engaging in the program provides learners with the opportunity to take corrective action such that later use of skills is aligned with the intended and proper use of the skills [32, 33]. Practice opportunities should seek to mimic key features of the learner's jobs in a realistic manner so that learners are immersed within the learning scenario. Creating a realistic simulated environment may not be sufficient for immersing participants within a scenario [34]; however, realism is important in this process in two ways. Identical elements theory highlights two potential avenues through which practitioners can create a sense of realism within simulation scenarios: that is through physical fidelity (i.e., closeness in appearance and function of simulator components to real-world devices, patients, equipment), and psychological fidelity (i.e., the believability of the scenario and chosen simulation techniques in the suspension of disbelief) [35]. Simulation can accomplish physical fidelity in a variety of ways; in particular, simulation equipment and technologies should seek to replicate the tasks and environment inherent in the work environment, such as incorporating realistic human patient simulators [36], which may assist in the transfer of skills by making recall of the proper use of learned skills less challenging [37]. While there is some debate as to whether the physical fidelity (i.e., believability of the physical replications in a learning program) carries importance in facilitating transfer, Hughes and colleagues [5] found that physical fidelity of the chosen patient simulator may not enhance effectiveness of educational programs which target teamwork related KSAs. Psychological fidelity has been noted to be of the utmost importance for ensuring simulation effectiveness [20]. Scenarios and break out activities disseminated in the IPE program should be crafted with forethought of the believability in the developed scenario. Specifically, scenarios should focus on the learning content related to transferrable teamwork related KSAs for interprofessional teams. The chosen clinical context for the scenario and patient case should reflect a likely case that the learners would experience on-the-job. Selection of a clinical context should align with the identified KSAs which emerged from a needs analysis used to formulate specific clinical problems (i.e., focus the content of IPE clinical context to tackle real-world human factors problems) for IPE context and educational content.

Simulation scenario flow, while also arguably important for psychological fidelity, should incorporate multiple opportunities to leverage a given KSA. While crafting a simulation scenario, it may be tempting to fit several KSAs (e.g. situation awareness, shared leadership, closed loop communication) linked to problem identification into a given scenario. However, this may reduce the number of opportunities as learners should demonstrate each of those skills within an IPE program, and subsequently, may mitigate the potential for meaningful feedback and learning [38]. Recommendations for IPE leveraging simulation scenarios are to include at least three opportunities to demonstrate each desired KSA. In this way, the evaluation of the learner's performance can be more complete (e.g., reduction of potential for human error on part of the learner as well as the facilitator or trainer) [39], and more diagnostic feedback can be provided [40]. In regards to feedback, the debriefer should seek to provide learners with constructive feedback immediately following practice sessions [40]. Feedback that is specific and non-punitive to correct mistakes [41, 42] and delivered by a reputable and credible source (i.e., one that learners' trust and respect [43]) can enhance learning and skill acquisition in IPE.

Interprofessional Education Implementation

Until this point, human factors theories were covered relevant to adult learning, motivation, and replicability of the work environment to create meaningful opportunities to practice within IPE programs. This next section will focus on implementation of learning activities which begins once the educational program has been created. The educator/education team should seek to maximize a smooth flow in the transitions (within the simulation scenario as well as any didactic content included) and that all equipment required to run the simulation scenario is available and functioning. It also follows that leveraging a "systems of redundancy" (i.e., having several back up materials necessary for the course's facilitation on hand) approach to maintaining simulation equipment is imperative.

Structure Learning Content

Learning content should be delivered in a manner which does not overwhelm trainees. This practice stems from cognitive load theory [44]. In the effort to maintain optimal levels of cognitive load (i.e., educators should consider the number of activities, length of the educational session and/or scenario, the number of KSAs embedded within the scenario, and length of the post-simulation after action review) [44]. Further, piloting the IPE simulation-based content allows time for potential changes such that the validity (i.e., simulation content disseminates the intended information to learners) of the education program is maximized. Prior research has indicated that learners who perceive content in education to be valid [45] and complementary or necessary to their work/job [46] are more motivated to engage in learning activities and reap greater benefits from engaging in the educational program. Trainees should be encouraged to ask questions during training; namely, this is so that information that is learned and retained is accurate and relatable to learner experiences. Providing specific time(s) (preferably before and after the scenario) should be allocated during the course of the simulation content to allow participants to share ideas, ask questions, and engage in discussion to increase their learning and ability to adapt the learning to different situations [47, 48]. Doing this in a group setting can foster support for learning from peers, which is critical for subsequent use of skills [49].

Interprofessional Education Evaluation

Evaluation Framework

A wide variety of frameworks are available to evaluate learning activities, such as those inherent within IPE; however, the first recommendation is to select a framework that best aligns with the IPE program's goals. Across the available and widely used frameworks at large (e.g., Holton [50]; Kirkpatrick [51]), there is agreement that effective educational programs enhance KSAs related to the education content and that improvements manifest in a type of behavioral change. Holton's [52] framework emphasizes the role of learner motivation and emphasizes behavioral change as a hallmark of an education program's success; Kirkpatrick [53] introduced a framework for training effectiveness which involves evaluating education along criteria at multiple levels. These levels or criterion include: trainees' reactions (i.e., does training surpass trainees' expectations?), learning (i.e., does IPE lead to gains in KSAs?), behaviors (i.e., does IPE-related content transfer to the work environment?), and results (i.e., does IPE result in improved organizational outcomes?). While Kirkpatrick's framework offers practical means by which training can be evaluated, meta-analytic estimates suggest that reactions may not play a substantive role in determining training effectiveness [5, 52]. Multi-level evaluations, however, may be helpful in determining the overall effectiveness of a given IPE program [53, 54]. To identify specific criteria (e.g., improved use of a suturing technique, increased knowledge in regards to management of post-partum hemorrhage) to be measured in the evaluation of IPE, the interprofessional needs identified prior to IPE development should be reviewed [19]. Ideally, evaluation of IPE should further strive to reveal portions of the educational program that should be changed or adapted for subsequent learners, particularly during the pilot phase of disseminating the program [21].

Assessment of IPE success can be performed in a variety of ways to evaluate IPE along multi-level criteria. Behaviorally anchored rating scales (BARS) can be developed to assess behaviors leveraged during simulation-based scenarios as well as use of skills on-the-job [55]. In these instances, it is most helpful to pilot the evaluation tools (should they be developed in-house for IPE needs rather than an available valid and reliable tool) separately from the piloting of the IPE program [56] as well as to train raters who complete the observational tool to ensure inter-rater reliability [57]. Self-report scales can also be leveraged to gauge learner reactions and perceptions of utility of the content, [58] and cognitive, affective, or skill-based assessments of learning [59]. However, self-report surveys and scales are subject to bias of the participant and should also be tested for reliability and validity if developed in-house [60]. The use of unobtrusive and objective measurement in the assessment of team-related education is possible and growing [61]. Therefore, to ensure IPE is impacting patient-related outcomes, it is suggested that evaluation of IPE further evaluate patient-outcome related data via patient chart information relevant to identified clinical context and specified problem area of focus (IOM) [9]. Through a multitude of methods, IPE evaluations can be robust, valid, and reliable to link IPE effectiveness to patient-related improvements.

Recommendations

Ongoing Support

Health care organizations wishing to reap the benefits of IPE should engage in supporting collaborative efforts. Recent evidence describes the essential role of organizational support in fostering use of skills on the job [62, 63], such that they become more typical in application [23] and a norm for the organization. Numerous studies, frameworks, and reviews have found that support can stem from peers (e.g., friendly reminders from colleagues on what was covered in IPE), peer networks, supervisors (e.g., supervisor provides feedback on use of a skill), and organizational level forms of support (e.g., top management creates and enforces policies and procedures which support IPE) [64] and have further sought to speak to the important support behaviors and resources at each prospective level [64–66], to provide successful support for integration of interprofessional teamwork on-the-job. One form of support includes enforcing policies, procedures, and rewards systems which incentivize use of KSAs related to IPE such that organizations are supportive [67] and learners are held accountable to integration of IPE's use in daily workflow [68].

A method by which organizations can stimulate support for IPE programs is to debrief and provide periodic feedback to learners in relation to the IPE KSAs. Peers, supervisors and members of top management can provide input; however, management should seek to foster an environment in which concerns related to IPE and its use can be discussed amongst learners or within management [41]. Receipt of feedback serves to assist learners in goal setting in relation to use of IPE-related KSAs [68]. Using the awareness of current level of use of KSAs from IPE, learners can connect with peers or integrate goals for IPE's use in professional development. Peer to peer mentorship, for instance, has been shown to increase use of skills as this supports ongoing discussions on IPE-related knowledge and skills [69, 70].

Practical Applications, Guidance, and a Way Forward

Simulation techniques for IPE show promise in advancing medical education across the continuum such that health care is moving toward a culture of collaboration [36]. However, the IOM suggests aligning IPE practices with competencies to impact patient care [9]. Potential avenues for future employment and research of simulation-based IPE include several applications.

Given the proliferation of team-based approaches to patient care and professional development, IPE programs should consider human factors methodologies for crafting, implementing and evaluating simulation based IPE opportunities such that the time and effort spent in educational program development is most effective. Therefore, the following recommendations are provided to create an action-oriented approach to developing and implementing effective IPE to enable alignment of IPE recommended core competencies [71] and the best practices from human factors theory.

Conduct a Needs Analysis To craft content that is contextual and motivating to learners, needs must first be identified. In the case of IPE, needs should be identified based on their overlap between professions or disciplines of interest for the learning activities. For instance, a learning activity intended to instruct clinicians from primary care should incorporate perceptions of learning needs from nurses, clerks, pharmacists, dieticians, and social workers in addition to primary care providers. In this way, IPE instructional simulation-based activities cover content relevant to all learners involved in the activities and motivation to learn and participate can be optimized.

Leverage Pre-existing Team-Based Learning Approach to Develop Content Core competencies of IPE incorporate KSAs relevant to improving team-based collaborations across professions and disciplines. To effectively address the need for cross-discipline communication and teamwork relevant KSAs, it makes sense to incorporate elements of teamwork training into IPE opportunities. Several agencies promoting patient safety provide slides and content for programs containing teamwork related learning activities online. One example of this is the Agency for Healthcare Research and Quality (AHRQ) developing the widely utilized program 'Team Strategies for Enhancing Performance and Patient Safety (TeamSTEPPS®) [72]. While I recommend modifying pre-existing content to meet the identified needs of interprofessional learners (e.g., teaching against use of field-specific jargon in handoffs and electronic health record notes), freely available team training programs provide a basis for educators to build a larger IPE program targeting teamwork skills.

Measure Effectiveness The purpose of this chapter was to translate the theory on effective learning and human behavior in context to actionable guidance for development of effective IPE. However, measurement plays a role in both determining IPE program effectiveness and communicating a message of importance related to IPE [73]. Taken together, it is best to perform baseline assessments of process and outcomes relevant to the IPE prior to its delivery and monitor improvements and/or declines over time.

As discussed earlier, IPE can and should be evaluated through a variety of assessment techniques (e.g., BARS, surveys) along multilevel criteria to ensure effectiveness. Developing content for evaluation strategies may pose challenges, particularly for institutions lacking an education specialist or education team. However, guidance exists on evaluation of criteria that are commonly embedded in IPE programs, such as teamwork-related skills (i.e., Teamwork Perceptions Questionnaire [TPQ]) [72], successful completion of tasks requiring interprofessional involvement (e.g., successful intubation of critical airway patient) [74]. To enable health care institutions with limited resources to overcome challenges related to assessment, I recommend utilizing pre-existing materials and further contextualizing metrics based on identified needs. For instance, if interprofessional communication arises as a need and focus for the IPE program, pre-existing metrics of teamwork should be leveraged and contextualized to evaluate IPE effectiveness.

Future Directions

Is Simulation Right for Me?

While I encourage incorporation of opportunities to practice leveraging a type of simulation-based education approach, not all institutions will have access to high fidelity equipment to mimic key patient responses and clinical contexts which may be of interest to IPE. While several academic institutions as well as hospitals are building their own simulation center(s) to foster simulation-based IPE opportunities for continuing education credits and resident programs, not all simulation requires equipment. In revisiting this chapter's section on crafting an effective simulation scenario, it is important to note that guidance from the literature states that psychological fidelity reigns supreme and is backed by evidence as being more critical to IPE-related activities than physical fidelity [5]. In this case, believable scenarios in which students, residents, or practicing clinicians can engage in role play may stimulate similar gains in interprofessionality than leveraging realistic high tech simulator equipment.

Not all IPE will require use of high fidelity manikins. By conducting a thorough analysis of the learner's needs, simulation scenario development can incorporate content, equipment, and clinical context that is most critical to learners identified IPE needs. In this way, health care organizations can spare time and resources in deciding whether to conduct the IPE program in a simulation center or whether role playing scenarios conducted in-situ or within the classroom will provide sufficient instruction, saving time and valuable resources.

Misdiagnosis

Misdiagnosis has been defined as "a failure to employ indicated tests; use of outmoded tests or therapy; or failure to act on results of monitoring or testing" [75] and is estimated to impact 12 million patients each year in the United States [75]. Yet, diagnosis is a team sport [76], which is currently lacking in interprofessional team development. In fact, estimates suggest that coordination failures in the follow up of test results and the lack of application of training and learning theory, including feedback on diagnostic performance, contribute to inflated confirmation bias (i.e., data is "selectively marshaled to support a favored hypothesis; [77], p., 1186) and self-pride in the accuracy of diagnosis. Thus, there has been a recent thrust toward understanding the role of IPE in addressing issues of misdiagnosis and coordination of care, particularly in the follow up of test results [78]. In the digital age of health care innovations and informatics, application of simulation-based IPE opportunities may foster collaborations and encourage use of team-based strategies which may help mitigate the impact of diagnostic error. For instance, IPE simulation which incorporates use of telemedicine to connect with other professionals or clinicians from other disciplines may improve the awareness of the need to connect or collaborate with other professionals. This principle stems from identical elements theory in that education which mimics the work environment is ultimately successfully in behavioral change. Future investigation is warranted on mechanisms for IPE to address the gap of stimulating interprofessional approaches to engage in more accurate diagnoses of chronic diseases across the care continuum.

Health Information Technology

One potential avenue for exploration in the future of IPE is how IPE related activities can be better coupled with newly approved HIT to support collaborative efforts in their use. For instance, findings on the utility of electronic health records (EHR) as a means for cross profession or cross discipline information exchange have resulted in several vital pieces of patient information falling through the cracks [79]. For instance, a patient in Dallas seen in the emergency room had described symptoms to the admitting nurse; however, these notes made in the electronic patient chart were unnoticed by the Emergency Room physician. The patient was sent home with a round of antibiotics and died several days later due to a missed diagnosis of Ebola. Simulation-based IPE which incorporates device training coupled with appropriate use of teamwork-related behaviors may enable standardized use of regularly used HIT, such as EHR. As health care transitions to the digital age of computing, human computer interaction principles of computer-supported cooperative work (CSCW; [80]) (e.g., team friendly interface design) should be tested within a simulation based IPE setting to ensure safety and proper use.

Conclusions

To conclude this chapter, evidence-based recommendations are provided to facilitate the next wave of IPE. Namely, considerations for simulation-based IPE should adopt a systems-based approach to understand interprofessional needs and contextual human factors problems to inform scenario development. Recommendations focused on evidence-based guidance can be completed before, during and after IPE implementation to ensure its success. Future research can apply the best practices of IPE to examine effectiveness of IPE and simulation-based approaches to enhance health care practices and reduce medical errors.

References

1. Kohn LT, Corrigan JM, Donaldson M. To err is human: building a safer health system. Washington, D.C.: National Academies Press; 1999.
2. Makary MA, Daniel M. Medical error—the third leading cause of death in the US. BMJ. 2016;353:i2139.
3. The Joint Commission. Sentinel event data: root causes by event type 2004–2014. 2014. Retrieved from: http://www.tsigconsulting.com/tolcam/wp-content/uploads/2015/04/TJC-Sentinel-Event-Root_Causes_by_Event_Type_2004-2014.pdf.
4. Beach S. Annual medical school graduation survey shows gains in team training. C.2013 [updated 2013 August]. www.aamc.org/newsroom/newsreleases/351120/080213.html. Accessed 5 May 2017.
5. Hughes AM, Gregory ME, Joseph DL, Sonesh SC, Marlow SL, Lacerenza CN, et al. Saving lives: a meta-analysis of team training in healthcare. J Appl Psychol. 2016;101(6):1266–304.
6. Hammick M, Freeth D, Koppel I, Reeves S, Barr H. A best evidence systematic review of interprofessional education: BEME guide no. 9. Med Teach. 2007;29(8):735–51.
7. Reeves S, Zwarenstein M, Goldman J, et al. The effectiveness of interprofessional education: key findings from a new systematic review. J Interprof Care. 2010;24(3):230–41.
8. D'amour D, Oandasan I. Interprofessionality as the field of interprofessional practice and interprofessional education: an emerging concept. J Interprof Care. 2005;19(1):8–20.
9. Institute of Medicine. Measuring the impact of Interprofessional education on collaborative practice and patient outcomes. Washington, D.C.: National Academy of Sciences; 2015.
10. Hammick M. Interprofessional education: evidence from the past to guide the future. Med Teach. 2009;22(5):461–7.
11. International Ergonomics Association. Definition and domains of ergonomics. http://www.iea.cc/whats/. 2017. Accessed 14 Jun 2017.
12. National Coordinating Council on Medication Error Reporting and Prevention. NCC MERP Taxonomy of medication errors. http://www.nccmerp.org/sites/default/files/taxonomy2001-07-31.pdf. 2001. Accessed 14 May 2017.
13. Carayon P, Bass EJ, Bellandi T, Gurses AP, Hallbeck MS, Mollo V. Sociotechnical systems analysis in health care: a research agenda. IIE Trans Healthc Syst Eng. 2011;1(3):145–60.
14. Sonesh SC, Gregory ME, Hughes AM, Lacerenza C, Marlow S, Cooper T, Salas E. An empirical examination of medication error in emergency medical systems (EMS): towards a comprehensive taxonomy. Orlando: Institute for Simulation & Training; 2013.
15. Carayon P, Karsh BT, Gurses AP, et al. Macroergonomics in health care quality and patient safety. Rev Hum Factors Ergon. 2013;8(1):4–54.
16. Holden RJ. Physicians' beliefs about using EMR and CPOE: in pursuit of a contextualized understanding of health IT use behavior. Int J Med Inform. 2010;79(2):71–80.
17. Holden RJ, Carayon P, Gurses AP, Hoonakker P, Hundt AS, Ozok AA, Rivera-Rodriguez AJ. SEIPS 2.0: a human factors framework for studying and improving the work of healthcare professionals and patients. Ergonomics. 2013;56(11):1669–86.
18. Carayon P, Hundt AS, Karsh BT, Gurses AP, Alvarado CJ, Smith M, Brennan PF. Work system design for patient safety: the SEIPS model. Qual Saf Health Care. 2006;15(Suppl 1):i50–8.
19. Goldstein RL, Ford K. Training in organizations: needs assessment, development and evaluation. 4th ed. Belmont: Wadsworth; 2004.
20. Salas E, Tannenbaum SI, Kraiger K, Smith-Jentsch K. The science of training and development in organizations: what matters in practice. Psychol Sci Public Interest. 2012;3(2):74–101.

21. Broad ML. Beyond transfer of training: engaging systems to improve performance. San Francisco: Pfeiffer; 2005.
22. Broad ML, Newstrom JW. Transfer of training: action-packed strategies to ensure high payoff from training investments. New York: Addison-Wesley Publishing Company; 1992.
23. Huang JL, Blume BD, Ford JK, Baldwin TT. A tale of two transfers: disentangling maximum and typical transfer and their respective predictors. J Bus Psychol. 2015;30:709–32. https://doi.org/10.1007/s10869-014-9694-1.
24. Baldwin TT, Ford KJ, Blume BD. The state of transfer of training research: moving toward more consumer-centric inquiry. Hum Res Dev Q. 2017;28(1):17–28.
25. American College of Obstetricians and Gynecologists (ACOG). Standards of obstetric-gynecologic services. 7th ed. Washington, D.C.: ACOG; 1989. p. 39.
26. Smith-Jentsch KA, Jentsch FG, Payne SC, Salas E. Can pretraining experiences explain individual differences in learning? J Appl Psychol. 1996;81(1):110–6.
27. Noe RA. Trainees' attributes and attitudes: neglected influences on training effectiveness. Acad Manage Rev. 1986;11(4):736–49.
28. Sankey KS. Sustaining proactive motivation for non-mandatory professional development: building self-determined employees. Unpublished doctoral dissertation. University of Southern Queensland; 2013.
29. Burke LA, Hutchins HM. Training transfer: an integrative literature review. Hum Res Dev Rev. 2007;6:263–97.
30. Meyer E, Lees A, Humphries D, Connell NA. Opportunities and barriers to successful learning transfer: impact of critical care skills training. J Adv Nurs. 2007;60(3):308–16.
31. Keith N, Frese M. Effectiveness of error management training: a meta-analysis. J Appl Psychol. 2008;93(1):59–69.
32. Zapp L. Use of multiple teaching strategies in the staff development setting. J Nurs Staff Dev. 2001;17:206–12.
33. Hays RT, Singer SJ. Simulation fidelity: definitions, problems, and historical perspectives. In: Hays RT, Singer SJ, editors. Simulation fidelity in training system design: bridging the gap between reality and training. New York: Springer; 1989. p. 1–22.
34. Cheng K, Cairns PA. Behaviour, realism and immersion in games. CHI. 2005:1272–5.
35. Kozlowski SW, DeShon RP. A psychological fidelity approach to simulation-based training: theory, research and principles. In: Salas E, Elliot LR, Schflett SG, Coovert MD, editors. Scaled worlds: development, validation, and applications. Burlington: Ashgate Publishing; 2004. p. 75–99.
36. Mitchell P, Wynia M, Golden R, et al. Core principles & values of effective team-based healthcare. Washington, D.C.: National Academies Press; 2012.
37. Issenberg SB, McGaghie WC, Petrusa ER, Lee Gordon D, Scalese RJ. Features and uses of high-fidelity medical simulations that lead to effective learning: a BEME systematic review. Med Teach. 2005;27:10–28.
38. Rosen MA, Salas E, Silvestri S, Wu TS, Lazzara EH. A measurement tool for simulation-based training in emergency medicine: the simulation module for assessment of resident targeted event responses (SMARTER) approach. Simul Healthc. 2008;3(3):170–9.
39. Weaver SJ, Dy SM, Rosen MA. Team-training in healthcare: a narrative synthesis of the literature. BMJ Qual Saf. 2014;23:359–72. https://doi.org/10.1136/bmjqs-2013-001848.
40. Tannenbaum SI, Mathieu JE, Salas E, Cannon-Bowers JA. Meeting trainees' expectations: the influence of training fulfillment on the development of commitment, self-efficacy, and motivation. J Appl Psychol. 1991;76:759–69.
41. Kluger AN, DeNisi A. The effects of feedback interventions on performance: a historical review, a meta-analysis, and a preliminary feedback intervention theory. Psychol Bull. 1996;119:254–84.
42. Hysong SJ. Meta-analysis: audit & feedback features impact effectiveness on care quality. Med Care. 2009;47(3):356.
43. Halperin K, Snyder CR, Shenkel RJ, Houston BK. Effects of source status and message favorability on acceptance of personality feedback. J Appl Psychol. 1976;61(1):85–8.

44. Sweller J. Cognitive load during problem solving: effects on learning. Cognit Sci. 1988;12:257–85.
45. Grohmann A, Beller J, Kauffeld S. Exploring the critical role of motivation to transfer in the training transfer process. Int J Train Dev. 2014;18(2):84–103.
46. Burke MJ, Salvador RO, Smith-Crowe K, Chan-Serafin S, Smith A, Sonesh S. The dread factor: how hazards and safety training influence learning and performance. J Appl Psychol. 2011;96(1):46–70.
47. Dornan T, Boshuizen H, King N, Scherpbier A. Experience-based learning: a model linking the processes and outcomes of medical students' workplace learning. Med Educ. 2007;41(1):84–91.
48. Kazbour RR, McGhee HM, Mooney T, Masica L, Brinkerhoff RO. Evaluating the impact of a performance-based methodology on transfer of training. Perform Improv Q. 2013;26(1):5–33.
49. Cromwell SE, Kolb JA. An examination of work-environment support factors affecting transfer of supervisory skills training to the workplace. Hum Res Dev Q. 2004;15(4):449–72.
50. Holton EF. The flawed four-level evaluation model. Hum Res Dev Q. 1996;7(1):5–21.
51. Kirkpatrick DL. Great ideas revisited: revisiting Kirkpatrick's four-level model. Train Develop. 1996;50:54–9.
52. Tharenou P, Saks AM, Moore C. A review and critique of research on training and organizational-level outcomes. Hum Res Manag Rev. 2007;17:251–73.
53. Alliger GM, Tannenbaum SI, Bennett BJ, Traver H, Shotland A. A meta-analysis of the relations among training criteria. Pers Psychol. 1997;50:341–58.
54. Arthur W, Bennett W, Edens PS, Bell ST. Effectiveness of training in organizations: a meta-analysis of design and evaluation features. J Appl Psychol. 2003;88:234–45.
55. Schwab DP, Heneman HG, DeCotiis TA. Behaviorally anchored rating scales: a review of the literature. Pers Psychol. 1975;28(4):549–62.
56. Jacobs R, Kafry D, Zedeck S. Expectations of behaviorally anchored rating scales. Pers Psychol. 1980;33(3):595–640.
57. Feldman M, Lazzara EH, Vanderbilt AA, DiazGranados D. Rater training to support high-stakes simulation-based assessments. J Contin Educ Health Prof. 2012;32(4):279–86.
58. Sitzmann T, Brown KG, Casper WJ, Ely K, Zimmerman RD. A review and meta-analysis of the nomological network of trainee reactions. J Appl Psychol. 2008;93:280–95.
59. Kraiger K, Ford JK, Salas E. Application of cognitive, skill-based, and affective theories of learning outcomes to new methods of training evaluation. J Appl Psychol. 1993;78(2):311–28.
60. Donaldson SI, Grant-Vallone EJ. Understanding self-report bias in organizational behavior research. J Bus Psychol. 2002;17(2):245–60.
61. Marlow SL, Hughes AM, Sonesh SC, Gregory ME, Lacerenza CN, Benishek LE, et al. A systematic review of team training in health care: ten questions. Jt Comm J Qual Patient Saf. 2017;43(4):197–204.
62. Burrow J, Berardinelli P. Systematic performance improvement-refining the space between learning and results. J Workplace Learn. 2003;15(1):6–13.
63. Blume BD, Ford JK, Baldwin TT, Huang JL. Transfer of training: a meta-analytic review. J Manag. 2010;36:1065–105.
64. Nijman DJJ, Nijhof WJ, Wognum AAM, Veldkamp BP. Exploring differential effects of supervisor support on transfer of training. J Euro Ind Training. 2006;30(7):529–49.
65. Hughes AM. A meta-analytic integration of what matters in training transfer. Unpublished doctoral dissertation. Orlando: University of Central Florida; 2016.
66. Thayer PW, Teachout MS. A climate for transfer model (AL/HR-TP-1995-0035). Retrieved from Brooks Air Force Base, Texas. 1995.
67. Burke LA, Hutchins HM, Saks AM. Best practices in training transfer. In: Paulidi MA, editor. Psychology for business success. Santa Barbara: Praeger; 2013. p. 115–32.
68. Grossman R, Salas E. The transfer of training: what really matters. Int J Train Dev. 2011;15(2):103–20.
69. Lim DH, Johnson SD. Trainee perceptions of factors that influence learning transfer. Int J Train Dev. 2002;6(1):36–48.

70. Putter SE. Making training stick: a close examination of how trainee readiness, supervisor support, and practice foster transfer in a mobile technology-based training program. Retrieved from ProQuest. (AAI3608415). 2014.
71. Interprofessional Education Collaborative (IPEC). Core competencies for interprofessional collaborative practice: 2016 update. https://ipecollaborative.org/uploads/IPEC-2016-Updated-Core-Competencies-Report__final_release_.PDF (2016). Accessed 16 Apr 2017.
72. King HB, Battles J, Baker DP, et al. TeamSTEPPSTM: team strategies and tools to enhance performance and patient safety. In: Henriksen K, Battles JB, Keyes MA, Grady ML, editors. Advances in patient safety: new directions and alternative approaches, Performance and tools, vol. 3. Rockville: Agency for Healthcare Research and Quality (US); 2008.
73. Rouiller JZ, Goldstein IL. The relationship between organizational transfer climate and positive transfer of training. Hum Resource Dev Q. 1993;4(4):377–90.
74. Fletcher G, Flin R, McGeorge P, Glavin R, Maran N, Patey R. Anaesthetists' Non-Technical Skills (ANTS): evaluation of a behavioural marker system. Brit J Anaesth. 2003;90(5):580–8.
75. Institute of Medicine (IOM). Patient safety: achieving a new standard for care. Washington, D.C.: The National Academies Press; 2004. p. 30.
76. Balogh EP, Miller BT, Ball JR. Improving diagnosis in health care. Washington, D.C.: National Academies Press; 2017.
77. Croskerry P. Achieving quality in clinical decision making: cognitive strategies and detection of bias. Qual Clin Decis Mak. 2002;9(11):1184–204.
78. Giardina TD, King BJ, Ignaczak AP, Paull DE, Hoeksema L, Mills PD, et al. Root cause analysis reports help identify common factors in delayed diagnosis and treatment of outpatients. Health Aff. 2013;32(8):1368–75.
79. Gregory ME, Bryan J, Mendez A. Educating interprofessional trainees to provide safe and effective team-based care: perspectives on curriculum development and implementation. A paper presented at the 2017 Human factors and ergonomics society annual symposium on human factors in healthcare. New Orleans. 2017.
80. Grudin J. Computer-supported cooperative work: history and focus. Computer. 1994;27(5):19–26.

Teamwork: Education and Training in Healthcare

4

Jennifer Feitosa and Adrian Fonseca

Introduction

As of 2015, medical errors are ranked third in leading causes of death in the United States, which roughly translates to around 440,000 patients [1], making it evident that team training is a necessity. A number of medical error cases result directly from coordination failures in healthcare [1]; for example, 37% of severe cases, that may result in the death of patients, have indeed been associated with communication issues among healthcare professionals [2]. Hospital discharges, appropriate medication handling, and patient handoffs are some of the most critical periods for a patient [3, 4] due to the fact that most of it relies on the effective teamwork that a healthcare team possesses. Albeit, these are professionals who have been highly trained and are indeed skilled in their jobs, the training of teamwork skills to better communicate, coordinate, and properly provide cohesive patient care is often overlooked [3]. Knowing that critical incidents may arise over an issue that can be minimized through effort and planning, healthcare professionals should ask themselves: Why avoid it?

Team training can be defined as the systematic acquisition of knowledge, skills, and abilities (KSAs) related to teamwork based on learning principles [5]. Considering how healthcare is an evidence-based practice, we cannot suggest to engage in team training without properly considering its effectiveness in enhancing performance. Fortunately, a recent meta-analysis that compiled over 146 effect sizes of team training in healthcare showed evidence of positive outcomes to not only trainees' reactions, learning, and transfer, but also to organizational results [6]. In other words, not only trainees perceived the training as useful, but the study also showed changes in teamwork KSAs, including enhanced team-related behaviors at work, which in turn led to better outcomes at the hospital-level. Besides this

J. Feitosa (✉)
Claremont McKenna College, Claremont, CA, USA

A. Fonseca
McKinsey & Company, San Jose, Costa Rica

J. T. Paige et al. (eds.), *Comprehensive Healthcare Simulation: InterProfessional Team Training and Simulation*, Comprehensive Healthcare Simulation,
https://doi.org/10.1007/978-3-030-28845-7_4

evidence, it is important to integrate this team based literature with concrete guidelines in order for practitioners to be able to implement effective team training techniques. This is true for actual practice in hospitals, but it starts with how medical professionals are trained (e.g., healthcare education) [7]. With this goal in mind, the purpose of this chapter is to highlight the theoretical underpinnings that can guide tangible actions to better educate and train healthcare professionals to be more effective team members.

Teamwork in Healthcare

Prior to extracting the theoretical underpinnings of teamwork, it is important to properly define what a team is. A team is defined as a set of individuals with specific functions who work interdependently and towards a shared goal [8]. From this definition, we can gather several resemblances to the medical field. First, for teams in healthcare systems, the daily interactions share the common objective of providing the best possible care and saving patients' lives [6]. Also, we recognize that healthcare professionals have very specific roles and functions: surgeons, emergency medicine physicians, radiologists, nurses, and a number of other professionals (e.g., therapist, administrative staff). Building from this, these roles lead to different provider functions which complement each other and require interdependent work to provide the proper patient care.

Studies have consistently found that team training generates overall positive team outcomes and up to a 20% overall improvement in team performance [7–9]. In the healthcare context, both the quality of decision making and interventions can improve when teams function properly, which ultimately improves patient outcomes [10]. Of course, we cannot assume that these results come easily, there are underlying factors that will influence the effectiveness of team training (e.g., training delivery, training methods, etc.) [11]. First of all, we have to consider that healthcare teams are not comprised of only one type of professional, but instead we see a constant interaction between a vast array of professionals with diverse specializations and educational backgrounds. Complimenting this, educational research has experienced many shifts throughout history and has evolved into what we know as traditional education today. For example, in recent times, there has been a distinction between pedagogy and andragogy, the latter being a focus entirely on adult education in order to contribute to training design [11]. Specifically, in the healthcare context, when examining these aforementioned factors, the adoption of interprofessional education (IPE) has seen a rise due to the increasing demand from professionals, from different educational backgrounds, to be able to carry out several tasks within a team context. Team training, as a discipline, has also experienced many advances that contribute to positive team-level outcomes, but is currently lacking the incorporation of IPE within their models in healthcare [12]. In order to counteract any divisions within teams and promote greater team performance, interprofessional education aims to close the perceived gap between professionals by having professionals learn together in order to enhance any future work as a team [13].

The EDUCA-TRAIN Model

There needs to be an integrated plan that invests in research to be able to portray adequate conditions and requirements for specific settings and situations [11] in order to properly design team training for healthcare, taking into account IPE. More specifically, organizations and hospitals alike need to open their doors to solidify working relationships with said schools to make these programs efficient [14]. Alongside more specific guidelines and requirements, medical school curricula need to be updated to include education and training on teamwork as a priority. Team training should be targeted at increasing teamwork competencies, and it is with such focus in mind that we developed the EDUCA-TRAIN model (Fig. 4.1). The purpose of this model is to clearly delineate evidence-based guidelines to enhance teamwork in the healthcare context. Albeit there are affective (i.e., team trust) and cognitive (i.e., shared mental models) processes that are beneficial to and can facilitate teamwork, this chapter focuses on the behavioral components of teamwork which are actionable and more easily observable (e.g., cooperation, conflict management, coordination, communication, coaching, and cognition) [8, 15].

Integrating education and team training means that a joint effort between practitioners and scholars must occur to bring upon meaningful changes to classrooms and hospitals alike [13].

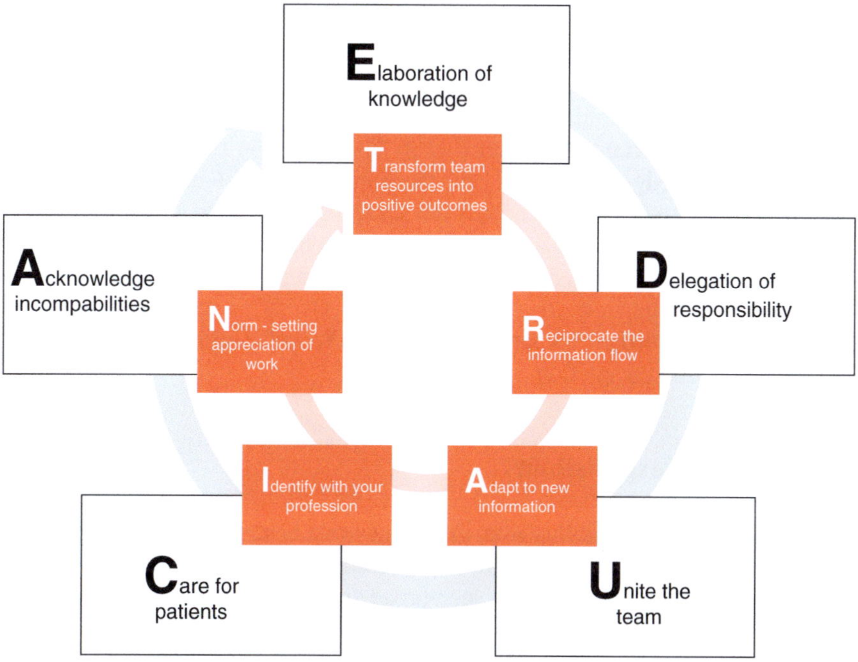

Fig. 4.1 EDUCA-TRAIN framework

To do so, we introduce the EDUCA-TRAIN model which is built on the constructs of elaboration of knowledge, delegation of responsibility, uniting the team, caring for patients, and acknowledgement of patients, in order to obtain the outcomes of transforming team resources into positive outcomes, reciprocating the information flow, members being able to adapt to new information, members identifying with their profession, and setting norms on appreciation of the work done. The EDUCA-TRAIN model is based on the relevant theoretical underpinnings of teamwork in healthcare that allows us to integrate and translate years of science into meaningful guidelines, to truly produce a positive impact on healthcare teams. Each element bases itself on a construct essential to team education and training directed at healthcare and reflects an aspired outcome.

Elaboration of Knowledge

Considering interprofessional teams such as those within the healthcare system, it is important to note that different perspectives, backgrounds of expertise, and unique skills are present. Because of such variability in knowledge, to succeed the team should focus on translating their specialized knowledge into a common language to allow communication flow [16]. This will require the elaboration of knowledge in order to effectively assign roles and tasks, as well as the strategies that are needed to succeed. This process consists of "members' exchange, discussion, and integration of ideas, knowledge, and insights relevant to the group's task" [17, p., 1010]. It is by engaging in this knowledge elaboration that team members can develop strategies, assign roles, establish norms, and agree on an overall approach to the task at hand. As the literature points out, the necessity of knowledge elaboration also shows how individuals often hold intergroup biases that can lead to knowledge silos or withholding of important information [16]. The transition from the individuals' expertise to knowledge sharing has been the center of many studies regarding team training because knowledge itself does not serve any purpose to a team unless it is distributed amongst members and utilized to benefit them [16, 17]. It is the core of interprofessional teams to have members from different professions with specific knowledge yet working towards a shared goal [18]. Overall, it can be agreed that the elaboration of knowledge is what allows expertise to spill over to other team members and aid in task completion.

Delegation of Responsibility

The delegation of responsibility is an important stride in healthcare as professionals can be responsible for care provision, care coordination, logistical help, to patients' socio-emotional support [19]. With such broad spectrum and highly consequential tasks, the need to properly delegate some of these responsibilities to those expert team members in order to accomplish the overall shared goal becomes a necessity. In actuality, we are now moving towards a flatter structure in which each member holds a role or a responsibility, that can include utilizing others' expertise to attain better outcomes [20]. Focusing on the education component, there needs to be knowledge previously acquired and continuously learned to be able to delegate responsibility in a productive way. Beyond holding their specific knowledge, the interaction of different healthcare professionals is required to coordinate their separate tasks that when combined contribute towards the patient's ultimate well-being through training. Different roles arise within a team, especially when teamwork needs to be facilitated in medical situations that are long-term or involve several teams working at the same time (i.e., multiteam systems). Therefore, no one member will be able to take care of a patient's case in its entirety without the help of others. With that being said, the delegation of responsibility –combined with other coordinating mechanisms– is what will lead to the most successful outcomes.

Unite the Team

A team divided is not a team, but merely subgroups. Consequently, efforts should be put into uniting the team. There are several factors that can be taken into consideration to ensure the members of a team feel as an entity. Drawing from social identity theory, it is common for individuals to categorize others as their ingroup or outgroup members, where they view these members differently [21]. According to this theory, individuals that identify with a group will try to favor and benefit their ingroup members above any outgroup member. In order for members to identify with their team, they should set common goals, share values, and other salient similarities [22]. When members identify with their team, unity starts building. Unity mostly relates to cooperation because of the functionality that team members can and must have between one another to be able to smoothly help each other and convey tasks. This obviously becomes more challenging when team members are in stressful situations, such as the healthcare context. Accordingly, a strong team identity has been identified as one of the differentiating factors of successful IPE [18]. Team members must identify their belonging in a team and the importance of each member within that team. When teams work together, we assume that there is a level of interdependence amongst members that leads to mutual help. By building mutual trust, healthcare professionals in a team start accepting reliance on other team members while also building an "openness" to receive help, making whatever cooperation that happens effective [23]. Thus, uniting the team should be a priority in which emergent states of team trust and behavioral indicators of cooperation, as opposed to conflict, becomes commonplace in these teams.

Care for Patients

Healthcare's central mission is the care for patients. Fortunately, patient outcomes have been proven to improve through team training in healthcare, [6, 13] whether it be in attitudes toward patient-centeredness [24] or simply in managing patients effectively minimizing critical incidents [25]. A functional consideration of patient care requires that all the actions and coordinated efforts, by multiple professionals, are combined for the well-being of an individual in need of medical help [26]. Many times, patients would like to be more involved in their treatment, and with limitations, they should. Simple trainable actions such as listening attentively to patients and encouraging any adequate participation, discussion, or decision-making can greatly benefit the patients' experience in the hospital. For example, many patients complain about a perceived lack of empathy towards their condition [27], thus a patient-centered approach can be adopted to counter this issue. More specifically, this approach can lead to smoother encounters between professionals and patients as well as more effective gains of important information, leading to correct diagnosis and treatment [13]. Patients are more satisfied when healthcare providers possess positive attitudes, provide relevant crucial information about their condition or treatment, respect the patient, show technical skills and can handle feedback [28]. Thus, it is important to train healthcare professionals to engage in more conversations, practice empathy, and understand patients' point-of-view.

Acknowledge Incompatibilities

A strong team can seek and find its flaws in order to continually better itself and its members. Unfortunately, it is common for organizations –especially in the healthcare industry– to want to repress any type of dissention among its employees [29]. However, acknowledging incompatibilities within a team will encourage team members to monitor each other, be cognizant of potential drawbacks, and work through ways to manage conflict. Conflict refers to any or all incompatibilities that may arise within a team between members, in the form of difference in interests, beliefs, or views [15]. We must establish that some conflict can have positive outcomes as it may save the team from overcommitting to a procedure that can result in hurting a patient [29]. When conflict relates to tasks, it is ideal to establish an environment in which professionals can swiftly make adjustments relating to events and situations that can emerge. It is important to identify the source of incompatibilities, such as whether they are relationship-focused or task-focused. Specifically, if members are paying attention to incompatibilities, they can also catch performance errors or deviations prior to becoming a more serious issue [30]. A common scenario, for instance, occurs with a discrepancy between nurses and the physician on-call regarding the initial treatment for an emergency patient. In this scenario, the roots of the incompatibility lie in how to best execute the task at hand and the professionals should now have a more thorough consideration regarding their next steps [31]. Accordingly, when a member can point out a lack of critical thinking poignantly, training itself can help him or her develop this skill. Mainly, acknowledging incompatibilities carries a negative tone because of the fact that we are detecting weaknesses, but in reality, it becomes a skill to be able to recognize areas for improvement personally and as a team.

Transform Team Resources

There is no purpose in identifying team weaknesses or detriments if the team is not looking for a way to overcome them. In this component of our model, the focus is not only on team's action but also whether they are able to convert their behaviors into meaningful outputs. Individual differences and skills can be converted or adjusted into a strength if the team can manage and utilize its resources effectively. More specifically, adjustments can range from knowledge, skills, and abilities [8], to any experience, possibility, physical tools, and contacts that different team members can gain through team training. A team needs to coordinate with each other to be able to fully benefit from whatever resources they may hold. Coordination refers to the execution of proper behaviors and management of resources that are necessary to carry out a task [15]. In simpler terms, a team "being on the same page" reflects what coordination is at its core. It is not a secret that a team in healthcare that lacks coordination is destined to put patients' lives at risk [4]. While a patient is going through an intense surgery, the healthcare professionals involved should engage in the proper team processes (e.g., coordination) and emergent states (e.g., information sharing) in order to truly transform team resources into positive patient outcomes. In other words, these professionals need to relay information amongst each other, transform their skills from an academic standpoint to a practical one, and have successful teamwork in order to attain an effective diagnosis and treatment, which relates back to preventing the different categories of errors mentioned earlier in the chapter [1]. Overall, there needs to be an efficient integration of the resources available to contribute towards solutions for complex problems or situations that may arise [32].

Reciprocate Information Flow

Communication should not flow exclusively in one direction but instead it should be reciprocated by the team members constantly. It is key to verify the meaning of the information received in addition to conveying information (i.e., closed-loop communication) in order to ensure everyone has a shared understanding of the case. For example, patient handover is a crucial part of the healthcare system where mistakes can lead to failure and critical incidents [3] due to ineffective communication among the surgeons, anesthesiologists, and nurses in the operating room that ultimately compromise patient safety. Furthermore, a critical incident study showed errors of communication (i.e., failing to disclose clear directions to patient or between providers) as one of the five main categories of errors in a hospital setting [1]. To counter this, teams need to be trained in effective communication that produces a reciprocate information flow amongst members, including knowing beyond *what* to say to incorporate *when*, *how*, and *to whom*. Research shows that effectively directing communication in combination with previously established roles results in enhanced quality of patient care [33]. Furthermore, the reciprocal process involves members acknowledging that information is being received while also reacting and shedding light on any discrepancies [15]. Acknowledging these interrupters, making adjustments, and constantly working towards a two-way information flow are key parts of communication's role in teams.

Adapt to New Information

Teams in healthcare will constantly face an array of novel situations that will present unexpected difficulties that team members must handle. A team's ability to react and adapt to all these constant changes defines its ability to maintain constant positive performance outcomes and reduce any problems or potential harm to patients. Adaptation refers to all changes in the team's behavior and strategy that come as a response to a salient event or cue, that in turn enhances performance and produces a desired outcome [34]. There are certain individual differences and interpersonal behaviors that can predict how one pays attention to certain situations (e.g., situational awareness) [35]. These can drive future selection and training procedures. Indeed, adapting standards of care are already being implemented in healthcare education (e.g., nurses' curricula) [36]. While medicine is continuously being updated with new discoveries, healthcare professionals need to maintain a high standard of patient care at the same time as they implement state of the art treatments. It can be argued that a medical team that lacks adaptability will have a very hard time and could potentially face critical situations because of the nature of task demands they may face that require versatility, flexibility, and attention to detail that can be the difference in their response time [34]. Of course, any enhancement in adaptive performance will greatly depend on the ability the team possesses to react in time to make any adjustments that are appropriate to the situation. Thus, adapting to new information is a key skill that should be included in the education and training of healthcare professionals.

Identify with Your Profession

Each member's roles must be perceived as important to themselves and to the team. Uncertainty of what they are doing, why they are doing it, and how they are doing it will deter the team's attempt to be efficient in their performance. The team's confidence when taking on a task relies heavily in each individual's identification with their role and profession. A professional identity defines itself through the context that education, interactions with colleagues, and the daily labor itself provides [37]. Because these professionals spend a large portion of their time engaging in their professional activities, it is important that they have a sense of belonging and pride in what they do. Furthermore, the identification with a profession goes beyond their specific role as they are part of overarching entities (e.g., team, unit, hospital) that can help with facilitation of their teamwork. This brings forth a development of their personality that is used to identify themselves within a team and for others to identify the team member [37]. For instance, albeit a surgeon's identity may consist of leading a successful team within the operating room and a triage nurse's identity may be more related to properly diagnosing the severity and accuracy of someone's complaints, these two professions have something in common: they both want to improve a patient's well-being. This example only shows a simplistic take on this concept, but in reality, the versatility in each individual's professional identity varies. However, one's identity can be combined into an overarching identity (i.e., superordinate) that drives their work as an effective team.

Norm-Setting Appreciation of Work

In addition to rules that are established and followed within a team, education and training need to teach teams to establish processes or systems to enable teamwork skills that are sustainable over time. Organized channels of communication, especially in debrief-format, can be effective in raising morale and in minimizing future mistakes. Norm-setting appreciation of work is not an easily implemented practice, but one that will take time for members to internalize these values that can shape their tasks, including sharing their input with the team. Team members need to feel safe to be able to express appreciation or even dissatisfaction with other members as well as questioning how a task is being handled in a contrastive manner [15]. Previously, we mentioned that mutual trust is essential for knowledge sharing, but what can create the proper climate for both the development of team trust and knowledge sharing is psychological safety. Psychological safety refers to the concern for other team members, the perceived respect, and the confidence emanated from and to other team members [38]. Its importance lies in the benefits that a team can gain through feedback, where improvements can be made when team members can point out mistakes in a positive light, but also team morale can increase by showing appreciation of the different team members of the strategies or work being done. Debriefs are critical because they serve as a review of what happened during training, therefore debriefs provide a means to learn from the experience as a whole or specifically [39]. Overall, team performance can additionally improve up to 25% by having an effective debriefing after training [38]. Participants will have an opportunity to really grasp what they have learned from each other, but at the same time, debriefing will also provide feedback regarding future updates to the model based on reactions and true outcomes perceived. Thus, it should be a healthcare institution's priority to establish norms that are conducive to information sharing, trust development, and constructive feedback.

From Education to Team Training

Education and team training, albeit different concepts, are not exclusive. As we have explored previously, in a general sense, education will aim to attain knowledge while training seeks to implement the acquired KSAs into the workplace [6, 9]. In order to bridge the gap between education and training, we must integrate only the best and most functional practices from each [14]. The principles and deliveries of both should be based on science, especially drawing from learning and motivational theories. First, the education and training of teamwork should focus on changes in attitude, behaviors, and cognition. These are underlying processes that can help convert inputs into positive outputs [40]. In order to make IPE training fluid, we consider a more cyclical Input-Mediator-Output-Input (IMOI) model that allows trainers to constantly update the program [41, 42]. More specifically, this model was an update of the simple input-process-outcome [43] since the IMOI model takes a more dynamic approach, consider the potential for variables to influence each other in a non-linear way, and how the outcome(s) can further shape inputs. Thus, as healthcare professionals acquire attitudinal, behavioral, and cognitive teamwork skills, it is important to closely consider other influencing variables (e.g., psychological safety, organizational culture) to ensure they will transfer and maintain such skills on the job.

Second, education and training programs should follow effective practices, such as the behavioral modeling, to focus on providing healthcare professionals with the necessary information about teamwork, followed by the demonstration of these behaviors, then allowing for professionals to engage in such behaviors themselves, and providing feedback in a timely and constructive manner [44, 45]. Third, a recent meta-analysis showed that these tactics when paired with setting goals, training the supervisors of these professionals. as well as establishing a reward system based on teamwork will make the transfer of acquired skills more likely [44]. Previously, programs like TeamSTEPPS® have brought systematics approaches to team training in healthcare settings [34] but have lacked incorporation of IPE. We need IPE to set forth a learning experience between interprofessional team members that also validates team training by incorporating all possible available knowledge into the KSAs training provides. Thus, designing the education and training program according to a needs analysis done within the context of healthcare is a necessity.

Last but not least, simulation presents trainees with real-life situations and serves as a method of team training that provides trainees with a reflection of what their decisions will result in if they were on the job [11]. Incorporating simulations into IPE team training provides the great benefit of allowing trainees to test their skills and decision making in a setting where errors will neither harm individuals' lives nor put the hospital's liability into question [46]. Yet, trainees can experience the impact of their actions in a situation of physical and psychological fidelity. This becomes even more useful when you consider high alert crisis situations that require great precision in how an ER team functions [13]. Through simulation-based training, all the steps in the EDUCA-TRAIN model can be applied in a real world setting and practiced in a way that participants will be more prepared when actually going through the situation. Incorporating simulations into IPE team training is not easy, it requires high accuracy in all aspects of the scenarios, tools, situations, people and patients involved, and any other potential condition in a medical setting [11]. Thus, we urge practitioners and researchers to pay careful attention to this step to maximize the learning during team education and training of healthcare professionals.

Future Research

While compiling the theoretical underpinnings of teamwork education and training, we uncovered a number of future research avenues. Although many studies have emphasized the positive impact of team training programs, more research is needed to understand how to properly design and deliver these programs specifically in different types of medical teams, such as ad-hoc or permanent teams [8, 44]. The team literature could greatly benefit from more nuanced studies in which the contextual boundaries that may influence the outcomes are disclosed. Also, the incorporation of other methods should be studied in order to facilitate learning and training, such as e-learning and mixed learning [11] that run parallel to courses found in the curricula of medical school. There are a number of technological advancements that should be taken into account to allow for a more paced and systematic delivery of training that maximizes learning. Alongside this, testing the effectiveness of each guideline set forth by the EDUCA-TRAIN model could inform managers in the healthcare setting what to pay the most attention to (e.g., is the elaboration of information more or less important than the level of reciprocity in the information flow?). Thus, we urge both researchers and practitioners to continue on this avenue of untangling how to make team education and training more effective as the positive consequences are numerous.

Conclusion

Even though education and training of teamwork has grown at an exponential rate within the healthcare industry, the integration of these findings is currently lacking. This chapter sets forth a framework to integrate the findings from these two literatures towards developing team skills. Teams are an essential pillar in healthcare, thus all components pertaining to its training and education have to be thoroughly studied to minimize any errors that can arise from the mismanagement of them. IPE's role in team training for healthcare teams unites and fortifies relationships across medical professionals, therefore allowing all team processes to flow smoothly and properly manage any conflict that may arise. The key in running a successful education and training program is not to focus in one component at a time (e.g., identify with your profession), but be sure to design a program that taps into multiple concepts simultaneously (e.g., norm-setting, acknowledging incompatibilities, adapting to new information). This will allow for the exposure of multiple facets necessary in education and training programs.

Furthermore, this chapter provided an overview of incorporating IPE in team training to further research and practice. However, this integration also brought to light the need for empirical studies to clearly establish the effectiveness of teamwork training and education in combination with contextual variables, especially when working on different types of teams (e.g., varying levels of familiarity). Finally, we identified several key avenues for future research, including the consideration of different pedagogies and their effectiveness evaluation. In doing so, we provided a foundation for researchers to continue advancing knowledge of teamwork in healthcare, while utilizing a framework that can be easily applied to this industry.

References

1. James J. A new, evidence-based estimate of patient harms associated with hospital care. J Patient Saf [Internet]. 2013 Sep. [cited 2017 Mar 31]; 9(3):122–8. Available from: http://journals.lww.com/journalpatientsafety/Fulltext/2013/09000/A_New,_Evidence_based_Estimate_of_Patient_Harms.2.aspx. https://doi.org/10.1097/PTS.0b013e3182948a69
2. Kern C. Healthcare miscommunication costs 2,000 lives and $1.7 billion [Internet]. 2006 [cited 2017 Mar 31]. Available from: https://www.healthitoutcomes.com/doc/healthcare-miscommunication-costs-lives-and-billion-0001.
3. Farber MA, Altman LK. A Great Hospital in Crisis. The New York Times [Internet]. 1988 Jan. [cited 2017 Mar 31]. Available from: http://www.nytimes.com/1988/01/24/magazine/a-great-hospital-in-crisis.html?pagewanted=all.
4. Rau J. Hospital discharge: it's one of the most dangerous periods for patients. The Washington Post [Internet]. 2016 Apr. [cited 2017 Mar 31]. Available from: https://www.washingtonpost.com/news/to-your-health/wp/2016/04/29/from-hospital-to-home-a-dangerous-transition-for-many-patients/?utm_term=.4259d177c379.
5. Salas E, Cannon-Bowers JA, Johnston JH. How can you turn a team of experts into an expert team? Emerging training strategies. In Zsambok CE, Klein G, editors. Naturalistic decision making. Mahwah: Erlbaum; 1997 [cited 2017 Mar 21]. p. 359–370.
6. Hughes AM, Gregory ME, Joseph DL, Sonesh SC, Marlow SL, Lacerenza CN, et al. Saving lives: a meta-analysis of team training in healthcare. Advance online publication. J Appl Psychol [Internet]. 2016 Sep. [cited 2017 Mar 7]; 101(9):1266–304. Available from: http://psycnet.apa.org/?&fa=main.doiLanding&doi=10.1037/apl0000120. https://doi.org/10.1037/apl0000120.
7. Weaver SJ, Dy SM, Rosen MA. Team-training in healthcare: a narrative synthesis of the literature. BMJ Qual Saf [Internet]. 2014 Jan. [cited 2017 Mar 4]; 23(5):359–72. Available from: http://qualitysafety.bmj.com/content/qhc/early/2014/02/05/bmjqs-2013-001848.full.pdf. https://doi.org/10.1136/bmjqs-2013-001848.
8. Salas E, DiazGranados D, Klein C, Burke CS, Stagl KS, Goodwin GF, Halpin SM. Does team training improve team performance? A meta-analysis. Human Factors [Internet]. 2008 Dec. [cited 2017 Mar 7]; 50(6):903–33. Available from: http://journals.sagepub.com/doi/pdf/10.1518/001872008X375009. https://doi.org/10.1518/001872008X375009.
9. Salas E, King HB, Rosen MA. Improving teamwork and safety: toward a practical systems approach, a commentary on Deneckere et al. Soc Sci Med [Internet]. 2012 Sep. [cited 2017 Mar 8]; 75(6):986–9. Available from: https://doi.org/10.1016/j.socscimed.2012.02.055.
10. Buljac-Samardzic M, Dekker-van Doorn CM, van Wijngaarden DH, van Wijk KP. Interventions to improve team effectiveness: a systematic review. Health Policy [Internet]. 2010 Mar. [cited 2017 Mar 8]; 94(3):183–95. Available from: https://www.researchgate.net/profile/Martina_Buljac/publication/241861618_Health_teams_Analyzing_and_improving_team_performance_in_long-term_care/links/54d9f6b60cf24647581fe721.pdf#page=119. https://doi.org/10.1016/j.healthpol.2009.09.015.
11. Noe RA. Introduction to employee training and development [Print]. New York: McGraw-Hill/Irwin; 2010 [cited 2017 Mar 4]; 5:2–52, 148, 270, 271, 305–37.
12. Thistlethwaite, J. Interprofessional education: a review of context, learning and the research agenda. Med Educ [Internet]. 2012 Jan. [cited 2017 Mar 8]; 46(1):58–70. Available from: https://doi.org/10.1111/j.1365-2923.2011.04143.x.

13. Brock T, Boone J, Anderson C. Health care education must be more of a team sport. Am J Pharm Educ [Internet]. 2016 Jan. [cited 2017 Mar 7];80(1): 1–3. Available from: http://www.ajpe.org/doi/full/10.5688/ajpe8011. https://doi.org/10.5688/ajpe8011.
14. King EB, Gulick L, Avery D. The divide between diversity training and diversity education: integrating best practices. J Manag Educ [Internet]. 2010. [cited 2017 Mar 22];34(6):891–906. Available from: https://doi.org/10.1002/job.728.
15. Salas E., Shuffler ML, Thayer AL, Bedwell WL, Lazzara EH. Understanding and improving teamwork in organizations: a scientifically based practical guide. Hum Resour Manag [Internet]. 2015 Jul. [cited 2017 Mar 21];54(4):599–622. Available from: https://doi.org/10.1002/hrm.21628.
16. Homan AC, Van Knippenberg D, Van Kleef GA, De Dreu CK. Bridging faultlines by valuing diversity: diversity beliefs, information elaboration, and performance in diverse work groups. J Appl Psychol [Internet]. 2007 Sep. [cited 2017 Mar 31]; 92(5):1189–99. Available from: https://doi.org/10.1037/0021-9010.92.5.1189.
17. Van Knippenberg D, De Dreu CK, Homan AC. Work group diversity and group performance: an integrative model and research agenda. J Appl Psychol [Internet]. 2004. [cited 2017 Mar 29];89(6):1008–22. Available from: https://doi.org/10.1037/0021-9010.89.6.1008.
18. Da Silva R, de Freitas F, de Araújo F, Ferreira M. A policy analysis of teamwork as a proposal for healthcare humanization: implications for nursing. International Nursing Review [Internet]. 2016 Dec. [cited May 20, 2017]; 63(4): 572–9. Available from: MEDLINE Complete.
19. Gorbenko KO, Fraze T, Lewis VA. Redesigning care delivery with patient support personnel: learning from accountable care organizations. Int J Care Coordination [Internet]. 2016 Sep. [cited 2017 May 21]; 19(3–4):73–83. Available from: https://doi.org/10.1177/2053434516676080.
20. O'Toole J, Galbraith J, Lawler EE. When two (or more) heads are better than one: the promise and pitfalls of shared leadership. California Manag Rev [Internet]. 2002 Jun. [cited 2017 Mar 31]; 44(4):65–83. Available from: http://www.jaygalbraith.com/component/rsfiles/downloadfile/files?path=whitepapers%2Ftwoheads.pdf.
21. Mannix E, Neale MA. What differences make a difference? The promise and reality of diverse teams in organizations. Psychol Sci Public Interest [Internet]. 2005 Oct. [cited 2017 Mar 29]; 6(2):31–5. Available from: https://doi.org/10.1111/j.1529-1006.2005.00022.x.
22. Liang L, Adair W, Hideg I. When should we disagree? The effect of relationship conflict on team identity in East Asian and North American teams. Negot Confl Manag Res [Internet]. 2014 Oct. [cited 2017 Mar 25]; 7(4):282–9. Available from: https://legacy.wlu.ca/documents/59640/When_should_we_disagree_The_effect_of_relationship_conflict_on_team_identity_in_East_Asian_and_North_American_teams.pdf. https://doi.org/10.1111/ncmr.12041.
23. Pinjani P, Palvia P. Trust and knowledge sharing in diverse global virtual teams. Inform Manag [Internet]. 2013 Jun. [cited 2017 Mar 15]; 50(4):144–53. Available from: http://www.sciencedirect.com/science/article/pii/S0378720613000141. https://doi.org/10.1016/j.im.2012.10.002.
24. Kowitlawakul Y, Ignacio J, Lahiri M, Khoo SM, Zhou W, Soon D. Exploring new healthcare professionals' roles through interprofessional education. J Interprof Care [Internet]. 2014 Jan. [cited 2017 Mar 22]; 28(3): 267–9. Available from: https://doi.org/10.3109/13561820.2013.872089.
25. Grymonpre RE, Ateah CA, Dean HJ, Heinonen TI, Holmqvist ME, MacDonald LL, et al. Sustainable implementation of interprofessional education using an adoption model framework. Can J Higher Educ [Internet]. 2016. [cited 2017 Mar 7]; 46(4), 76–93. Available from: http://journals.sfu.ca/cjhe/index.php/cjhe/article/view/186571/pdf.
26. Moyer MR, Brown RD. Medical team training: using simulation as a teaching strategy for group work. J Special Group Work [Internet]. 2011 Oct. [cited 2017 Mar 22]; 36(4):330–51. Available from: https://doi.org/10.1080/01933922.2011.613900.
27. Jamison L. The empathy exams. Minneapolis: Graywolf Press [Print]; 2014[cited 2017 Mar 22].
28. Lori J, Munro M, Moore J, Fladger J. Lessons learned in Liberia: preliminary examination of the psychometric properties of trust and teamwork among maternal healthcare workers. BMC

Health Ser Res [serial on the Internet]. 2013 Apr. [cited May 20, 2017]; 13:134–45. Available from: http://www.biomedcentral.com/1472-6963/13/134.
29. Sarkar, S. P. The dance of dissent: managing conflict in healthcare organizations. Psychoanal Psychother [Internet]. 2009. [cited on 2017 Mar 30]; 23(2):121–35. Available from: https://doi.org/10.1080/02668730902920389.
30. Flin R, Yule S. Leadership for safety: industrial experience [Internet]. Qual Saf Health Care. 2004 Dec. [cited May 20, 2017]; 13(2):45–51. Available from: http://qualitysafety.bmj.com/content/13/suppl_2/ii45.long.
31. Dwyer CP, Boswell A, Elliott MA. An evaluation of critical thinking competencies in business settings. J Educ Bus [Internet]. 2015 May [cited 2017 Mar 30]; 90(5):260–9. Available from: https://doi.org/10.1080/08832323.2015.1038978.
32. Gardner HK, Gino F, Staats BR. Dynamically integrating knowledge in teams: transforming resources into performance. Acad Manag J [Internet]. 2012 Aug [cited 2017 Mar 31]; 55(4):998–1022. Available from: https://doi.org/10.5465/amj.2010.0604.
33. Mundt MP, Agneessens F, Tuan W, Zakletskaia LI, Kamnetz, SA, Gilchrist VJ. Primary care team communication networks, team climate, quality of care, and medical costs for patients with diabetes: a cross-sectional study. Int J Nurs Stud [Internet]. 2016 Jun [cited 2017 Mar 29]; 581–11. Available from: https://www.ncbi.nlm.nih.gov/pubmed/27087293. https://doi.org/10.1016/j.ijnurstu.2016.01.013.
34. Bedwell WL, Ramsay S, Salas E. Helping fluid work: a research agenda for team adaptation in healthcare. Transl Behav Med [Internet]. 2012 Oct [cited 2017 Mar 30]; 2(4):504–9. Available from: https://doi.org/10.1007/s13142-012-0177-9.
35. Stubbings L., Chaboyer W., McMurray A. Nurses' use of situation awareness in decision-making: an integrative review. J Adv Nurs [Internet]. 2012 Mar [cited 2017 Mar 24]; 68(7):1443–53. Available from: https://doi.org/10.1111/j.1365-2648.2012.05989.x.
36. Cusack L, Gebbie K. Call for National Dialogue: Adapting Standards of Care in Extreme Events. We are not Ready. [Internet]. Science Direct; 2015 Sep. [cited May 20, 2017]. Available from: https://www.researchgate.net/profile/Lynette_Cusack/publication/284006962_Call_for_national_dialogue_Adapting_standards_of_care_in_extreme_events_We_are_not_ready/links/564d4cff08ae1ef9296a9562.pdf.
37. Koskiniemi A, Perttula J, Syväjärvi A. Existential–experiential view of self-sourced (in) authentic healthcare identity. J Leader Stud [Internet]. 2015 Sep [cited 2017 Mar 22]; 9(2):6–18. Available from: https://doi.org/10.1002/jls.21360.
38. Koopmann J, Lanaj K, Wang M, Zhou L, Shi J. Nonlinear effects of team tenure on team psychological safety climate and climate strength: Implications for average team member performance. J Appl Psychol [Internet]. 2016 Jul [cited 2017 Mar 15]; 101(7): 940–957. Available from: https://doi.org/10.1037/apl0000097.
39. Tannenbaum SI, Cerasoli CP. Do team and individual debriefs enhance performance? A meta-analysis. Hum Factors [Internet]. 2013 Feb [cited 2017 Mar 27]; 55(1):231–45. Available from: https://doi.org/10.1177/0018720812448394.
40. Kozlowski SW, Ilgen, DR. Enhancing the effectiveness of work groups and teams. Psychol Sci Public Interest [Internet]. 2006 Dec [cited 2017 Mar 24]; 7(3):77–124. Available from: https://doi.org/10.1111/j.1529-1006.2006.00030.x.
41. Henriksen K, Battles JB, Keyes MA, Grady, ML, editors. Advances in patient safety: new directions and alternative approaches. Rockville: Agency for Healthcare Research and Quality [Internet]; 2008 Aug. [cited 2017 Mar 27]; 3. Available from: https://www.ncbi.nlm.nih.gov/books/NBK43665/?report=classic.
42. Ilgen DR, Hollenbeck JR, Johnson M, Jundt D. Teams in organizations: from I-P-O models to IMOI models. Annu Rev Psychol [Internet]. 2005 Jan [cited 2017 Mar 28]; 56:517–44. Available from: https://pdfs.semanticscholar.org/56f2/43e998be2e6c73ff1015f105def0b10654f9.pdf. https://doi.org/10.1146/annurev.psych.56.091103.070250.
43. McGrath JE. Social psychology: a brief introduction [print]. New York: Holt, Rinehart & Winston; 1964 [cited 2017 May 21].

44. Taylor PJ, Russ-Eft DF, Chan DWL. A meta-analytic review of behavior modeling training. J Appl Psychol [Internet]. 2005 Jul [cited 2017 Mar 30]; 90:4:692–709. Available on: https://doi.org/10.1037/0021-9010.90.4.692
45. Gregory ME, Feitosa J, Driskell T, Salas E, Vessey WB. Designing, delivering, and evaluating team training in organizations: principles that work. In Salas E, Tannenbaum SI, Cohen D, Latham G, editors. Developing and enhancing high-performance teams: evidence-based practices and advice. San Francisco: Jossey-Bass; 2012 [cited 2017 May 21]. p. 481–487.
46. Reader TW, Flin R, Mearns K. Developing a team performance framework for the intensive care unit. Critical Care Medicine, PubMed [Internet]. 2009 May [cited 2017 Mar 22]. Available from: https://doi.org/10.1097/CCM.0b013e31819f0451.

Best Practices for Interprofessional Education Debriefing in Medical Simulation

5

Kristen L. W. Webster and Joseph R. Keebler

Introduction

Debriefing is the constructive review of performance for the purpose of forming and preserving effective team coordination [1]. In order to provide this feedback, the trainee's observed performance is compared against a provided standard to encourage performance improvement to encourage performance improvement. Within interprofessional education, debriefing is a powerful tool that aligns individuals from differing backgrounds and perspectives. Team debriefing has been shown to have positive influences within both simulated and real-world training [2]. Though there is some disagreement about the details of appropriate delivery of debriefs, the literature overwhelmingly supports the use of debriefing for technical and nontechnical skills (communication, collaboration, decision making) [3]. Throughout this chapter, we will expand upon the reasons behind employing debriefs after simulation based training and how best to implement debriefs to include the elements and environment required for successful IPE training.

Why Debrief?

Simulation-based training allows healthcare providers the opportunity to master knowledge, skills, and attitudes in an immersive learning environment without real world consequences that can directly impact the patient [4]. Specifically, debriefing in simulation should be "designed to synergize, strengthen and transfer learning from an experiential learning exercise" [5 p., 91]. Specific to IPE, debrief should

K. L. W. Webster
Johns Hopkins Hospital, Department of Anesthesiology and Critical Care Medicine and Department of Surgery, Baltimore, MD, USA

J. R. Keebler (✉)
Embry-Riddle Aeronautical University, Daytona Beach, FL, USA

J. T. Paige et al. (eds.), *Comprehensive Healthcare Simulation: InterProfessional Team Training and Simulation*, Comprehensive Healthcare Simulation,
https://doi.org/10.1007/978-3-030-28845-7_5

focus on enhancing the relationships between the professionals to foster knowledge, behaviors, and teamwork [6]. By doing so, communication, collaboration, and teamwork can be improved [6]. When practiced properly in simulation, these skills readily transition into the real world [7, 8]. It is important to note that debriefing is only one component of the feedback process, meaning that word "debriefing" and "feedback" are not synonymous terms [9]. While feedback includes any form of comment about the trainee's performance, debriefing particularly focuses on comparing that performance with a set criterion or standard and generating changes in behavior so that the performance adheres to that standard. Further, participants must actively engage in self-learning and self-discovery.

Debriefing is an essential part of simulation-based learning, allowing maximum learning and performance change [9–11]. Some have even stated that it is "unethical" to not debrief after experiential-learning exercises such as a simulation [11 p. 168]; [12, 13]. Debriefing encourages thoughtful discussion so that the team can self-evaluate and make sense of simulation events in order to self-diagnose what happened and why. While it may be slower than a lecture and not all material can be taught through simulation [14], debriefing after experiential learning, like simulation, has been demonstrated that debriefs could improve performance between 20% and 26% for both teams and individuals [2]. This improvement can extend to both simulated and real-world settings. These results highlight the effect debriefing has on team and individual performances demonstrating the skills, knowledge and behaviors learned in simulation-based training extend into the real-world. This same outcome should be expected for simulations that combine individuals of differing backgrounds/experiences, ie interprofessional education participants. Now that we have briefly discussed why debriefing is so important, we will discuss the varying elements of debriefing and the appropriate application of each.

How to Debrief – Structural Elements

There are many approaches to debriefing, although little evidence has been published regarding the effectiveness of each approach or the differences between them [15]. These approaches revolve around Bloom's taxonomy, Kolb's learning model, and Greenaway's refinement of Kolb's model [16]. Many consider debriefing an essential part of simulation-based training [17–19]. Within healthcare, debriefing has focused on improving learning, performance, and patient outcomes [15]. Lederman [20] dilineated debriefing into seven elements: (1) facilitator, (2) participants, (3) experience, (4) impact of the experience, (5) recollection, (6) mechanisms for reporting, and (7) the timing (Table 5.1).

Facilitator As the person responsible for leading debrief and assisting in organizing the participants from varying backgrounds, the role of the facilitator is paramount [22–24]. Adequate preparation by the facilitator was cited as a critical component to the students' learning in Cantrell's [21] study as well as appropriate demeanor, meaning that the facilitator must be polite, non-judgmental and encouraging of participation. A facilitator does not necessarily have to be an expert in what

Table 5.1 Seven elements of debriefing [20]

Element	Process	Outcome
Facilitator	Conduct facilitator training if needed Facilitator should be polite, non-judgmental, encouraging Strive to achieve a low level of involvement in discussion	Creates an open and safe culture for learning to take place
Participants	Participants should also be open and non-judgmental Come from varying backgrounds, roles, professions	Participants and facilitator gain more experience and learn more during the simulation and discussion
Experience	Follow a common model of debriefing Include reflection, discussion, expression, and application	Ensures that all necessary parts of a effective debrief are met
Impact of the experience	Compare the performance to a standard without judgment Assist participants in creating a plan to improve performance	Removes the possibility of opinion and supports the purpose of simulation be striving to reach a goal
Recollection	Encourage accurate and opinion-less list of actions Encourage participants to compare their action to that of the standard	Removes the possibility for opinion and ensures participants self- assess their own performance
Mechanisms for reporting	Use video play back, audio-visual feedback, and/or verbal discussion where appropriate	Provides insight into mistakes, good practices, and ways to improve
Timing	Provide adequate time for participants to decompress, self-examine and compose thoughts Debrief after every simulation Debrief long enough to cover important discussion points and create a full assessment and plan for performance enhancement	Provides adequate time for self-analysis Provides the ability to learn from mistakes in every scenario

they are training, though they are often chosen for their expertise is a specific area. However, facilitators should be well versed in clinical and nontechnical skills [22]. As the guide and a co-learner in the debrief, the facilitator must have emotional intelligence skills (e.g. patience, listening skills) that can assist him/her in the actual facilitation of the debrief [23]. The guide must be able to drive a conversation, create a safe environment that encourages participation, and provide feedback without lecturing or being disrespectful [24]. The facilitator must be able to engage and maintain a learning environment while providing organization and structure for debriefing. The facilitator must help identify and explore performance gaps and assist participants in moving toward a predetermined and standardized performance goal [25]. These performance goals are established based upon the needs of the organization, in accordance with regulations and rules of the facility and healthcare regulatory bodies (e.g. The Joint Commission, Accreditation Council for Graduate Medical Education (ACGME)).

With all the recommended standardized performance goals, the ability for a facilitator to be accomplished in all the required areas is not always an option given the chosen facilitator's skill set, so facilitator training can be instrumental in preparing the facilitator for the difficult conversations that can arise during debriefs [24]. Depending upon the goal of the simulation, the chosen facilitator can be a superior or a peer, but will act as a co-learner in the debriefing. The facilitator can interact with the participants at any one of the three levels: high facilitation, intermediate facilitation or low facilitation [9, 26]. High facilitation encourages participants to engage in a high level of self-reflection in order to problem solve and address issues in their own performance. The facilitator acts as a guide in this situation and has a low level of involvement. If high level facilitation is not achievable, then an intermediate facilitation level requires the facilitator to assist in guiding the conversation and reflection so that a deeper understanding of the goals/outcomes is obtained. Within IPE, the facilitator may need to help participants overcome the existing hierarchy structure that exists within the healthcare setting in order to ensure equity between participants [6]. Last, within a low facilitation level, the facilitator drives the conversation and reflection of performance by asking questions and directly engaging the participants. High facilitation is supported as effective by the literature, suggesting that the facilitator should organize the discussion but also continuously prompt participants to provide the majority of the conversation and reflection [22, 26, 27], by asking open-ended questions specific to the behaviors manifested in the simulation [28].

Participants Agreement among the literature about who should be involved in a debrief and the number of participants does not exist. Wagner et al. [29] suggests that four participants is best while others suggest that debriefing can still be achieved through self-assessment without an instructor if video play back is used [30]. Because IPE simulation training focuses on training professionals from differing backgrounds together, participants can learn from one another's expertise and experience. The simulation and debrief can encourage participants from multiple professions to learn from one another about each other's roles in order to improve quality of care for the patient by improving teamwork [31]. The most commonly combined professions for simulation-based training in healthcare included nursing and medicine [31].

Experience One of the most commonly cited ways to organize a debrief is based upon Kolb's Experiential Learning model which involves using concrete experimentation (active participation in an experience), reflective observation, abstract conceptualization, and active experimentation where the concrete experimentation is conducted in the simulation scenario while the rest is composed of the debrief [32, 33]. Greenaway reduced the Kolb model by developing a four-stage model with reflection/discussion, emotions, detachment from the experience, and application for the future [16]. Another approach, Bloom's taxonomy, highlights the knowledge and comprehension sections of the taxonomy followed by discussion by the participants regarding the application and analysis of the simulation to the real world [16]. Drifuerst [3] lists reflection, emotion, reception, and integration/assimilation as the defining criteria for debriefing. Over all, the differing models most frequently contained a section for reflection, discussion, expression of emotions, and application for real world scenarios. These sections recommended when structuring a debrief for IPE simulation-based training, one must consider the goal of the training and adapt the debrief accordingly.

Impact of the Experience One of the first considerations for developing and implementing an effective debrief is to focus on the measurement and tools. These tools should be developed based upon the goals and objectives of the simulation. In order to provide an adequate debrief, the facilitator and participants must be able to compare the performance with the predetermined standard. One of the easiest ways to achieve this is by measuring and scoring the performance. This is not meant to be used as punitive action or to be compared to other participants in the simulation, but as a way to compare that student to the standard. By comparing the participant's performance with the predetermined standard, the facilitator and rest of the participants can provide appropriate feedback regarding performance improvement [22].

Culture/environment for debriefing is also important for setting the stage for a positive simulation based scenario and debrief. Positive and non-threatening environments which are separate from the simulation experience are best for debriefing [9, 25, 33]. Trust, respect, and confidentiality are necessary so that all participants can speak freely without fear of judgment or punishment [25, 33, 34]. To further encourage participation, asking participants to sit in a circle at eye-level creates the feeling of equality and community [9, 25, 33].

Debriefing outcomes include non-technical and technical skills. Non-technical skills include, but are not limited to the following: situational awareness, communication skills, teamwork, knowledge acquisition, psychomotor skills [15], team working, decision-making, and task management [30, 36, 37]. Technical skills, on the other hand, are behaviors that are based upon automated data collection (e.g. chest compression rate/depth [39], vital sign monitoring [40]). The selection of technical data that can be used for assessment of participant behavior must align with the scenario and goals of the simulation. For example, one would not measure hand washing behavior if the simulation's goal is to improve performance of cardiopulmonary resuscitation. For your convenience, an in depth analysis of the outcome assessment tools can be found in Levett-Jones and Lapkin's [15] review.

Recollection Recalling and recollecting the memory of the simulation during a debrief provides the ability for the participants to compare their actions to the discussed standard and allows for discussion of actual events rather than subjective opinions. By facilitating the recollection of a simulation, the facilitator emphasizes objectivity. To promote an objective view of the simulation, sometimes it is helpful to recreate the scenario verbally by having participants discuss first the step-by-step actions/behaviors of the simulation, avoiding emotion so that the discussion is factually based upon the events, not performance [42]. In particular, this allows the participants to hear each other's view of the simulation before discussing their own views in depth [42].

Mechanisms for Reporting The mechanisms for recording/reporting observations of performance and suggestions for performance improvement during debrief vary dependent upon many variables. Some of the most common types of debrief reporting mechanisms include video play back, verbal discussion/analysis, audio-visual feedback (e.g., from a defibrillator), or a combination of these, all with different success rates [17, 39–41, 43, 44]. In particular, those exposed to videos of the performance episode are more likely to demonstrate desirable behaviors [17, 39–41, 43, 44]. Chronister and Brown [43] demonstrated that nursing skills (assessment and psychomotor) and response times were positively affected by video-assisted verbal debriefing, while knowledge retention was positively affected by traditional verbal debriefing. Others have compared multimedia instruction with video-assisted oral debriefing and found no significant difference between the two suggesting that multimedia instruction is just as effective as oral debriefing [37]. In opposition to this, some studies did not find a significant difference for participants who viewed a video play back [38] and some even suggested "video review did not offer any advantage over oral feedback alone" [36]. Meta-analytic evidence by Tannenbaum and Cerasoli [2] suggested that multimedia was not necessarily indicative of improvement but did not negate the possibility of video/audio recording usefulness during debriefing.

Timing The ideal timing of when to debrief is debated. Some suggest that debriefings should take place immediately after the simulation episode [21, 45, 46] and that the timing of the debrief was more essential than the medium through which was delivered [21]. The students in Cantrell's [21] study stated that it was best to review the simulation when it was still "fresh in their mind and they were still engaged in the learning activity" [p. e21]. Further, debriefing should take place as often as logically necessary. For example, debriefing should take place after every simulation or after every critical event. Engaging in debriefs more often makes it easier for personnel to discuss these issues [46].

Debrief length is also disputed. Arafeh et al. [17] posits that an ideal debrief should be three times the length of the scenario event. On the other hand, Cantrell [21] suggests limiting the amount of debrief time, citing for example that a 45-minute simulation scenario should be debriefed in 10 minutes or less. Furthermore, debriefing after the simulation provides participants the opportunity to decompress after the stress of running through a simulation as well as the ability to integrate what they have learned into knowledge [21]. Due to the nature of simulations, student emotions can be triggered. These emotional responses have been demonstrated to impact the retention of knowledge [9]. Allowing time to decompress provides the student the ability to acknowledge the emotion and redirect attention to the experience and knowledge gained [4, 17, 21, 23, 34, 35, 47, 48]. However, Arafeh et al. [17] suggest limiting the time spent on emotions to only 5 minutes with the rest of the time being dedicated to analysis of the events in the simulation.

How to Debrief – Elements of Debriefing Events

Debriefs should include active self-learning and developmental intent, be focused on specific events, and utilize multiple information sources [2], as well as a set of core elements including: critique, correction, evaluation of performance, and discussion of experience [3]. *Active self-learning* involves participants using an iterative process of self-examination to assess their own performance [2]. Rather than having others explain the pros/cons of individual performance that is passive in nature, active self-examination engages insight [49], thus enforcing learning [50]. Debriefs traditionally include a discussion between the facilitator and the participants. The discussion should be guided but be as open as possible so that participants contribute freely while engaging with their peers and the facilitator. Further, the discussion should avoid judgmental critiquing. While it is positive to critique behavior and performance, the demeanor in which this is done must be neutral and devoid of judgment. To accomplish this, the developmental intent becomes imperative. Creating an open environment devoid of judgment or any form of punitive actions provides a safe environment that facilitates learning. During debriefs, the administration/organization should not be conducting any form of performance review as this can cause participants to be defensive and apprehensive, dampening the ability to learn or improve [2].

The facilitator can encourage an open, safe environment and elicit the team by providing a structure driven toward self-correction that provides positives and negatives of the performance. Further, the facilitator can reach performance/behavior correction by encouraging individuals to be critical of their own performance and behavior [51]. By asking directional but neutral questions (e.g., Give an example of when effective communication was used), the facilitator can direct the conversation for the purpose of performance correction while remaining non-judgmental [28]. Additionally, the facilitator can focus on specific events that allow for direct comparison between the performance and the predetermined standard [2]. Instead of generalizing goals, the debriefing can pinpoint specific goals and create an individualized or team-oriented action plan for future performance improvement [52]. Last, debriefs should encourage the utilization of information from other participants in the simulation, the facilitator, and other external sources when available, in order to expose participants to other viewpoints and perspectives [2].

In summary, debrief through active self-learning drives effective developmental experiences [53], and contributes to learning by encouraging experimentation with knowledge and performance [50]. Next, debriefs must be used to foster learning and development rather than judgment or evaluation. Through focusing on performance improvement, not punitive action, trainees are more receptive to the debriefing, less defensive, and more willing to participate by sharing information [54, 55]. Debriefs should also focus on specific events. By concentrating on one event, an action plan with goals can be created [56], in turn inspiring motivation [52]. Last, the use of multiple information sources allows for a breadth of coverage for the providers performance, combining diverse accounts in order to form a complete picture of behaviors/actions [2]. When a combination of the elements are properly aligned, the effects of the debrief are heightened. For example, Tannenbaum and Cerasoli's [2] meta-analysis demonstrated that when participants' intent and measurement were aligned, this combination resulted in the greatest improvement in performance. However, the study also demonstrated that this alignment was not necessary to reach efficacy.

Conclusion

Throughout this chapter, we have addressed what, why, and how to debrief in regards to IPE simulation based training. It is important to note that when employing simulation based training for an interprofessional team, the facilitator of a debrief must ensure that all roles are encouraged to speak and that collaboration between professionals as peers takes place. To achieve this, facilitators may need to become aware of the professionals' relationships with each other, or lack thereof, before attempting to debrief the team. Having familiarity with the team may encourage high-level facilitation where all participants actively and openly engage with one another as peers. Participants should be open to the experience and be willing to share experiences from their own backgrounds capitalizing upon the shared knowledge present during interprofessional education. Debriefs should encourage active self-learning in a safe and open environment, devoid of judgment or punitive action. When all these items are taken under consideration, an effective debrief has the capability to improve performance and increase skills, knowledge, and attitudes of all involved team members. Within an IPE environment, providers develop relationships that foster communication, collaboration, coordination and teamwork by sharing and listening to other experiences and viewpoints.

References

1. Helmreich RL, Merritt AC. Culture at work in aviation and medicine: national, organizational and professional influences. Vermont: Ashgate Publishing Brookfield; 1998.
2. Tannenbaum SI, Cerasoli CP. Do team and individual debriefs enhance performance? A meta-analysis. Hum Factors. 2013;55(1):231–45.
3. Dreifuerst KT. The essentials of debriefing in simulation learning: a concept analysis. Nurs Educ Perspect. 2009;30(2):109–14.
4. Lateef F. Simulation-based learning: just like the real thing. J Emerg Trauma Shock. 2010;3(4):348–52.
5. Warrick DD, Hunsaker RL, Cook CW, Airman S. Debriefing experiential learning exercises. J Exp Learn Simul. 1979;1:91–100.
6. Boet S, Bould MD, Burn CL, Reeves S. Twelve tips for a successful interprofessional team-based high-fidelity simulation education session. Med Teach. 2014 Oct;36(10):853–7.
7. Galloway S. Simulation techniques to bridge the gap between novice and competent healthcare professionals. Online J Issues Nurs. 2009;14(2):1–9.
8. Rothgeb M. Creating a nursing simulation laboratory: a literature review. J Nurs Educ. 2008;47(11):489–94.
9. Fanning RM, Gaba DM. The role of debriefing in simulation-based learning. Simul Healthc. 2007;2(2):115–25.

10. Dieckmann P, Molin Friis S, Lippert A, Ostergaard D. The art and science of debriefing in simulation: ideal and practice. Med Teach. 2009;31(7):287–94.
11. Gardner R. Introduction to debriefing. Semin Perinatol. 2013;37(3):166–78.
12. Kriz WC. Systemic-constructiveist approach to the facilitation and debriefing of simulations and games. Simul Gaming. 1992;41(5):663–80.
13. Stewart LP. Ethical issues in postexperimental and postexperiential debriefing. Simul Gaming. 1992;23(2):196–211.
14. Phrampus P, O'Donnell JM. Debriefing in simulation education – using a structured and supported model. A special presentation at the symposium on nursing simulation at the Peter M. Winter Institute for Simulation, Education & Research.
15. Levett-Jones T, Lapkin S. A systematic review of the effectiveness of simulation debriefing in health professional education. Nurs Educ Today. 2014;34(6):58–63.
16. Nicholson S. Completing the experience: debriefing in experiential educational games. Proceedings of the 3rd international conference on society and information technologies. Winter Garden: International Institute of Informatics and Systemics; 2012. p. 117–121.
17. Arafeh J, Hansen S, Nichols A. Debriefing in simulated-based learning: facilitating a reflective discussion. J Perinat Neonatal Nurs. 2010;24(4):302–9.
18. Issenberg SB, Mcgaghie WC, Petrusa ER, Gordon DL, Scalese RJ. Features and uses of high-fidelity medical simulations that lead to effective learning: a BEME systematic review. Med Teach. 2005;27(1):10–28.
19. Shinnick MA, Woo M, Horwich TB, Steadman R. Debriefing: the most important component in simulation? Clin Simul Nurs. 2011;7:105–11.
20. Lederman LC. Debriefing: toward a systematic assessment of theory and practice. Simul Gaming. 1992;23(2):145–60.
21. Cantrell M. The importance of debriefing in clinical simulations. Clin Simul Nurs. 2008;4(2):19–23.
22. Lyons R, Lazzara EH, Benishek LE, Zajac S, Gregory M, Sonesh SC, et al. Enhancing the effectiveness of team debriefings in medical simulation: more best practices. Jt Comm J Qual Patient Saf. 2015;41(3):115–25.
23. Tannenbaum SI, Goldhaber-Fiebert SN. Medical team debriefs: simple, powerful, underutilized. In: Salas E, Frush K, editors. Improving patient safety through teamwork and team training. New York City: Oxford University Press; 2013. p. 249–53.
24. Johson-Pivec CR. Debriefing after simulation: guidelines for faculty and students. Master theses published at St. Catherine University; 2011.
25. Ghauri, B. Debriefing with your pants on. Presentation. Presented at the Drexel University conference: Simul Healthc, Orlando; 2011, March.
26. McDonnell LK, Jobe KK, Dismukes RK. Facilitating LOS debriefings: a training manual. Aldershot: Ashgate; 2000. p. 26–49.
27. Overstreet M. Ee-chats: the seven components of nursing debriefing. J Contin Educ Nurs. 2010;41(12):538–9.
28. Smith-Jentsch KA, Cannon-Bowers JA, Tannenbaum S. Guided team self-correction: impacts on team mental models, processes, and effectiveness. Small Gr Res. 2008;39:303–29.
29. Wagner D, Bear M, Sander J. Turning simulation into reality: increasing student competence and confidence. J Nurs Educ. 2009;48:465–7.
30. Boet S, Bould MD, Bruppacher HR, Desjardins F, Chandra DB, Naik VN. Looking in the mirror: self-debriefing versus instructor debriefing for simulated crises. Crit Care Med. 2011;39(6):1377–81.
31. Zang C, Thompson S, Miller C. A review of simulation-based interprofessional education. Clin Simul Nurs. 2010;7(4):117–26.
32. Burns CL. Using debriefing and feedback in simulation to improve participant performance: an educator's perspective. Int J Med Educ. 2015;6:118–20.
33. Kolb DA. The Kolb learning style inventory (version 3.1). Boston: Hay Group; 2005.
34. Anderson M. Debriefing and guided reflection. 2008. From: http://sirc.nln.org/mod/resource/view.php?id=168.

35. Waxman K. The development of evidence based clinical simulation scenarios: guidelines for nurse educators. J Nurs Educ. 2010;49:29–35. https://doi.org/10.3928/01484834-20090916-07.
36. Savoldelli GL, Naik VN, Park J, Joo HS, Chow R, Hamstra SJ. Value of debriefing during simulated crisis management. Anaesthesia. 2006;105(2):279–85.
37. Welke TM, LeBlanc VR, Savoldelli GL, Joo HS, Chandra DB, Crabtree DB, et al. Personalized oral debriefing versus Standardized multimedia instruction after patient crisis simulation. Anesth Analg. 2009;109(1):183–9.
38. Byrne A, Sellen A, Jones J, Aitkenhead A, Hussain S, Gilder F. Effect of videotape feedback on anaesthetists performance while managing simulated anaesthetic crises: a multicentre study. Anaesthesia. 2002;57:176–9.
39. Dine C, Gersh R, Leary M, Riegel B, Bellini L, Abella B. Improving cardiopulmonary resuscitation quality and resuscitation training by combining audiovisual feedback and debriefing. Crit Care Med. 2008;36:2817–22.
40. Grant JS, Moss J, Epps C, Watts P. Using video-facilitated feedback to improve student performance following high-fidelity simulation. Clin Simul Nurs. 2010;6:177–84.
41. Van Heukelom J, Begaz T, Treat R. Comparison of postsimulation debriefing versus in-simulation debriefing in medical simulation. Simul Healthc. 2010;5:91–7.
42. Jaye P, Thomas L, Reedy G. 'The diamond': a structure for simulation debrief. Clin Teach. 2015 Jun;12(3):171–5.
43. Chronister C, Brown D. Comparison of simulation debriefing methods. Clin Simul Nurs. 2012;8(7):281–8.
44. Morgan P, Tarshis J, LeBlanc V, Cleave-Hogg D, DeSousa S, Haley M. Efficacy of high-fidelity simulation debriefing on the performance of practicing anaesthetists in simulated scenarios. Br J Anaesth. 2009;103:531–7.
45. Decker S. Integrating guided reflection into simulated learning experiences. In: Jeffries P, editor. Simulation in nursing education: from conceptualization to evaluation, 2007. New York: National League for Nursing. p. 73–85.
46. Flanagan B. Debriefing: theory and techniques. In: Riley R, editor. Manual of simulation in healthcare. New York: Oxford University Press; 2008. p. 155–70.
47. Jeffries PR. Simulation in nursing education: from conceptualization to evaluation. New York: National League for Nursing; 2007.
48. Wotton K, Davis J, Button D, Kelton M. Third-year undergraduate nursing students' perceptions of high-fidelity simulation. J Nurs Educ. 2010;49(11):632–9. https://doi.org/10.3928/01484834-20100831-01.
49. Ron N, Lipshitz R, Popper M. How organizations learn: post-flight reviews in a F-16 fighter squadron. Organ Stud. 2002;27:1069–89.
50. Kolb D. Experiential learning: experience as a source of learning. Englewood Cliffs: Prentice Hall; 1984.
51. Kolbe M, Weiss M, Grote G, Knauth A, Dambach M, Spahn DR, Grande B. TeamGAINS: a tool for structured debriefings for simulation-based team trainings. BMJ Qual Saf. 2013;22(7):541–53.
52. Locke EA, Latham GP. Building a practically useful theory of goal setting and task motivation: a 35-tear odyssey. Am Psychol. 2002;57:705–17.
53. Eddy ER, D'Abate CP, Tannenbaum SI, Givens-Skeaton S, Robinson G. Key characteristics of effective and ineffective developmental interations. Hum Resource Dev Rev. 2006;17:59–84.
54. Jawahar IM, Williams CR. Where all the children are above average: the performance appraisal purpose effect. Pers Psychol. 1997;50:905–25.
55. Murphy KR, Cleveland JN. Understanding performance appraisal: social, organizational, and goal-based perspectives. Thousand Oaks: Sage; 1995.
56. Locke EA, Latham GP. A theory of goal setting and task performance. Englewood Cliffs: Prentice Hall; 1990.

Part II

Nuts and Bolts

Challenges to Conducting Simulation-Based Interprofessional Education for Non-technical Skills

6

Lauren E. Benishek, Elizabeth H. Lazzara, and Shirley C. Sonesh

Introduction

Healthcare is increasingly complex and ever-changing [1–3]. Medical knowledge is doubling at continuously faster rates, from 50 years in 1950 to 3.5 years in 2010 to a projected 73 days in 2020 [4]. So quickly is this body of knowledge increasing that no single clinician could cultivate and maintain universal medical expertise. As a result, healthcare practice is shifting away from the traditional model of a single physician as the sole practitioner overseeing all aspects of patient care. Now, healthcare is an inherently multidisciplinary task where the welfare of patients is contingent upon the interactions of individuals from diverse backgrounds and varying degrees of expertise, training, and experience [5, 6]. It is nearly universal for patient care to be provided by teams of healthcare professionals, each contributing their own specialized and unique skills and knowledge throughout the patient's health journey. As such, effective collaboration among individuals of different professions (i.e., teamwork) is a critical factor in patient care and safety. Indeed, interactions among healthcare workers are intrinsically linked to effective and ineffective performance [7]. These realities have prompted national organizations to recognize the

L. E. Benishek (✉)
Johns Hopkins University School of Medicine, Armstrong Institute for Patient Safety and Quality, Baltimore, MD, USA
e-mail: lebenishek@jhu.edu

E. H. Lazzara
Department of Human Factors and Behavioral Neurobiology, Embry-Riddle Aeronautical University, Daytona Beach, FL, USA
e-mail: lazzarae@erau.edu

S. C. Sonesh
Organizational Psychologist Sonnenschein Consulting, LLC, New Orleans, LA, USA
e-mail: ssonesh1@tulane.edu

J. T. Paige et al. (eds.), *Comprehensive Healthcare Simulation: InterProfessional Team Training and Simulation*, Comprehensive Healthcare Simulation,
https://doi.org/10.1007/978-3-030-28845-7_6

importance of interprofessional interaction in patient care and promote the use of interprofessional training and education (IPE). The Institute of Medicine (IOM) listed the ability to work in interprofessional teams as one of its core competencies for healthcare professionals [8] and called for transforming continuing education into an interprofessional endeavor focused on professional development [2]. Interprofessional collaborative practice is such a critical component of modern healthcare that prominent healthcare organizations and associations have begun defining key competencies and requirements for effective care [9]. Therefore the need for effective IPE using well-designed curricula is essential.

Given its importance for the future of healthcare practice, it is useful to understand exactly what is meant by IPE. The concept of interprofessionality has been described as the process through which representatives of different professions reflect on and develop ways of practicing that meet the demands and needs of the client, or, in the case of healthcare, patients [10]. As such, interprofessional activities are inherently patient-centered and are intended to better serve patients by integrating and capitalizing on expertise from disparate knowledge backgrounds [11]. By this definition, the practice of modern healthcare practice is intensely interprofessional. However, cross-professional teamwork and coordination is often challenging given different cultures, expectations, attitudes, terminology, and skills of multiple professions. Thus, interprofessional education is one mechanism for improving interpersonal and communication skills (i.e., teamwork) across professions.

To clarify what interprofessional education is and inform curriculum development, several definitions have been offered. Reeves and colleagues [3] consider IPE to be any type of educational training, teaching, or learning opportunity in which two or more health and social care professions learn interactively. Yet, what is interactive learning? The World Health Organization (WHO) suggests that IPE occurs when students from two or more professions learn *about*, *from*, and *with* each other [12]. As such, information-based training modalities alone are not enough to qualify as true IPE, even when the training audience is multidisciplinary or multiprofessional.

Simulation-based training (SBT), however, is one learning modality that meets the criteria for interactive learning. Following its success in aviation and the military [13–15], SBT has been adopted to train healthcare providers in many contexts [16]. SBT is a practice-based instructional paradigm in which learners apply knowledge, skills, and attitudes (KSAs) in a safe and controlled environment [17, 18]. There are several advantages to simulation. First, clinicians can make and learn from mistakes without causing harm to real patients. Second, situations that may not arise with regularity on-the-job but require effective interprofessional performance can be replicated, allowing more numerous practice opportunities. Furthermore, SBT creates a learning environment predicated on practice and feedback, which are necessary supplements to didactics as they hone providers' practical capabilities for successful performance of non-technical KSAs on-the-job [19].

The particular case in which simulation is used with the explicit aim of accelerating the acquisition of non-technical teamwork skills, attitudes, and cognitions underlying effective team communication, cooperation, and coordination is known as *simulation-based team training* (SBTT) [20]. SBTT can be used within the context of IPE to ensure that interprofessional clinical teams are capable of enacting effective interpersonal and communication skills within the high-stakes and often fast-paced environment characteristic of patient care. However, there are also staple challenges associated with conducting SBTT for IPE. The purpose of this chapter is to describe some of these challenges and offer recommendations for how to address them.

Challenges in SBTT for IPE

In the sections that follow we present challenges to designing and conducting SBTT in IPE settings. Although logistical challenges are sure to present constraints and difficulties in conducting simulation-based IPE [11], within this chapter we address challenges to providing a well-designed learning curriculum focused on enhancing non-technical competencies within interprofessional teams. We detail what makes each a challenge to SBTT for IPE and offer evidence-based recommendations for managing each challenge during the engineering and execution of simulation scenarios. The challenges and their respective recommendations are summarized in Table 6.1. The order in which we present these challenges is not meant to be indicative of their complexity. To illustrate, focusing scenarios on multiple learner needs does not necessarily present a greater challenge than appropriately debriefing participants. Instead, we present the challenges in an order that loosely follows the chronology of SBT development and implementation [21].

Focusing Simulation Events on Team-Based Competencies Instead of Task-Based Competencies

SBTT is targeted at accelerating the acquisition of team competencies – the KSAs required for optimal team performance (e.g., communication, coordination, cooperation, and leadership) [22]. Despite the explicit focus on nontechnical skills, practitioners often resort to selecting the clinical context prior to identifying the purpose and team objectives for the scenario. Implementing this approach presents the danger of concentrating scenario content on technical knowledge and skills as opposed to teamwork KSAs. Introducing new technical skills during training substantially limits its validity as a mechanism for developing teamwork [20]. Attempting to learn any new KSA can be cognitively and even physically demanding; thus, requiring learners to acquire new technical KSAs as well as non-technical KSAs may be overly burdensome. Also, incorporating new technical KSAs detracts from the primary purpose of accelerating the acquisition of team competencies. Finally, leveraging a pre-existing scenario that previously targeted taskwork is vulnerable to being unable to capture enough opportunities for learners to exhibit sufficient mastery of teamwork. Indeed, scenarios focusing on technical KSAs can already be challenging and complex, and incorporating additive team competencies can compound the complexity of the overall scenario while still not necessarily providing enough instances for the learners to demonstrate the targeted team competencies. More simply stated, the best design meets the needs of the learner while also accomplishing the educational objectives [23]. Further, technical scenarios adapted to

Table 6.1 Recommendations for addressing SBTT-specific challenges

Challenge	Recommendations
Focusing on team-based competencies instead of task-based competencies	1. Generate scenarios with the sole intent of training teamwork KSAs 2. Establish collaborations between clinical experts and team and instructional experts
Meeting the needs of multiple learners and individual learners' multiple needs	3. Target the same KSAs in multiple events 4. Purposefully aim to script scenarios so each learner has the opportunity to practice each KSA at least once 5. Rotate learners through each learner role targeted by the scenario to cultivate interpositional knowledge
Anticipating learner responses to events	6. Design independent scenario events that are not contingent on earlier learner behaviors 7. Create a flowchart to account for different contingency plans
Measuring teamwork successfully	8. Employ multiple observers to rate performance 9. Rate videotaped performance during SBTT sessions 10. Align performance measurement with instructional objectives
Debriefing and providing feedback on teamwork KSAs	11. Tailor debriefs and feedback with measurement content and the targeted performance level 12. Debrief immediately following SBTT 13. Enlist video recordings to present specific examples of performance 14. Align feedback to measurement content 15. Provide individual-level feedback to participants privately 16. Rely on multi-source feedback

include additional team competencies can become overly complex and burdensome on the raters when trying to account for all technical and team aspects of performance.

To ensure that practitioners do not fall into some of these common traps, we offer several recommendations. First, although it may be more time consuming initially, we strongly recommend generating simulation scenarios with the *sole* intent of teaching interprofessional teamwork. Optimal learning starts with scenarios that are driven with the purpose of enhancing team competencies and not clinical context [24]. Thus, we suggest that the purpose and nontechnical competencies are established early in scenario development [25]. In the event that the only option is to leverage a pre-existing technical scenario and transition it towards teamwork, we encourage ample opportunities for learners to practice as well as corresponding measurement tools that can capture teamwork proficiency.

Second, we recommend collaborations to ensure that the curriculum development group represents varied perspectives and possesses expertise in the clinical domain as well as the team and instructional domains [24]. A diverse yet experienced curriculum development group ensures that the scenarios and tasks are clinically relevant and feasible while also appropriately and sufficiently tapping into the focal construct, teamwork. Preferably, these collaborations will include representatives from the clinical professions for whom the training is intended. Further, including instructional designers in curriculum development helps safeguard that practice activities are guided, which literature has shown to be more effective than unguided practice experiences [26]. Implementing such recommendations positions SBTT to be a successful tool for acquiring team KSAs.

Meeting the Needs of Multiple Learners and Individual Learners' Multiple Needs

Training multiple learners simultaneously may reduce the benefit any individual learner derives from participation. Ideally, each learner will have multiple opportunities to demonstrate teamwork competencies throughout the scenario. Multiple opportunities not only provide additional practice but also allow raters to assess the current capability level of each individual with better accuracy. Yet, increasing the number of learners will likely reduce the number of practice opportunities afforded to each learner within a scenario, a tradeoff that could have consequences for providing sufficient learning opportunities to each individual.

Though perhaps obvious, care must be taken to ensure that no learner is overlooked or receives lower quality practice opportunities than any other learner. When scripting scenarios, designers should purposefully aim to allow each learner to practice each KSA at least once, though multiple practice opportunities per KSA are ideal. However, the presence of practice opportunities alone is not sufficient to ensure learning. Practice opportunities must be structured and guided [25]. Specifically, the scenario must be systematically designed to elicit responses that will indicate whether or not the learner(s) possess the KSA(s) of interest.

Requiring participants to practice teamwork in different roles representative of their job responsibilities is another way to expose learners to multiple KSAs during simulation. Clinicians often perform various roles on the job. For instance, a nurse may find himself in a leadership role as charge nurse one day but acting as a bedside nurse during his next shift. One method to ensure that participants are able to practice relevant KSAs is to administer a single scenario multiple times but rotate participants through the learner roles (i.e., cross-training). While such a tactic may not be appropriate cross-professionally (e.g., swapping nurses with residents), when appropriate it would allow learners to perform KSAs most applicable to a given role within a scenario. Doing so would help to develop learners' interpositional knowledge (i.e., knowledge of multiple roles) [27–29], which facilitates the development of shared expectations among team members. Shared expectations empower team members with the knowledge of when team members may require assistance and cross-training provides learners with the experiences necessary to know the best way to provide support when it is needed.

Anticipating Learner Responses to Events

A marker of effective simulation entails realistically replicating real-world circumstances. Given the dynamic nature of patient care, realistic SBTT can also become multiplex. For instance, scenario events (i.e., changes in the scenario originating from those controlling the scenario) [25] can have one or even multiple appropriate learner responses. To illustrate, when the human patient simulator is in ventricular fibrillation during a resuscitation case, the appropriate learner responses could include defibrillation, cardiac compressions, or intravenous access. Much like a *Choose Your Own Adventure* book, the decisions of the team could change how scenario events unfold, and scenario scripts must be ready to meet those taxing requirements. Hopefully this example demonstrates that scenarios can become exceedingly complex with multiple events and especially with multiple learners. Despite this complexity, multiple events are necessary to accurately demonstrate proficiency. Consequently, it can become challenging to develop triggers and flawlessly script out the flow of the scenario [30].

The simplest recommendation to overcome this obstacle is to design independent events. In other words, no event should be completely contingent upon the learner's behaviors. Independent events provide those responsible for the simulator as well as observer evaluations with a priori guidance and expectations as to how the scenario will proceed, making adjustments and assessments less cognitively taxing. However, we realize that is not always obtainable. As such, another recommendation is to consider a spectrum of potential responses to each event and script a scenario "flow chart" that would account for different contingency plans. Irrespective of the approach (independent events vs. flow chart of contingency plans), it is fundamental that the demands of the scenario and in particular the difficulty of the events are matched to the learner's level of proficiency [24]. This pairing between events and learners is critical for the progression of the actual scenario. Learners facing a scenario above and beyond their knowledge and abilities may freeze or get lost, making it exceedingly difficult for the simulation to logically proceed to the next event. One method to determine if the matching between scenario difficulty and learner is suitable is to assess each learner's proficiency *before* the simulation scenario. In addition to fostering such pairings, evaluating individuals prior to SBTT also offers a means to identify the extent that the KSAs were acquired as a result of the scenario. The following section will discuss assessments and measurements in greater detail.

Measuring Teamwork Successfully

Measuring teamwork is crucial to ensuring that simulation-based IPE is effective in its aims to improve non-technical skills [31]. Accurate assessments serve as a mechanism to inform feedback and improve subsequent learning. However, interprofessional teams make measurement complex. First, each learner may choose to respond to a given scenario in different but equally effective ways, thereby challenging how 'correct' and 'incorrect' responses should be recorded. Moreover, as briefly mentioned earlier, IPE scenarios increase the cognitive load of observers and instructors tasked with assessing teamwork. Not only must assessors be vigilant to subtle team behaviors that are not always observable [32], but they must also attend to multiple learners at once, in a context characterized by high activity. As such, the complexity of team performance makes meaningful measurement difficult [33].

Second, the decision must be made on *what* to measure. Facilitators may have difficulty determining whether to conduct global team assessment (i.e. overall team success) or measure individual performance (i.e. how well each individual demonstrates teamwork). Along the same lines, another challenge lies in the fact that while the clinical outcome of a SBTT may be negative (e.g. the patient dies), the teamwork exhibited throughout the scenario may be optimal. As such, it is important to measure the specific KSAs that are being trained and not only the clinical outcomes that might result from patient acuity rather than team performance. Third, it is difficult to develop and maintain the reliability of observer team performance ratings [21, 34–36]. Designing valid and reliable measurement tools to provide diagnostic and corrective feedback requires explicitly defining what to measure [37]. However, the more complex the performance to be trained, the more difficult it is to determine what and how to measure it [32].

We propose several recommendations to address these challenges. First, to overcome the issue of trying to capture subtle teamwork in a fast-paced scenario, we propose using more than one observer to evaluate teamwork during a scenario, as feasible. When resource constraints make employment of multiple observers impractical, an alternate solution is to audio and video record simulation performance. Video records can be replayed so that a single observer may witness details of the action missed during prior viewings. Second, just as we would require reliability of a paper and pencil scale, when using observers to evaluate teamwork, it is crucial that the observations are reliable [33]. Observer training, as well as the use of behaviorally anchored rating scales (BARS) are ways to ensure that evaluations are accurate, consistent, valid, and useful. BARS offer a solution to the need for tailoring measures to the desired learner responses as they explicate specific and observable pre-determined behaviors that should be elicited from each scripted SBTT event [38, 39]. Observers can assess whether or not each expected behavior was enacted as well as document the variation in quality of those behaviors. Another option to overcoming the challenge of capturing the multiple nuances of teamwork in a short period of time is to videotape learners engaging in SBTT scenarios so that they may be (re)coded for details that can be easily missed during live observations of highly complex and interactive scenarios.

Finally, a solution for whether or not to evaluate individual performance, global team performance, or both, lies in asking oneself what the SBTT is meant to improve and what is most pertinent to the goals of training. Measures should be linked to specific learning objectives [37]. That is, it is necessary to focus the measurement on the level (i.e. team or individual) that the SBTT facilitator would most like to improve. If improvement of an intact team is a concern, measurement should target global team performance. Such an evaluation should address the embodiment of teamwork: the behavioral, cognitive, and affective processes that teams engage in to coordinate and achieve shared goals [37, 40]. If individual effectiveness is of greater importance, measurement should target individual-level team performance. Finally, it is recommended to measure both individual- and team-level behaviors if both outcomes are desired equally [41].

Debriefing and Providing Feedback on Teamwork KSAs

Feedback is an integral component of the learning process [19]. Indeed, meta-analytic empirical evidence has demonstrated that feedback assists skill development during medical simulation [42]. Feedback associated with healthcare simulation is most frequently delivered during debriefs (i.e., after action reviews). Debriefs are facilitated discussions of training performance that serve to improve future performance by reinforcing good behavior and providing corrective guidance for subpar behavior. According to a recent meta-analysis, properly conducted debriefs can improve both individual and team effectiveness by approximately 25% [41], indicating that debriefing as a tool can be hugely valuable. Guided team self-correction is one debrief approach associated with enhanced teamwork and team effectiveness [43]. However, the effectiveness of debriefs largely depends on how well aligned feedback is with IPE objectives as well as when and how it is delivered.

To capitalize on the potential benefits of feedback, facilitators should tailor the points addressed during debriefing to the targeted performance level. Feedback is more effective for teams and individuals when it focuses on team- and individual-level performance, respectively [41]. Overemphasis of team-level processes may be distracting when the intention is to improve individual team member capabilities. Similarly, group discussions facilitate a shared understanding among team members and cultivate commitment to the team's strategy. Thus, when seeking to improve overall team performance, discussion should focus on team activities rather than individual team member behaviors. Deconstructing individual performance in a group can prevent the team from learning how to function as a unit and overcome future obstacles similar to those presented in the SBTT scenario. Moreover, discussing personal shortcomings publically may unnecessarily embarrass participants, particularly if there is no major benefit to discussing individual performance as a group. Instead, facilitators might consider providing individual-level feedback to participants separately. Separate feedback is especially important when it is of a sensitive nature. Individual-level feedback should be strictly behavior-based. It is inappropriate to use debriefing as an opportunity to present personal criticisms.

The applicability of feedback diminishes with time as learners forget their performance or gain additional experience in the meantime. Thus, dedicating time immediately following SBTT will generate more productive debriefing sessions. Allowing participants to view video recorded examples of their performance can aid the delivery of specific feedback. Participants can see exactly what they did right or wrong in a particular instance and the instructor can strategically pause the recording at critical moments to facilitate discussion. Barring video records of performance, specifics drawn from measurement tools may be leveraged to guide feedback. We recommend addressing both strengths and weaknesses during debriefs as it important to reinforce good behavior as much as it is to correct poor performance. Lastly, to further strengthen its impact, instructors might consider drawing from multiple sources when delivering feedback. Multi-source feedback has been shown to be better than single-source feedback for enhancing learning outcomes [42].

Conclusion

Interprofessional teams are currently the standard in modern healthcare practice and there is no reason to believe that the future of healthcare will not become increasingly complex. It will continue to require the collective knowledge and expertise of multiple physical and social health professionals to provide individualized, integrated care plans for patients. In order to provide top-rated, safe care, healthcare professionals must learn to collaborate efficiently and effectively across professional boundaries. Therefore, it is crucial to provide healthcare professionals with opportunities to practice and improve their teamwork KSAs in a safe and controlled interprofessional setting. Well-designed simulation-based IPE is an excellent modality for providing these educational opportunities.

References

1. Beaubien JM, Baker DP. The use of simulation for training teamwork skills in health care: how low can you go? Qual Saf Health Care. 2004;13:51–6.
2. Institute of Medicine (IOM). Redesigning continuing education in the health professions. Washington, DC: The National Academies Press; 2010. 276 p.
3. Reeves S, Rice K, Conn LG, Miller KL, Kenaszchuk C, Zwarenstein M. Interprofessional interaction, negotiation and non-negotiation on general internal medicine wards. J Interprof Care. 2009;23(6):633–45.
4. Densen P. Challenges and opportunities facing medical education. Trans Am Clin Climatol Assoc. 2011;122:48–58.
5. Epstein NE. Multidisciplinary in-hospital teams improve patient outcomes: a review. Surg Neurol Int. 2014;5(Suppl 7):S295–303.
6. Heinemann GD. Teams in health care settings. In: Heinemann GD, Zeiss AM, editors. Team performance in health care: assessment and development. New York: Kluwer Academic; 2002. p. 3–17.
7. Alonso A, Dunleavy DM. Building teamwork skills in healthcare: the case for communication and coordination competencies. In: Salas E, Frush K, Baker DP, Battles JB, King HB, Wears RL, editors. Improving patient safety through teamwork and team training. New York: Oxford; 2013. p. 41–58.
8. Greiner AC, Knebel E. Editors. Health professions education: a bridge to quality. Washington, D.C.: Institute of Medicine, National Academies Press; 2003. 176 p.
9. Interprofessional Education Collaborative Expert Panel. Core competencies for interprofessional collaborative practice: report of an expert panel. Washington, D.C.: Interprofessional Education Collaborative; 2011.
10. D'Amour D, Oandasan I. Interprofessionality as the field of interprofessional practice and inteprofessional education: an emerging concept. J Interprof Care. 2005;19(Suppl 1):8–10.
11. Paige JT, Garbee DD, Brown KM, Rojas JD. Using simulation in interprofessional education. Surg Clin N Am. 2015;95(4):751–66.
12. World Health Organization (WHO) [Internet]. Framework for action on interprofessional education & collaborative practice. Geneva: World Health Organization; 2010. [cited 2017 Jun 2]. Available at http://apps.who.int/iris/bitstream/10665/70185/1/WHO_HRH_HPN_10.3_eng.pdf.

13. Oser R, Cannon-Bowers JA, Salas E, Dwyer D. Enhancing human performance in technology-rich environments: guidelines for scenario-based training. In: Salas E, editor. Human/technology interaction in complex systems, vol. 9. Greenwich, CT: JAI Press; 1999. p. 175–202.
14. Prince C, Salas E. Training and research for teamwork in the military aircrew. In: Wiener EL, Kanki BG, Helmreich RL, editors. Cockpit resource management. San Diego: Academic; 1993. p. 337–66.
15. Salas E, Priest HA, Wilson KA, Burke CS. Scenario-based training: improving military mission performance and adaptability. In: Adler AB, Castro CA, Britt TW, editors. Minds in the military: the psychology of serving in peace and conflict, Operational stress, vol. 2. Westport: Praeger Security International; 2006. p. 32–53.
16. McGaghie WC, Issenberg SB, Petrusa ER, Scalese RJ. A critical review of simulation-based medical education research: 2003-2009. Med Educ. 2010;44(1):50–63.
17. Gaba DM, Howard SK, Fish KJ, Smith BE, Sowb YA. Simulation-based training in anesthesia crisis resource management (ACRM): a decade of experience. Simul Gaming. 2001;32(2):175–93.
18. Lateef F. Simulation-based learning: just like the real thing. J Emerg Truama Shock. 2010;3(4):348–52.
19. Salas E, Tannenbaum SI, Kraiger K, Smith-Jentsch KA. The science of training and development in organizations: what matters in practice. Psychol Sci Public Interest. 2012;13(2):74–101.
20. Weaver SJ, Salas E, Lyons R, Lazzara EH, Rosen MA, Diazgranados D, et al. Simulation-based team training at the sharp end: a qualitative study of simulation-based team training design, implementation, and evaluation in healthcare. J Emerg Trauma Shock. 2010;3(4):369–77.
21. Rosen MA, Salas E, Silvestri S, Wu T, Lazzara EH. A measurement tool for simulation-based training in emergency medicine: the simulation module for assessment of resident targeted event responses (SMARTER) approach. Simul Healthc. 2008;3(3):170–9.
22. Salas E, Rosen MA. Beyond the bells and whistles: when simulation-based team training works best. Harvard CRICO RMF Forum. 2008;26(4):6–7.
23. Bremner MN, Aduddell K, Bennett DN, VanGeest JB. The use of human patient simulators: best practices with novice nursing students. Nurse Educ. 2006;31:170–4.
24. Rosen MA, Salas E, Tannenbaum SI, Pronovost PJ, King HB. Simulation-based training for teams in healthcare: designing scenarios, measuring performance, and providing feedback. In: Carayon P, editor. Handbook of human factors and ergonomics in health care and patient safety. Boca Raton: Taylor and Francis Group; 2012. p. 573–94.
25. Rosen MA, Salas E, Wu TS, Silvestri S, Lazzara EH, Lyons R, et al. Promoting teamwork: an event-based approach to simulation-based teamwork training for emergency medicine residents. Acad Emerg Med. 2008;15(11):1190–8.
26. Kirschner PA, Sweller J, Cark RE. Why minimal guidance during instruction does not work: an analysis of the failure of constructivist, discovery, problem-based experiential, and inquiry-based training. Educ Psychol. 2006;41(2):75–86.
27. Cooke NJ, Salas E, Kiekel PA, Bell B. Advances in measuring team cognition. In: Salas E, Fiore SM, editors. Team cognition: understanding the factors that drive process and performance. Washington, D.C.: American Psychological Association; 2004. p. 83–106.
28. Gum L, Greenhill J, Dix K. Clinical simulation in maternity (CSiM): interprofessional learning through simulation team training. Qual Saf Health Care. 2010;19(5):e19–24.
29. Matheson L, Levi E. Optimal utilization of registered nurses through all phases of care in the cardiac cath lab. Cardiac Cath Lab Director. 2011;1(3):110–2.
30. Blum RH, Raemer DB, Carroll JS, Dufresne RL, Cooper JB. A method for measuring effectiveness of simulation-based team training for improving communication skills. Anesth Analg. 2005;100(5):1375–80.
31. Shapiro MJ, Gardner R, Godwin SA, Jay GD, Lindquist DG, Salisbury ML, et al. Defining team performance for simulation-based training: methodology, metrics, and opportunities for emergency medicine. Acad Emerg Med. 2008;15(11):1088–97.
32. Salas E, Wilson KA, Lazzara EH, King HB, Augenstein JS. Simulation-based training for patient safety: 10 principles that matter. J Patient Saf. 2008;4(1):3–8.

33. Rosen M, Weaver SJ, Lazzara EH, Salas E, Wu T, Silvestri S, et al. Tools for evaluating team performance in simulation-based training. J Emerg Trauma Shock. 2010;3(4):353–9.
34. Baker DP, Salas E. Principles for measuring teamwork skills. Hum Factors. 1992;34(4):469–75.
35. Baker DP, Salas E. Principles for measuring teamwork: a summary and a look toward the future. In: Brannick MT, Salas E, Prince C, editors. Team performance and measurement. Mahwah: Erlbaum; 1997. p. 331–55.
36. Valentine MA, Nembhard IM, Edmondson AC. Measuring teamwork in healthcare settings: a review of survey instruments. Med Care. 2015;53(4):e16–30.
37. Rosen MA, Salas E, Wilson KA, King HB, Salisbury M, Augenstein JS, et al. Measuring team performance in simulation-based training: adopting best practices for healthcare. Simul Healthc. 2008;3(1):33–41.
38. Fowlkes JE, Dwyer DJ, Oser RL, Salas E. Event-based approach to training (EBAT). Int J Aviat Psychol. 1998;8:209–21.
39. Nguyen N, Watson WD, Dominguez E. An event-based approach to design a teamwork training scenario and assessment tool in surgery. J Surg Educ. 2016;73(2):197–207.
40. Mathieu J, Maynard MT, Rapp T, Gilson L. Team effectiveness 1997-2007: a review of recent advancements and a glimpse into the future. J Manage. 2008;34(3):410–76.
41. Tannenbaum SI, Cerasoli CP. Do team and individual debriefs enhance performance? A meta-analysis. Hum Factors. 2013;55(1):231–45.
42. Hatala R, Cook DA, Zendejas B, Hamstra SJ, Brydges R. Feedback for simulation-based procedural skills training: a meta-analysis and critical narrative synthesis. Adv Health Sci Educ. 2014;19(2):251–72.
43. Smith-Jentsch KA, Cannon-Bowers JA, Tannenbaum SI, Salas E. Guided team self-correction: impacts on team mental models, processes, and effectiveness. Small Gr Res. 2008;39(3):303–27.

Establishing a Sustainable, Integrated Pre-professional Interprofessional Simulation Program

7

Erik W. Black, Heather A. Davidson, and Nicole M. Paradise Black

Introduction

In 1998 the Pew Health Professions Commission published a study entitled "Recreating Health Professional Practice for a New Century"; this study identified nearly two dozen clinical skills and competencies for the contemporary health professional [1]. Paramount among these skills and competencies was the ability to work as a member of an interprofessional team of diverse healthcare providers. The authors drew from the original definition of interprofessional education (IPE) by the Centre for the Advancement of Interprofessional Education (CAIPE):

> …involv(ing) educators and learners from two or more health professions and their foundational disciplines who jointly create and foster a collaborative learning environment. The goal of these efforts is to develop knowledge, skills and attitudes that result in Interprofessional team behaviors and competence. Ideally, Interprofessional education is incorporated throughout the entire curriculum in a vertically and horizontally integrated fashion." ([6, 7], p. 19)

Since the publication of the Pew report and a successive number of other reports, health science accrediting bodies have incorporated many of the Pew recommendations by requiring health professional schools to offer

E. W. Black (✉)
UF Health Shands Children's Hospital, Department of Pediatrics, Gainesville, FL, USA
e-mail: ewblack@ufl.edu

H. A. Davidson
Vanderbilt University Medical Center, Center for Patient and Professional Advocacy, Nashville, TN, USA
e-mail: heather.a.davidson@vanderbilt.edu

N. M. Paradise Black
UF Health Shands Children's Hospital, Department of Pediatrics, Gainesville, FL, USA
e-mail: blacknm@peds.ufl.edu

J. T. Paige et al. (eds.), *Comprehensive Healthcare Simulation: InterProfessional Team Training and Simulation*, Comprehensive Healthcare Simulation,
https://doi.org/10.1007/978-3-030-28845-7_7

interprofessional learning experiences to all students. The number of accreditation bodies requiring collaboration between professions has mirrored the trends and has resulted in creativity and new models for the delivery of education through IPE offerings [2]. These recommendations challenge schools to expand on their traditional methods of supporting only faculty from their home profession to be central to student learning (in the many instructional methods from lecturing to bedside teaching) to including faculty from other professions to participate in student learning. In a short matter of time, IPE transformed from an obscure practice to an institutional priority that, in some institutions and for some licensing bodies, now encompasses training for pre-professional, graduate-professional, and practicing professional learners [3].

Just 5 years after its initial formation, the Interprofessional Education Collaborative (IPEC), an organization created to facilitate the development of core competencies for health professions, more than tripled in size, growing from 6 to 20 professional organizations [4, 5]. The collaborative now includes membership from across the health professions spectrum (Table 7.1).

IPEC's collaborative reach and professional development activities have included professions from outside of the current 20 member organizations, such as architecture, law and basic science, genetics and microbiology [5]. IPEC's initial role was to establish a set of competencies that provides a basis for IPE across campuses and professions (Table 7.2). These four competencies, each with between eight to ten sub-competencies, emphasize a community- and population-oriented viewpoint and a patient- and family-centered perspective (Fig. 7.1). These competencies reflected recommendations from other professional organizations advocating for healthcare reform [6].

Addressing these Interprofessional competencies while at the same time assuring the education needs of a diverse body of individuals from across the learning continuum, each with robust curricula and/or working schedules, is a formidable challenge.

IPE involves many learners, diverse professional cultures and, at present, very few experienced faculty leaders with the expertise to share critical knowledge. Institutions often find themselves inventing their own IPE programs from scratch [7]. This process of invention has commonly resulted in coursework and intersession activities for pre-professional learners or other often-brief experiences to meet the benchmarks established by accreditors or stakeholders, but it offers little opportunity to promote systemic cultural change. Some institutions have built complex experiences that provide learners with early access to clinics and patients (e.g., Vanderbilt's Program in Interprofessional Learning (VPIL), The University of Florida's Putting Families First, Florida International University's Neighborhood-HELP™) [8, 9]. These institutions are the exception. Several other institutions have led efforts to incorporate simulation activities for pre-professional learners (e.g. University of Washington, Ohio State University) [10, 11]. Unfortunately, given the nascent and rapidly evolving nature of IPE, many academic institutions, both large and small, continue to struggle to establish sustainable IPE programs, much less incorporate simulation-based activities [12].

Table 7.1 Current IPEC members (January, 2017)

Organization	Profession(s) represented
Accreditation Council for Education in Academy of Nutrition and Dietetics (ACEND)	Registered Dietician, Nutrition and Dietetic Technician
American Speech-Language-Hearing Association (ASHA)	Audiologist, Speech-Language Pathologist
Association of Academic Health Sciences Libraries (AAHSL)	Librarian
Association of Chiropractic Colleges (ACC)	Chiropractor
National League of Nursing (NLN)	Nurse
American Association of Colleges of Nursing (AACN)	Nurse
American Association of Colleges of Osteopathic Medicine (AACOM)	Physician
American Association of Colleges of Pharmacy (AACOP)	Pharmacist
American Association of Colleges of Podiatric Medicine (AACPM)	Podiatrist
American Association of Veterinary Medical Colleges (AAVMC)	Veterinarian
American Council of Academic Physical Therapy (ACAPT)	Physical Therapist
American Dental Education Association (ADEA)	Dentist
American Occupational Therapy Association (AOTA)	Occupational Therapy
American Psychological Association (APA)	Psychologist
Association of American Medical Colleges (AAMC)	Physician
Association of Schools and Colleges of Optometry (ASCO)	Optometrist
Association of Schools and Programs of Public Health (ASPPH)	Public Health
Association of Schools of Allied Health Professions (ASAHP)	Diverse professionals including technicians, mental health counselors and therapists, and assistants in full scope of care
Council on Social Work Education (CSWE)	Social Work
Physician Assistant Education Association (PAEA)	Physician Assistant

Simulation and simulators provide opportunities for learners to realistically experience tasks and situations without risk to patients, equipment, themselves or others. Simulation has emerged as a valuable methodology for clinical instruction as it provides a safe learning environment that is standardized and reproducible [13, 14]. Importantly, simulations can be delivered at varying levels of challenge and complexity based upon the needs of the learner and the evaluator [14, 15]. Simulation in medical and health sciences education traces its roots back to mannequins used to train eighteenth century midwives in Europe [14]. During the subsequent 150 years, simulation has advanced to include multiple modalities including standardized patients or actors who play scripted roles for learners, task-specific trainers

Table 7.2 IPEC competencies

Competency	Definition
Competency 1: Values/ ethics for Interprofessional practice	Work with individuals of other professions to maintain a climate of mutual respect and shared values
Competency 2: Roles/ responsibilities	Use the knowledge of one's own role and those of other professions to appropriately assess and address the health care needs of patients and to promote and advance the health of populations
Competency 3: Interprofessional communication	Communicate with patients, families, communities, and professionals in health and other fields in a responsive and responsible manner that supports a team approach to the promotion and maintenance of health and the prevention and treatment of disease
Competency 4: Teams and teamwork	Apply relationship-building values and the principles of team dynamics to perform effectively in different team roles to plan, deliver, and evaluate patient/population-centered care and population health programs and policies that are safe, timely, efficient, effective, and equitable

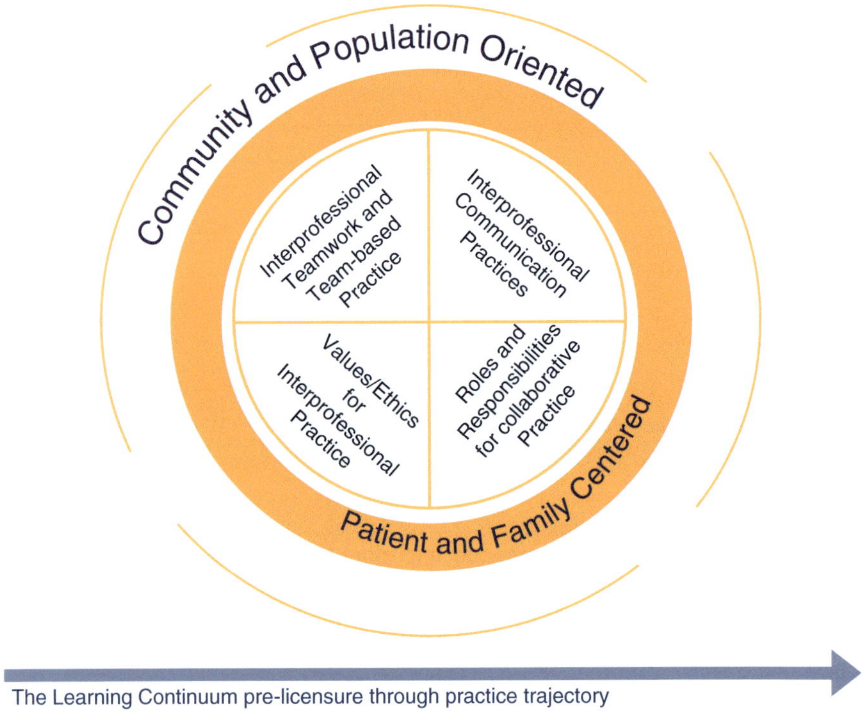

Fig. 7.1 IPEC collaborative competency domains. (Reproduced with permission of the American Medical Colleges, on behalf of IPEC [5])

(e.g. Laerdal's Blood Pressure Arm), high fidelity mannequins which can emulate human biological functions, and screen-based simulations (e.g. Shadow Health's Digital Clinical Experiences™) [14].

Simulation in IPE: What Does the Contemporary Landscape Related to Pre-professional IPE Simulation Look Like?

Perhaps it is the breadth associated with IPE that presents one of its biggest obstacles. As Edwards, Stoyan-Rosenzweig and Hahn describe, and the aforementioned competencies (see Table 7.2) provide evidence of, IPE can encompass many topics and ideals, all of which are salient to future and current healthcare providers [16].

Contemporary healthcare delivery is an interprofessional endeavor involving practitioners, non-clinical staff, patients and families. The team-based interplay between these groups of individuals is influenced by cultural and societal norms and stereotypes [17]. While the historical delivery of healthcare could be described as inherently interprofessional, the training of healthcare professionals has been predominantly uniprofessional. Graduating professionals were expected to possess the ability to work effectively with one-another by virtue of their general intelligence and the communicative abilities demonstrated within their respective uniprofessional domains. This was the status quo, with some minor exceptions, until the early 2000s [2, 18].

Not quite two decades later, Gottlieb et al. describe the present healthcare delivery system as one that has departed from a model that focused on and rewarded exceptional individuals to one that ascribes increasing value to team-based, high-value care [19]. Even in academic scholarship, team-based scholarly works are the new norm. Gottlieb et al. astutely recognize that the historical and societal norms associated with healthcare delivery, which, often, placed a physician in a leadership role, may need to be revised based upon the situation. A rigid hierarchical model may not be appropriate in instances when the healthcare team's psychological conceptualization doesn't support it or the defacto leader lacks the skills to address the problem at hand. In fact, forcing this structure may serve as a barrier to positive outcomes [19].

Published academic literature describing interprofessional simulation activities go as far back as 1947 [20]. Yet, as Dickie describes, IPE's history is not well documented within the peer-reviewed literature [3]. It wasn't until the 1990s, with the incorporation of team training and crisis resource management activities associated with the military and aviation industry, that interprofessional simulation became an area of interest [21, 22].

Palaganas' review of IPE simulation literature provides a discussion of 22 preprofessional peer reviewed articles describing outcomes-based IPE that incorporates simulation [18]. The studies included a range of simulation modalities, including mannequin-based simulation and standardized patients in both low and high fidelity settings, and a majority of studies incorporated formal debriefing of participants. Palaganas' review asserts that outcomes associated with these studies were primarily anecdotal, often incorporating non-validated assessments and multiple confounding variables that remained unadjusted in analysis. More pointedly, Palaganas describes common challenges associated with IPE simulation, including lack of equipment, meeting the needs of learners from disparate disciplines, a lack of simulation knowledge, divergent learning objectives among participating programs, and inadequate assessment of team performance [18].

Reeves et al.'s 2016 best evidence in medical education (BEME) systematic review of outcomes in IPE, provides a more global review that incorporates both simulation and non-simulation modalities and supports Palaganas' conclusions [22]. The conclusions include that: (1) IPE is generally well-received by participants; (2) IPE can be used to enhance the development of practice and service improvement; (3) learners involved in IPE bring unique perspectives and experiences which create complexities in educational delivery; (4) authenticity and customization of the IPE experience is an important component of positive learning experiences; (5) successful IPE experiences incorporate adult learning theory; and (6) faculty development is needed to promote best practices.

Two contemporary MedEdPORTAL curricula provide an opportunity to review the present state of IPE simulation. MedEdPORTAL is the Association of American Medical College's online learning artifact repository. Learning artifacts, which include curricula, are submitted to MedEdPORTAL for peer review by a panel of domain and content experts. Authors receive feedback and revision instructions in a manner like a peer reviewed manuscript. Following acceptance, the artifact can be accessed and used by other professionals under a creative commons licensing agreement [23].

A cursory review of MedEdPORTAL provides 27 different artifacts that include the keywords 'Interprofessional', 'pre-professional' and 'simulation'. The curricula range in publication date from 2009 to present. Richmond et al.'s published curriculum, "Discharging Mrs. Fox: a Team-Based Interprofessional Collaborative Standardized Patient Encounter", provides an example of contemporary interprofessional simulation using a standardized patient [24]. Learning objectives associated with this experience include demonstration of effective communication and conflict resolution, comparing professional scopes of practice, effectively communicating profession-specific perspectives and priorities, and verbalizing the way each profession contributes to quality care. In this example, nursing, pharmacy and medical students collaboratively establish a care plan that includes five different discharge decisions for a standardized patient.

Sanders, Richards and Panahi's published curriculum, "Interprofessional Education in a Pediatric Simulation: Case of an Infant with Fever", provides a second example [25]. This experience focuses on the application of effective inteprofessional communication, demonstrating the ability to practice effective patient-centered care, utilizing communication tools and time-outs, demonstrating procedural skill, formulation and prioritization of assessment and care for a sick child, and analyzing roles as salient to the care of the child. This either high or low-fidelity simulation experience incorporates nursing, medicine and pharmacy students. Students must collaboratively progress through a series of stations, which encourage collaborative practice and problem-solving in the context of a febrile infant. The simulation begins with a case presentation that promotes collaborative clinical care decision making and proceeds through three different stations including an infant lumbar puncture; medication selection and order writing and finally medication preparation and administration. Prior to the simulation experience pertinent uniprofessional background content is covered by each profession independently.

Both curricula examples incorporate affective self-assessment and qualitative evaluative guidelines, including checklists to evaluate learner performance. Both are formative in nature, requiring students to demonstrate the application of knowledge in a contextualized setting, and, finally, both acknowledge the importance and emphasize the role of debriefing.

Due to many logistical and financial factors, simulations using standardized patients are often designed as a one-time case. With longitudinal programs, there is also the opportunity to design cases with multiple time points. Therefore, faculty have the ability to identify developmental growth of individuals and team dynamics. An example of a multiple time point, longitudinal simulation experience is embedded in (VPIL) VPIL admits first-year students from medicine, advanced practice nursing, pharmacy, and social work and assigns them as a team to clinical environments to work and learn together one half day each week over a 2 year time period. In addition to clinic and seminar components, the program also includes a three-part standardized patient encounter over their first year. VPIL faculty collaborated with Vanderbilt's Center for Experiential Learning and Assessment (CELA) to develop a standardized patient case of Walter Adkins, a man with congestive heart failure. The case takes place over three sessions (time points) spanning the first year of the 2 year curriculum. Students interview Mr. Adkins individually from the perspective of their own professions then gather as a team to develop an interprofessional care plan and finally present the plan to Mr. Adkins for shared decision making. In each new encounter, Mr. Adkins's situation becomes more complicated (specifically through declining physical health indicators and psychosocial factors), thus stretching and testing student abilities to think longitudinally about this patient's situation. All sessions are videotaped, and faculty members from one of the four professions provides immediate feedback. The actor (standardized patient) also provides feedback to the students based on his patient point of view. Students are asked to view their performance and identify areas where they can improve.

This exercise allows students to discuss differences and similarities in their perspectives on Mr. Adkin's situation, and to practice collaborative care planning [26, 27]. In addition to their real patient experience in the clinic, the Mr. Atkins case is one of the highest-ranking experiences from the student perspective. Students and faculty are able to discuss their growth over time – both individually and as their team develops. Other curricular content taught during VPIL, such as motivational interviewing, assessing behavioral stages of change, and appropriate medication reconciliation interview skills, are also incorporated into the case. Therefore, students are given formative feedback on how they integrate these skills into a "regular" clinic visit with Mr. Atkins.

Additional simulation activities are being submitted to MedEdPORTAL and cataloged in IPE repositories, such as the National Center for Interprofessional Practice and Education with each passing year [28]. The cases and structure of the learning activities provide for a wonderful opportunity to come up with creative solutions to IPE needs. However, the administrative needs of sustaining these programs require faculty with creative ideas to plan strategically.

Sustainable IPE and Simulation

Prior to discussing sustainability, it is worth defining it. By adapting Brundtland and Khalid's definition, we could assert that sustainability incorporates meeting the economic, social and educational needs of present and future learners [29]. As such, sustainable IPE would include programs and initiatives that address the curricular, institutional, and practice-based needs of individual learners in an economically feasible manner, while at the same time complying with their professional graduating competencies. Sustainable IPE also includes institutional requirements that mandate participation; relegating IPE to extracurricular or optional curriculum delegitimizes it. While students do not need to participate in the same IPE activities, all students need to engage in IPE [30]. Yet, a "one size fits all" approach may not be appropriate for all programs. For example, incorporating biomedical science students into a clinical IPE scenario may not result in optimal learning. Instead, it might be more valuable to design an experience with business or engineering students that provide opportunities to think about emergent issues in contemporary drug and device discovery.

While a body of literature describes IPE and interprofessional practices, there are few documented models of successful, broad IPE implementation strategies that allow for systemic generalization to the diverse institutions and organizations challenged to implement IPE [10–13, 15, 18, 20, 24–27]. Adding to the complexity is the fact that relatively few institutions have IPE programs that meet the aforementioned definition of sustainability [3]. One institution that meets the definition is the University of Utah, and it's Interprofessional Education Program. Utah's IPE program provides six simulation-based courses set in multiple care settings that involve more than 1200 students annually from dentistry, health science, medicine, nursing, pharmacy and social work [31]. Another example is The College of Health Disciplines at the University of British Columbia's Interprofessional Education Passport model (http://www.health.ubc.ca/students/interprofessional-education-passport). They have developed a register for students to keep track of and meet requirements for their IPE activities that include earning "points" for participation and a portal for signing up for various events [32]. Allowing for institutions to develop a wide variety of activities and promoting a high quality standard could help mitigate the challenges related to context. Shipman et al. describe the conceptualization of IPE programs as highly contextually based, which may inhibit generalization [31]. They assert, however, there are some important points from which other institutions seeking to establish sustainable programs could benefit, including obtaining leadership support, establishing a dedicated IPE team (inclusive of salary support for efforts), and developing a conceptual model that guides the design process from the beginning. They also recommend understanding the institutional curricular landscape, including plans for programmatic evaluation from the start, exploration of shared curricular needs among health science programs, taking into account the challenges associated with logistics, planning for effective faculty development and engaging in thoughtful documentation and dissemination [31].

Sustainable Best Practices in IPE Simulation

Shipman et al.'s experiences are echoed in the general academic literature describing successful non-simulation IPE implementations where research had identified several common factors critical to IPE programmatic success [21, 30–37]. These factors are quite congruent to those described by Salas et al. when describing the successful implementation of team-training initiatives in healthcare and other high-risk institutions [38]. When synthesized, these factors provide a potential roadmap for successful IPE simulation development and adoption (Table 7.3).

Implied within these guidelines is cost. Implementing any IPE program, much less a simulation-based program is a time intensive undertaking, requiring buy-in at multiple organizational levels and commitment. West et al. report that financial support represents a considerable barrier for many institutions with current and emergent IPE programs [37]. While extramural funding opportunities that encourage curricular development and advancement are available (e.g., Josiah H. Macy Fund, Robert Wood Johnson Foundation), these funds may dictate the strategic direction of an institution's IPE efforts, rather than allowing the institution's strategic and organizational goals to influence the nature of IPE [30]. We encourage institutions to adequately fund central Offices of Interprofessional Education to facilitate the curricular, logistic and evaluative challenges associated with IPE. Geographical regions could also consider developing a network to facilitate opportunities and support each other through shared resources. For example, 38 institutions and organizations in British Columbia, Canada have developed a network for simulation to not only promote collaborative opportunities for their trainees during simulated learning activities but also share the resources and expense of high quality simulation centers in order to meet the need for training at different level of professional work [40]. Further, we advocate that institutions consider existing and new simulation practices in a situated fashion, that is, by first considering institutional objectives, then common instructional objectives shared across disciplines, before considering the core IPEC competencies [5, 41]. Regardless of profession, faculty and administrators will be challenged to find available time within their curricula to implement new activities. Instead, they should focus on replacing existing learning objectives and materials that are suitable for interprofessional instruction. Ideally,

Table 7.3 Convergent guidelines (IPE and Team Training)

Convergent Guideline	Definition
1. Top-down leadership commitment	Senior leadership must facilitate a climate that is conducive to change, and it must dedicate time and personnel to the effort. Grassroots IPE efforts often encounter challenges that cannot be overcome unless they obtain senior leadership buy-in [32–38]
2. Establish dedicated resources as well as organizational structure	Dedicated resources including space and instructional time in the curriculum must be allocated for IPE to be successful. An organizational structure that exists outside of a college or colleges (that is, an Office of Interprofessional Education) can also help to facilitate collaboration by mediating the needs of all professions involved [30, 32–38]
3. Establish an awareness and common understanding of IPE	Promoting a campus-wide understanding of the importance of IPE to the future of health delivery can increase adoption and provide context for learning activities which may be new or different from extant educational experiences [30, 32–38]
4. Open and regular communication to stakeholders	An operational communications infrastructure that encourages responsible resource allocation and reporting of success metrics via open and regular communications is a critical factor promoting efficient adoption and greater success [35–37]
5. Student engagement in the design and delivery of the implementation	Incorporation of students in the initial needs assessment, design and evaluation of an emergent program increases success [32–37]
6. Facilitate early student and faculty involvement	Similar to # 5 above. Incorporation of disparate faculty in the initial needs assessment, design and evaluation will also facilitate greater campus-wide adoption and participation [32–37]
7. Alignment with institutional strategic objectives	IPE programs that are aligned with institutional strategic goals are, by definition, relevant to the mission of the entire institution. For example, the UF Health Science Center's strategic plan emphasizes community engagement, quality improvement and specifically mentions the goal to "become a national model of Interprofessional Education". IPE program development emphasizes these goals [21, 30, 31, 33, 36, 38, 39]
8. Measure the effectiveness of the program	Program measurement and evaluation begins with a comprehensive needs assessment and includes process and outcome measures that are established apriori [38]

these interprofessional instructional activities progress from simple non-contextually based experiences to more complex hands-on, team-based practices allowing for scaffolded, progressive learning [42]. For example, non-contextually based experiences may include case based activities where students come together in a one-time seminar environment. More complex, involved hands-on activities may require design and implementation of projects. For VIPL, interprofessional student teams design, implement and test quality improvement projects in their assigned clinical environment over the course of their second year. Since the teams are embedded in their respective clinics for a year prior to beginning their project, they not only have developed trust with the clinical team but also have a deeper understanding of the needs of the patient populations [11].

Finally, institutions should consider their peers and establish collaborative relationships with other local institutions and similar institutions nation-wide. For example, satellite campuses presented a challenge for the University of Florida with its three satellite pharmacy college sites in Orlando, Jacksonville and St. Petersburg, Florida. Meeting the institutional and graduating competencies required partnerships with St. Petersburg College, the University of North Florida and the University of Central Florida. Fostering these collaborations was surprisingly simple; cold calls to faculty at each institution produced rapid results. UF satellite campuses assist their partner institutions to meet similar accreditory requirements. In each case, UF is able to provide curriculum and pharmacy students, the partnering institution provides space and their own health professions students. A common assessment and evaluation is used by all participating programs [42]. Similarly, the VPIL program is a partnership between Vanderbilt University's Schools of Medicine and Nursing, Lipscomb University's College of Pharmacy, and the Master of Social Work programs at University of Tennessee and Tennessee State University. Administrative and strategic decisions allowed the institutions to develop their shared goals [43]. Each of these partnerships has proven to be incredibly valuable for faculty and students, encouraging rapid innovation and economies of scale [42].

Looking Forward

Sustainable IPE Practices

This chapter makes the assertion that simulation in pre-professional interprofessional health science education is an emergent topic with relatively few examples of sustainable practices. Yet, the general practices associated with establishing a sustainable IPE program that does not include simulation provides a roadmap for those wishing to establish or expand their program to include simulation. Resources, such as MedEdPORTAL and the National Center for Interprofessional Practice and Education, can accelerate the rate at which institutions can implement and improve on existing infrastructure, including simulation infrastructure, but faculty and administrators should expect to have to customize aspects of any curriculum obtained from another institution to meet their unique needs [25, 28].

Logistical Challenges

Logistical challenges associated with IPE are often underestimated, even on the most conservative of campuses. Campuses may need to adapt programs to meet the needs of distance and online learners or to address a lack of participation on their own campuses by potentially looking outside their institution for willing partners, which could include local community colleges or institutions with differing professional programs [42, 44].

Technological Opportunities

Technology offers some intriguing opportunities for enhancing interprofessional simulation. Emergent screen-based simulation has demonstrated the capacity to address logistical challenges. For example, research by Robb et al. describe the use of screen-based virtual humans as a substitute for absentee team members in team simulation experiences [45, 46]. Increasingly 'academic' electronic medical records (EMRs) are incorporated into learning experiences to provide students with opportunities to use screen-based technology to interact in real and non-real time around simulated patient experiences [47, 48].

Conclusion

Even with a concerted effort to develop and implement pre-professional IPE experiences over the past 20 years, institutions continue to encounter challenges when implementing meaningful and sustainable curricula and programs. Within the context of interprofessional simulation, there are an unfortunately small number of exemplars that have developed comprehensive sustained programs (e.g. University of Utah). A majority of those considered leaders in the field are currently working towards the systematic incorporation of simulation into IPE (e.g. Vanderbilt University, the University of Florida, University of British Columbia). Yet, achievement of the vision for a compressive simulation program to drive IPE curriculum is still relatively far away.

Fortunately, by drawing upon known successes and practices that have resulted in the establishment of successful non-simulation based programming (Table 7.3) it is anticipated that programs will continue to evolve to include simulation as an essential methodology for preparing learners for future practice.

References

1. Barr H, Gray R, Helme M, Low H, Reeves S. Interprofessional education guidelines. Fareham: Center for the Advancement of Interprofessional Education; 2016.
2. VanKuiken DM, Schaefer JK, Hall MF, Browne FR. Integrating interprofessional education into the curriculum: challenges and solutions for a university without a medical center. J Interprofessional Educ Pract. 2016;2:5–11.
3. Dickie R. The history of Interprofessional education. In: Edwards ME, editor. Interprofessional education and medical libraries: partnering for success. Lanham: Rowman and Little Field; 2016.
4. Collaborative IE. Core competencies for interprofessional collaborative practice: 2016 update. Washington, D.C.: Interprofessional Education Collaborative; 2016.
5. Panel IE. Core competencies for interprofessional collaborative practice: report of an expert panel. Washington, D.C.: Interprofessional Education Collaborative Expert Panel; 2011.

6. Plsek P. Redesigning health care with insights from the science of complex adaptive systems. In: Crossing the quality chasm: a new health system for the 21st century. Washington, D.C.: National Academies Press (US); 2001. p. 309–22.
7. Buring SM, Bhushan A, Broeseker A, Conway S, Duncan-Hewitt W, Hansen L, et al. Interprofessional education: definitions, student competencies, and guidelines for implementation. Am J Pharm Educ. 2009;73(4):59.
8. Barr H. Interprofessional education: today, yesterday and tomorrow. London: Learning and Teaching support Network: Centre for Health Sciences and Practice; 2002.
9. Hall LW, Zierler BK. Interprofessional education and practice guide no. 1: developing faculty to effectively facilitate interprofessional education. J Interprof Care. 2015;29(1):3–7.
10. Blue AV, Zoller J, Stratton TD, Elam CL, Gilbert J. Interprofessional education in US medical schools. J Interprof Care. 2010;24(2):204–6.
11. Black EW, Stetten N, Blue AV. Engaging service learning in interprofessional education. In: Edwards ME, editor. Interprofessional education and medical libraries: partnering for success. Lanham: Rowman and Little Field; 2016.
12. Thomas EM, Rybski MF, Apke TL, Kegelmeyer DA, Kloos AD. An acute interprofessional simulation experience for occupational and physical therapy students: key findings from a survey study. J Interprof Care. 2017;31(3):317-24.
13. Grymonpre RE, Ateah CA, Dean HJ, Heinonen TI, Holmqvist ME, MacDonald LL, et al. Sustainable implementation of interprofessional education using an adoption model framework. Can J High Educ. 2016;46(4):76.
14. Singh H, Kalani M, Acosta-Torres S, El Ahmadieh TY, Loya J, Ganju A. History of simulation in medicine: from Resusci Annie to the Ann Myers Medical Center. Neurosurgery. 2013;73:S9–14.
15. Brock D, Abu-Rish E, Chiu CR, Hammer D, Wilson S, Vorvick L, et al. Interprofessional education in team communication: working together to improve patient safety. BMJ Qual Saf. 2013;22(5):414–23.
16. Edwards ME, Stoyan-Rosenzweig N, Hahn P. Preface. In: Edwards ME, editor. Interprofessional education and medical libraries: partnering for success. Lanham: Rowman and Little Field; 2016.
17. Buck GH. Development of simulators in medical education. Gesnerus. 1990;48:7–28.
18. Palaganas JC. Exploring healthcare simulation as a platform for interprofessional education [Doctoral dissertation]. [cited 2013 Nov 28]. Available from http://gradworks.umi.com/3547895.pdf
19. Gottlieb M, Grossman C, Rose E, Sanderson W, Ankel F, Swaminathan A, et al. Academic primer series: five key papers about team collaboration relevant to emergency medicine. West J Emerg Med. 2017;18(2):303–10.
20. Jantsch E. Inter-and transdisciplinary university: a systems approach to education and innovation. High Educ Q. 1947;1(1):7–37.
21. Davidson RA, Waddell R. A historical overview of interdisciplinary family health: a community-based interprofessional health professions course. Acad Med. 2005;80(4):334–8.
22. Reeves S, Fletcher S, Barr H, Birch I, Boet S, Davies N, et al. A BEME systematic review of the effects of interprofessional education: BEME Guide No. 39. Med Teach. 2016;38(7):656–68.
23. Reynolds RJ, Candler CS. MedEdPORTAL: educational scholarship for teaching. J Contin Educ Health Prof. 2008;28(2):91–4.
24. Richmond A, Burgner A, Green J, Young G, Gelber J, Bills J, Parker DL, Ridinger HA. Discharging Mrs. Fox: a team-based interprofessional collaborative standardized patient. MedEdPORTAL Publications. 2017;13:10539.
25. Sanders M, Richards D, Panahi L. Interprofessional education (IPE) in a pediatric simulation: case of an infant with fever. MedEdPORTAL Publications. 2013;9:9515.

26. Cole S, Waynick Rogers P. Utilizing standardized patients to promote interprofessional education: a case study using Mr. Atkins. Oral abstract presented at the Tennessee Simulation Alliance, Nashville; 2016, p. 18.
27. Cole S, Waynick Rogers, P. Utilizing standardized patients to promote interprofessional education: a case study using Mr. Atkins. Oral abstract presented at the American Association of Colleges of Nursing, Orlando; 2015 Nov 19.
28. NEXUS Learning System [Internet]. Minneapolis: National Center for Interprofessional Education and Practice c2015 [cited 2017 May 16]. Available from https://nexusipe.org/engaging/learning-system
29. Brundtland GH, Khalid M. Our common future. New York: Oxford University Press; 1987.
30. Wernicke A, LeMaster J. Centers for interprofessional education: structure and role in establishing Interprofessional health curricula. Washington, D.C.: Educational Advisory Board; 2012.
31. Shipman JP, Chase-Cantarini S, Wilson RD, Weber AI. Designing an Interprofessional education program from planning to implementation. In: Edwards ME, editor. Interprofessional education and medical libraries: partnering for success. Lanham: Rowman and Little Field; 2016.
32. Birnbaum D, Gretsinger K, Ellis U. The new frontier of public health education. Leadersh Health Serv. 2017;30(1):3.
33. MacKenzie D, Merritt BK. Making space: integrating meaningful interprofessional experiences into an existing curriculum. J Interprof Care. 2013;27(3):274–6.
34. Blue AV, Mitcham M, Smith T, Raymond J, Greenberg R. Changing the future of health professions: embedding interprofessional education within an academic health center. Acad Med. 2010;85(8):1290–5.
35. Djukic M, Fulmer T, Adams JG, Lee S, Triola MM. NYU3T: teaching, technology, teamwork: a model for interprofessional education scalability and sustainability. Nurs Clin N Am. 2012;47(3):333–46.
36. Evans CH, Cashman SB, Page DA, Garr DR. Model approaches for advancing interprofessional prevention education. Am J Prev Med. 2011;40(2):245–60.
37. West C, Graham L, Palmer RT, Miller MF, Thayer EK, Stuber ML, et al. Implementation of interprofessional education (IPE) in 16 US medical schools: common practices, barriers and facilitators. J Interprofessional Educ Pract. 2016;4:41–9.
38. Salas E, Almeida SA, Salisbury M, King H, Lazzara EH, Lyons R, et al. What are the critical success factors for team training in health care? Jt Comm J Qual Patient Saf. 2009;35(8):398–405.
39. UFHealth Newsroom [Internet]. Gainesville, Florida: UFHealth; c1953 [cited 2017 May 16]. Available from: https://ufhealth.org/news/2015/uf-health-launches-new-five-year-strategic-plan.
40. Qayumi K, Donn S, Zheng B, Young L, Dutton J, Adamack M, et al. British Columbia interprofessional model for simulation-based education in health care: a network of simulation sites. Simul Healthc. 2012;7(5):295–307.
41. Black EW, Blue AV, Davidson R, McCormack WT. Using team based learning in a large interprofessional health science education experience. J Interprofessional Educ Pract. 2016;5:19–22.
42. Barr H, Gray R, Helme M, Low H, Reeves S. Steering the development of interprofessional education. J Interprof Care. 2016;30(5):549–52.
43. Buerhaus P. Spreading like a wildfire: Interprofessional Education – The Vanderbilt Experience. Health Affairs Blog. [Internet] 2014. Available from http://healthaffairs.org/blog/2014/11/20/spreading-like-a-wildfire-interprofessional-education-the-vanderbilt-experience/.
44. Schorn MN, Wu A, Davidson HA, Black E, Rockhold R. Interprofessional education (IPE): synchronous, asynchronous, clinical practice, simulation across disciplines, across universities. Med Sci Educ. 2014;24(1):9–11.
45. Robb A, Kleinsmith A, Cordar A, White C, Wendling A, Lampotang S, et al. Training together: how another human trainee's presence affects behavior during virtual human-based team training. Frontiers ICT. 2016;3:17.

46. Robb A, Cordar A, Lampotang S, White C, Wendling A, Lok B. Teaming up with virtual humans: how other people change our perceptions of and behavior with virtual teammates. IEEE Trans Vis Comput Graph. 2015;21(4):511–9.
47. Robinson MV, Estes KR, Knapfel S. Use of technology in the classroom to increase professional preparation. J Nurse Pract. 2014;10(10):e93–7.
48. Curry RH. Meaningful roles for medical students in the provision of longitudinal patient care. JAMA. 2014;312(22):2335–6.

8 Optimizing Interprofessional Education with In Situ Simulation

Aimee Gardner, Stephanie DeSandro, M. Tyson Pillow, and Rami Ahmed

Introduction

Interprofessional teams are at the core of healthcare delivery. We know that care delivered by highly functioning teams is better than care provided by health professionals practicing without coordination [1–5]. We also know that the existing educational system is not equipping health professionals with all of the requisite and critical teamwork competencies [6]. Simulation has been shown to be a beneficial solution to developing and honing these core competencies among interprofessional teams as it allows teams to work together and refine skills central to high-level performance. The literature has presented many examples of simulation improving procedural skills, communication skills, and team dynamics [4–7]. Evidence of the impact of simulation-based interprofessional education (IPE) has been evaluated and can be seen in the literature as well, as shown in Box 8.1.

A. Gardner (✉)
School of Health Professions, Baylor College of Medicine, Houston, TX, USA

Department of Surgery, Baylor College of Medicine, Houston, TX, USA
e-mail: aimee.gardner@bcm.edu

S. DeSandro
School of Health Professions, Baylor College of Medicine, Houston, TX, USA
e-mail: desandro@bcm.edu

M. T. Pillow
Department of Emergency Medicine, Baylor College of Medicine, Houston, TX, USA
e-mail: pillow@bcm.edu

R. Ahmed
Department of Emergency Medicine, Summa Health System, Akron, OH, USA
e-mail: ahmedr@summahealth.org

J. T. Paige et al. (eds.), *Comprehensive Healthcare Simulation: InterProfessional Team Training and Simulation*, Comprehensive Healthcare Simulation,
https://doi.org/10.1007/978-3-030-28845-7_8

Box 8.1 Outcomes in Simulation-enhanced IPE

Perceived improvement areas:

1. Knowledge, skills, attitudes, and behaviors related to teamwork
2. Appreciation of other professionals, their patient care roles, and skills
3. Awareness regarding the effective use of resources
4. Communication and collaboration
5. Self-confidence as it related to teamwork
6. Clinical reasoning
7. Shared mental model
8. Understanding the importance of patient safety initiatives

Observed/measured improvement areas:

1. Understanding professional health care roles
2. Identifying effective team performance supporting the best interest of patients and families
3. Improving team communications
4. Increasing awareness and acknowledgment of patients' needs and conditions
5. Improving patient outcomes and experiences

Adapted from Decker [8]

Unfortunately, there are many barriers and logistical burdens for implementing off-site simulation programs (i.e., in a simulation center) for healthcare teams in practice, including team availability, travel time to and from locations, and limited realism [9]. In situ simulation, which utilizes a functional clinical environment with real staff, equipment, and systems to provide rehearsal and training for clinical teams, has been touted as one possible solution to ensure that healthcare providers can train together on simulated patients to develop and examine core team competencies [9]. Thus, in situ simulation offers enhanced realism (as team members are in real clinical settings often using real equipment), convenience, and offers opportunities for systems-based improvement.

This chapter provides an overview of how in situ simulation is being used for IPE to enhance teamwork and team effectiveness. Going through the lifecycle of interprofessional teams, we first describe how in situ simulation-based IPE can be used for onboarding and orientation to new workspaces. We then describe how it offers unique opportunities for quality improvement initiatives and ongoing skill maintenance for interprofessional teams. Finally, we conclude with an overview of advantages and disadvantages of in situ simulation, provide the reader with our "Top Ten" takeaways of implementing in situ simulation for improving healthcare team effectiveness, and offer opportunities for further exploration.

In Situ Simulation-Based IPE for Onboarding

New employees of hospitals or medical clinics, whether they are a part of the medical team or ancillary staff, must participate in a formal orientation process. Medical team members include, but are not limited to, registered nurses (RNs), medical doctors (MDs), residents, medical students, advanced practice providers (APPs), APP students, technicians, and pharmacists. Historically, new employees are usually given written materials and may attend an orientation that covers details specific to departments or care units with an overview of hospital policies and procedures, privacy and confidentiality, clinical practice expectations, ethics and codes of conduct, patient safety and quality care – just to name a few. Unfortunately, these materials and meetings may aide in the cognitive component of learning but do not truly explore the psychomotor and affective skills needed for developing a confident and competent employee in their specific environment/work place.

In situ simulation, however, can be a unique complement to traditional onboarding processes for teams. In fact, there have been a number of studies [10–14] investigating the role of in situ simulation-based IPE during the orientation stages where staff can learn in a risk free environment. Such training can provide hospital teams a better understanding of roles, increase comfort with the clinical environment, and help with collaboration as well as communication. The need for in situ IPE simulation has been recognized and recently introduced into the orientation process of some medical institutions not only to develop these necessary skills but also to act as a catalyst for important socialization within the healthcare team [10, 11]. For example, Adler et al. [12] found that a majority of participants who attended an early orientation that included simulation had an easier transition to a new hospital. Other work has similarly demonstrated that team-based simulations can increase team members' knowledge and skill competencies along with perceived confidence levels with both other team members and the workspace itself [13, 14].

In Situ Simulation-Based IPE for Orientation to New Workspaces

In situ simulation can also play a critical role for introducing healthcare teams, who may or may not have previous work experience together, to newly created workspaces in which they will be working. By having members of the team within the unit run the case scenario together, insight into team and space readiness can be examined.

Kerner, Gallo, Casara, et al. [11] used interprofessional in situ simulation as a part of establishing an orientation curriculum for experienced clinicians before opening a new large urban freestanding emergency department (ED). This comprehensive IPE curriculum set out to assess and ensure competencies, enable team work, validate protocols, detect any latent safety threats (LSTs), and optimize patient flow [11]. The curriculum was multi-method, and consisted of didactic courses for team building and orientation activities, laboratory simulation to assess and refresh technical skills, and in situ simulation to look at preoperational logistics including patient flow, layout/design, access, and team communication [11].

Participants included emergency medicine physicians and physician assistants, nurses, and patient care technicians. A pre-activity briefing on the first full day of in situ simulation was followed by post- simulation debriefing. During the in situ simulation several LSTs, including staff roles, physical layout, flow, and protocol-based errors, were detected. Along with these findings, participants indicated that they found this methodology encouraged collaboration, sharing of ideas, and that it made them more comfortable caring for patients in the new ED setting.

In situ simulation-based IPE has also been shown to improve new team communication during patient resuscitation efforts. Ventre et al. [15] used in situ simulation to understand and explore communication among new teams who would be working together in a children's hospital unit. From these simulations, this group was able to test the communication skills within teams to help them identify areas that may delay or impede patient care. As a result of this work, the administration put measures in place to ensure clarification of roles and expected behaviors among teams.

Researchers have similarly been able to implement in situ simulation to examine critical team dynamics for teams transitioning to new facilities. Specifically, Villamaria et al. [16] found similar deficiencies among newly-formed teams, including lack of clarity among roles and members not identifying themselves during mock codes within a new facility. Fortunately, these and other studies [11, 17] have shown positive outcomes in members' perceptions of communication within the team after in situ simulation programs. Increases in ability to communicate within a new work space, established trust, getting to know team members and their capabilities, and better closed loop communication have all been documented benefits of using in situ simulation for examining and enhancing interprofessional team competencies in new work settings [11, 17].

These studies have shown that in situ simulation-based IPE can improve a number of team competencies within a new work environment. Unfortunately, there is a dearth of published evidence specifying best practices in this area. Obstacles such as resource constraints, cost, time, and planning have been cited as reasons for lack of utilization on a larger scale for new team orientation and onboarding [18]. Institutions may be wise to consider how the specific use of simulation may prove valuable for both new hires and newly formed teams or departments, thus expanding understanding of the value proposition of simulation [19]. There may be many opportunities for measuring the return on investment of this methodology, such as quicker time to productivity, increased team member collaboration, and improved worker morale. Administrators will likely agree that the benefit of these elements on positive patient outcomes can outweigh any associated financial costs. Future work needs to be done in this area to confirm the return on investment for such practices.

In Situ Simulation-Based IPE for Quality Improvement

One of the core drivers for simulation-based IPE is quality improvement (QI). The need for systems-based QI has been highlighted by literature and media demonstrating healthcare's failings to provide quality in the US healthcare system. For

Box 8.2 Example Simulation-based Interprofessional Education Activities for Quality Improvement

- Table-top discussions
- Team training (TeamSTEPPS™)
- Team-based objective structured clinical exams
- Crisis resource management training
- Patient hand-offs
- Telemedicine
- Operating room communications
- Procedural guideline adherence
- Error reporting
- Mock codes/resuscitations
- Online training
- Leadership training
- Ethical/professional behavior training
- Conflict management training
- Disaster preparedness
- Maintenance of certification

example, in 2000, the Institute of Medicine report, To Err is Human: Building a Safer Health System, revealed that up to 98,000 hospital deaths each year were due to medical error [20]. Prior to 2000, reports citing similarly high rates of error and harm existed in the literature [8, 21]. For these reasons, organizations are constantly seeking opportunities to implement ongoing QI activities to ensure high-quality patient care [22–24]. Examples of the use of in situ simulation for QI are noted in Box 8.2.

In situ simulation has been frequently utilized to help teams identify LSTs both prior to openings of new facilities and also to ensure continued improvement for established clinical settings [17, 25]. In order to decrease medical errors and increase patient safety, identifying these issues before conducting real-time patient care gives the hospital organization a more directed approach to revise and reconstruct the system, environment, and examine team collaboration. For example, by having interprofessional teams perform two simultaneous critical trauma scenarios together in a new trauma bay, Gardner et al. [17] were able to identify several equipment issues including missing monitors near the trauma bay, lack of supplies within the resuscitation carts, and difficulty locating equipment due to inadequate labeling. In a similar study, researchers used multiple emergent scenarios including cardiac arrest, multitrauma, uroseptic shock, and pediatric toxicology to test processes within a new ED [25]. From these scenarios, serious equipment issues were noted such as airway equipment easily knocked off pillar shelves, airway management devices not readily available, missing laryngoscope blades and endotracheal tubes, and unclear location of several vital kits. Without all team members present in the actual clinical space, these critical LSTs may not have been discovered until actual patients were being cared for. Fortunately, these issues were identified in the simulation scenario and corrected before the new departments opened preventing any harm to actual patients.

Ongoing Development

Deeper dives into the question of quality and the call to provide better healthcare in our country have shown that the core issues lie in both the systems of medical education training and delivery of healthcare. Students in a particular discipline largely learn from instructors in that same discipline, frequently referred to as "learning in silos." Exposure to other professionals in the realm of patient care occurs only in parallel and generally, protected by a bubble made of both real and perceived barriers to collaboration. Upon completion of training, healthcare professionals are expected to possess expert communication and collaboration skills, and the fault for any deficiencies are usually placed on the individual. The solution to these problems must incorporate training throughout the education and delivery continuum, and must have a systems approach. In situ simulation is well-suited to achieve each of these aims.

Because of the temporal proximity to the real clinical setting, in situ simulation is ideal for "just in time" training, wherein team members simulate low-frequency events prior to the occurrence of these events. This may occur in an ad hoc fashion (e.g., a trauma team rehearsing roles and responsibilities just prior to a trauma victim's arrival) or in a planned fashion (e.g., a simulated "dress rehearsal" of a complex surgical procedure scenario involving all involved team members prior to implementation of a planned procedure).

In situ simulation can also ensure ongoing maintenance of skills for interprofessional teams with utilization as a spontaneous teaching tool. For example, Sutton et al. [26] used high-frequency episodes of brief bedside CPR training with a task trainer simulator to improve CPR skill retention among hospital providers. Used in this manner, in situ simulation can be implemented with brief snippets of teaching when team members have even a few moments free to ensure competency of interprofessional teams.

Simulation-based IPE is also ideal for maintaining interprofessional teamwork skills. Work has shown that in situ simulations for interprofessional teams can enhance teams' self-efficacy and readiness to perform [17]. Additionally, other work examining emergency department teams has shown that even two in situ simulations can be enough to significantly improve team cognition, thereby improving team performance [27]. Given the importance of team cognition and shared understandings on team effectiveness [28–30], these findings can have important implications for patient safety outcomes. For example, teams that are on the same page with patient indicators and plans of action may have enhanced ability to communicate and coordinate activities, and thus be better suited to engage in more effective and efficient patient care activities [28].

Despite research demonstrating its value, accrediting bodies have yet to formalize requirements specific to IPE. One such area where simulation-based IPE can provide formative assessment is maintenance of certification (MOC). Multiple organizations, including the American Heart Association (Basic Life Support, Advanced Cardiac Life Support) and the American College of Surgeons (Advanced Trauma Life Support), may benefit from simulation-based IPE during certifications, but they do not necessarily measure team performance dynamics as requirements for passing. Few specialties, like Anesthesiology, utilize simulation-based assessments in maintenance of certification, but none seem to utilize simulation-based IPE in MOC [31]. Another area of ongoing development is disaster training. Anecdotally, many institutions incorporate simulation-based IPE into disaster response training, but few measure outcomes or require this training. Convincing literature supporting simulation-based disaster training can be found in nursing, surgery, and pre-hospital medicine [32–35]. The findings and recommendations from the disaster literature reflect that simulation-based IPE helps prepare teams to perform in "unique and challenging high-risk situations." [23]

Advantages and Disadvantages of In Situ Simulation for IPE

Given the many benefits and outcomes of implementing in situ simulation for IPE mentioned above, it is important to consider how and when this methodology is most impactful, and to also consider any potential limitations to this approach. As noted by an array of authors [36–38], in situ simulation to enhance team competencies and effectiveness can have many advantages. One of the most simple, but critical, benefits of in situ simulation for healthcare teams is that participants are more comfortable in their own healthcare setting. In their review of in situ simulation versus off site simulation, Sorensen et al. [39] found that in situ simulation had a stronger effect on multiple disciplines of postgraduate healthcare professionals. In situ simulation allows teams to practice the actual activity they are most likely to experience in a real event; healthcare teams favor in situ simulation over off site simulation [38] and perceive it as more authentic [39].

There may also be conceptual frameworks to support the use of in situ simulation over training performed off site. Specifically, research within cognitive psychology suggest that learners are more likely to recall newly learned information and techniques when they have been encoded or learned in the same physical environment [40]. This phenomenon termed *"context-dependent memory"* [40] suggests that healthcare teams will be more likely to apply newly-honed skills in the clinical arena if they were learned in that environment. Transfer of training theory also supports this proposition, suggesting that the more similar a learning environment is to the environment in which learners will be performing, the more likely they are to apply those skills in a real setting. Finally, in situ simulation can also allow for just-in-time training as mentioned above, wherein training is performed when it is needed rather than as part of a structured curriculum, allowing for optimal performance. For example, once a trauma team receives an alert that a patient is in route, the team can gather together to assign roles and run through a mock code to ensure all team members understand their responsibilities and are on the same page about patient care goals.

In addition, In situ simulation has many logistical advantages over off site or center-based simulation. As described earlier, simulating team activities in the actual clinical environment can allow unique opportunities for orienting new staff to their workspace as well as identifying LSTs in a newly-created facility. Implementing these training activities in the real patient care environment can also increase efficiency of training. Not only is it logistically more feasible to get healthcare teams to participate because of the proximity of training, but it also decreases time needed for travel and setup. It is easier to have personnel released for learning opportunities in their own clinical setting than sending staff off site. Finally, and most practically, in situ simulation does not require expensive real estate, dedicated areas or specific structures for simulation, as they are unnecessary to re-create a clinical environment. Instead, healthcare teams can practice where they work.

Finally, with in situ simulation comes a unique opportunity for institutions to create and reveal their unique culture. For example, an institution with ongoing simulation activities that are conducted in the least burdensome manner for clinical staff can signal not only that continued professional development is important, but that the organization is also considerate of worker schedules and needs. These activities can be strategically crafted to impact an organization's reputation as well, by demonstrating to patients and family members that the organization strives for excellence and is dedicated to ensuring continued and high quality training of its employees.

Despite these numerous advantages, in situ simulation for healthcare teams does have some drawbacks. The first is just the practical – by implementing training programs for staff in close proximity to the clinical environment, their training activities may be more likely to be interrupted when patient care needs arise. These interruptions may include distractions such as pages, phone calls, or provider inquiries. In extreme circumstances, they might also include complete abandonment of training activities due to critical patient care needs or heavy patient loads.

Another potential drawback may be the inability to create a completely safe psychological environment that is necessary for optimal learning. For example, in situ training for healthcare teams does not inherently allow for privacy, as staff are performing with others and in a physical environment in which other providers and patients may be able to observe. Thus, educators and administrators need to ensure that all available steps are taken to ensure a safe learning environment so that healthcare teams feel comfortable putting their professional identities on the line.

Although one of the most frequently cited advantages of in situ simulation is enhanced logistical feasibility [37], training in the clinical arena may also be a constraint. For example, there may be limited opportunity to re-create some clinical scenarios when real patients and providers are in close proximity, such as the use of smoke, fire, belligerent family members, and screaming patients. Specific cases may also take considerable time and effort to set up in standard clinical rooms, whereas dedicated simulation space could allow for unique scenarios to remain in place for extended periods of time. Further, many hospital settings are not equipped with the necessary video recording capabilities that are ideal for performance review and debriefing. Setting up for technological capabilities and solving technical issues may be an additional constraint if technicians do not have easy access to clinical space. Finally, for those who use simulated medication and/or equipment in clinical environments to conduct in situ training, there is increased potential for adverse events. If simulated medications or fake equipment are inadvertently used on real patients, serious consequences may occur [36].

Fortunately, measures can be taken to reduce these disadvantages and potential threats of in situ simulation. These may include establishment of specific policies and procedures for in situ training, labeling simulation equipment and medication, keeping simulation-specific materials and equipment in separate and locked spaces, educating staff and instructors, and informing patients, staff, and other non-involved parties about planned simulation activities via signage and other announcements [36]. Further, in situ simulation has a multitude of advantages, but educators must consider potential drawbacks of this methodology and proactively put processes in place to reduce any trainee or patient harm.

Tips for Implementing In Situ Simulation

Whether developed as a relatively inexpensive way to start a hospital-based simulation program or an added expansion to a centralized simulation center, in situ simulation can present unique obstacles for implementation and return on investment. An overview of the "Top Ten" tips for instituting a high-quality in situ simulation program are presented below and in Box 8.3.

Box 8.3 Ten Tips for Conducting Interprofessional In Situ Simulations

1. Implement scenarios and protocols across a wide range of staff constituents.
2. Focused debriefing sessions must take place immediately after the simulation.
3. Prioritize and immediately correct latent safety threats.
4. Cognitive aids may need to supplement simulation activities.
5. Surprise in situ simulations need to be carefully coordinated and have support from senior administration.
6. Include ancillary staff when performing full-scale simulations to "stress the system."
7. Obtain senior leadership approval to open crash carts and use real supplies.
8. Standardized patient actors are sometimes best for in situ simulations.
9. In some circumstances, consider using a physician champion to serve as the team leader who has no clinical responsibility during the simulation
10. Align training initiatives with comparisons to high performing teams in other industries.

1. *Implement scenarios and protocols across a wide range of staff constituents.*
   When investigating the performance of a large interprofessional group, it is important to obtain an adequate number of staff across various specialties before conclusions are made and resources are spent to "fix the problems." For example, a typical large level one trauma center can easily have over 50 credentialed Emergency Medicine physicians, over 100 nurses on staff, and several hundred ancillary staff. Performing a single in situ simulation with one group of clinicians may not accurately reflect the performance or capability of the larger group. As a simulation educator, any report of performance to senior administration will be more accurate if you have multiple sessions that include personnel during morning, afternoon, and evening shifts. You may identify high variability in adherence to established protocols which may need to be further investigated. Additionally, it is critically important to repeat simulations within a period of time (6–12 months), which is suggestive of the highest rates of skill decay [41, 42]. This will ensure improvements are sustained or may identify if new problems arise that were not anticipated with new policies or modifications to existing policies.
2. *Focused debriefing sessions must take place immediately after the simulation.*
   Many providers participating in in situ simulations during a shift feel the added pressure of knowing there are new patients being added to their area of clinical responsibility. Although they understand the importance of training, they feel an overwhelming need to return and address their patient's immediate needs. Simulation faculty must recognize when this is occurring and put processes in place to adjust the length and focus of their debriefing to address the most critical aspects of the simulation. The most beneficial part of simulation exercises for healthcare teams is overwhelmingly during the debriefing period, in which a facilitator prompts reflection of the participants to reflect upon what just happened and why [43]. This requires effective self-reflection on interprofessional communication, self-identified areas of strength, self-identified areas needing improvement and a self-identified plan for improved performance [44]. The powerful role of debriefing should not be underestimated, as meta-analyses have demonstrated that individual and team performance can improve by 20–25% by using properly conducted debriefs [45].
3. *Prioritize and immediately correct latent safety threats.*
   Simulation educators must serve as content experts, curriculum developers, expert debriefers, and process engineers [46]. The focus of any focused debriefing should be to reinforce positive behaviors and identify areas needing improvement. LSTs that immediately put patients at risk if not corrected must be addressed during the debriefing and reported to senior administration. The development of a timely action plan is imperative. These threats cannot be left unresolved not only for patient safety reasons, but also because they leave the hospital at increased medicolegal risk, especially if it is discovered that such threats were identified and no corrective action was taken [37].
4. *Cognitive aids may need to supplement simulation activities.*
   Some processes, no matter how much practice is conducted, requires the use of cognitive aids (e.g., structured pieces of information designed to improve

adherence to a protocol) for successful completion [47, 48]. Rarely used equipment and high-risk/low-frequency clinical presentations need checklists or clinical informatics alerts to ensure successful completion of all necessary tasks. For example, at one of the author's institutions, an in situ mass casualty incident (MCI) training session allowed multi-disciplinary staff 10 minutes to prepare for an influx of victims. They focused their preparation on the materials they would need immediately for the care of patients (e.g., airway equipment, chest tube setup, warmed intravenous fluids). Despite several simulations in which activation of a disaster protocol and communication with other departments about the influx of a large number of patients was repeatedly emphasized, the staff could not complete all the critical items needed. Staff repeatedly forgot to call the blood bank, prepare trauma blood, alert the operating room, and did not mobilize additional ventilators, trauma carts, and ultrasound machines. Once a cognitive aid, a checklist, was provided by the charge nurse, the completion of all critical items was near 100% (unpublished data).

5. *Surprise in situ simulations need to be carefully coordinated and have support from senior administration.*

   Surprise in situ simulations can be very disruptive to the normal work flow of the real clinical environments. While they can provide very useful information on the preparedness of healthcare teams at any moment without notice, simulation educators must be prepared for the charge physician or nursing leadership to re-schedule the simulation if staffing is too low or the volume and/or acuity of the patients is too high [36]. Simulation faculty also need to prepare for pushback from staff who may feel overwhelmed or irritated with a sudden unexpected training in the middle of a work day. This pushback is best handled with participation from senior leadership observing the simulations and stressing the importance of effective training in the actual practice environment. If this is not possible, an additional strategy is a uniform message to all staff from senior leadership on the importance of participation in such training before the onset of the surprise simulations. Additionally, simulation educators need to make sure to have very focused objectives for each simulation covering one or two succinct topics to allow for more streamlined debriefings. Consideration of staff time can help ensure continued buy-in from staff and minimize the disruption on actual patient care.

6. *Include ancillary staff when performing full-scale simulations to "stress the system."*

   Assessing the medical staff's ability to handle a large surge of patient's medical needs in a MCI simulation is only one piece of the puzzle necessary to truly test the system. Involving staff from patient registration, security, radiology technicians, respiratory therapists, the blood bank, patient transport, social workers and even pastoral care may be critical to assess the ability of the facility/staff. For example, a simulation scenario of an explosion at a nearby factory will result in multiple ambulatory victims presenting in triage. Ambulances with critical victims can start to fill up the trauma bays within 10 minutes. In this example unanticipated logistical issues may arise that impact the healthcare team's ability to provide care to patients. With the large surge of patients in triage, resources such as wheelchairs to transport patients back to the ED may become constrained, charge nurses can become overwhelmed with clinical duties and can no longer assist staff, and the blood bank may be unsure who to provide blood to because registration is unable to register patients and provide wrist identification bands amidst the chaos. These are critical issues frequently overlooked during simulations and must be addressed to ensure a high level of fidelity and readiness.

7. *Obtain senior leadership approval to open crash carts and use real supplies.*

   In situ simulations, especially those that require staff to use and open equipment and supplies from the clinical departments, can be costly. These costs must be discussed with the appropriate leadership as part of the pre-simulation preparation. As noted earlier, if simulation equipment, supplies, or medication are used for in situ simulations, it is imperative that these items do not get into the circulation of equipment utilized for actual patients, potentially causing patient harm (e.g., expired saline, simulated medications, chest tubes) [35]. If real materials are to be used during in situ simulations, the responsible parties must ensure that those items are re-stocked and ready should they be needed for actual patient care.

8. *Standardized patient actors are sometimes best for in situ simulations.*

   Some simulations can feel much more real to trainees when performed in the in situ environment and with standardized patient (SP's) actors rather than simulators. For example, simulations intended to test stroke protocols with physical exam findings critical to the evaluation (facial droop or weak extremities) are nearly impossible to demonstrate with the current generation of simulators. Utilizing a volunteer standardized patient actor, especially one with residual neurologic deficits (e.g., flattened nasolabial fold, chronic hemiparetic extremity) can provide an extremely high level of realism. A simulation case may involve a standardized patient actor presenting with stroke symptoms who is quickly determined to have a stroke by staff and is then quickly rushed to the CT scanner. Depending on the objectives of the case, this actor can be easily switched out when they return from the CT scanner with a high fidelity simulator. This switch can be facilitated by a confederate nurse reporting that the patient aspirated or is unresponsive following maneuvers like intubation or CPR on the simulator. Many times these actors can be found within the volunteer office of your hospital and need minimal training from simulation staff.

9. *In some circumstances, consider using a physician champion to serve as the team leader who has no clinical responsibility during the simulation.*

   "Attitude reflects leadership" is an old adage that carries substantial merit in busy clinical departments. The demeanor of the team leader can significantly improve (or ruin) the *esprit de corps* of the rest of the team. If you plan to do an in situ simulation during a time when you know a certain physician is working who doesn't understand or appreciate the importance of simulation training, it may be beneficial to recruit a physician with a positive attitude to participate in the simulations with no clinical responsibility [37]. This simple move can change the entire demeanor of the staff, which can thus improve the effectiveness of the simulation. This can also help maintain the flow of patients through the department and reinforce the importance of these simulations to staff. After training episodes, sharing the results of simulation activities and associated outcomes on patient safety can also be a strategic method to increase buy-in among staff.

10. *Align training initiatives with comparisons to high performing teams in other industries.*

    The most successful and high functioning teams train the hardest [49]. Most medical providers take a lot of pride in their ability to handle "whatever comes through the door." Part of the preparation for that ability requires frequent and challenging training to maintain a high-level of readiness [50]. Incorporation of anecdotes during debriefing from previous clinical experiences that were successful because of training in simulation or stories of success from other elite teams as a result of rigorous training (e.g., military special forces, olympians, professional sports teams, aviation) may help to inspire and provide greater internal motivation to participate in such training.

Next Steps

While many benefits of in situ simulation have been discussed in this chapter, many opportunities still exist to demonstrate benefits of this method of instruction. While many institutions have begun using simulation as part of the onboarding process for new hires to decrease the time necessary for independent practice and to increase retention [51], there is a dearth of research into the time and cost savings associated with using simulation, especially in situ simulation, compared to more traditional onboarding (clinical shadowing) strategies. These investigations need to compare objective performance and reported errors in the first several months of independent staff practice with and without in situ simulation. Additionally, as healthcare teams continue to play a major role in the delivery of care, the need for further investigation and standardization into the best practices of using in situ simulation for IPE is essential.

Another area requiring further exploration is the value of "surprise" or unannounced simulations in the in situ environment in comparison to announced or planned simulations regarding differences in confidence, knowledge, and performance. The true cost of these must be assessed with an understanding that a significant percentage of these surprise simulations are cancelled or delayed [52] resulting in wasted time and effort by simulation staff as well as taking into consideration the potential disruption to patient care in the clinical environment.

Conclusions

In situ simulation-based IPE has been shown to be a valuable solution for developing and honing core competencies among interprofessional teams, as it allows healthcare providers an opportunity to work together and refine skills central to high-level performance. This chapter provided an overview of how in situ simulation is being and can be used for IPE to enhance teamwork and team effectiveness through the lifecycle of an interprofessional team. Though in situ simulation for IPE involves a variety of techniques, it provides realism, flexibility, and convenience, with less expense and fewer space requirements than off-site simulation. As detailed in this chapter, in situ simulation can also provide unique opportunities for administrative and systems improvement, such as onboarding, orientation, and examination of new clinical workspaces. Regardless of use, in situ simulation is an important tool for entry, development, and continued improvement of any healthcare team.

References

1. Shortell SM, Zimmerman JE, Rousseau DM, Gillies RR, Wagner DP, Draper EA, et al. The performance of intensive care units: does good management make a difference? Med Care. 1994;32(5):508–25.
2. Stevenson K, Baker R, Farooqi A, Sorrie R, Khunti K. Features of primary health care teams associated with successful quality improvement of diabetes care: a qualitative study. Fam Pract. 2001;18(1):21–6.
3. Mukamel DB, Temkin-Greener H, Delavan R, Peterson DR, Gross D, Kunitz S, et al. Team performance and risk-adjusted health outcomes in the Program of All-Inclusive Care for the Elderly (PACE). Gerontologist. 2006;46(2):227–37.
4. Capella J, Smith S, Philip A, Putnam T, Gilbert C, Fry W, et al. Teamwork training improves the clinical care of trauma patients. J Surg Educ. 2010;67(6):439–43.
5. Marr M, Hemmert K, Nguyen AH, Combs R, Annamalai A, Miller G, et al. Team play in surgical education: a simulation-based study. J Surg Educ. 2012;69(1):63–9.
6. Interprofessional Education and Healthcare Simulation Symposium. Interprofessional Healthcare in Simulation [White paper]. [Internet]. Retrieved on [Cited 2017 May 10]. Available from http://www.nln.org/professional-development-programs/teaching-resources/interprofessional-education-(ipe).
7. Levine AI, DeMaria S Jr, Schwartz AD, Sim AJ, editors. The comprehensive textbook of healthcare simulation. New York: Springer; 2013.
8. Gawande AA, Thomas EJ, Zinner MJ, Brennan TA. The incidence and nature of surgical adverse events in Colorado and Utah in 1992. Surgery. 1999;126:66–75.
9. Raemer DB. Ignaz Semmelweis Redux? Sim Healthcare. 2014;9:153–5.
10. Will KK, Stepanak J, Brewer KK, Colquist JA, Cruz JE, Donald CB, et al. Interprofessional orientation for health professionals using simulated learning: findings from a pilot study. J Interprof Care. 2016;30:254–6.
11. Kerner RL, Gallo K, Cassara M, D'Angelo J, Egan A, Simmons JG. Simulation for operational readiness in a new freestanding emergency department: strategy and tactics. Simul Healthc. 2016;11:345–56. https://doi.org/10.1097/SIH.0000000000000180.
12. Adler MD, Mobley BL, Eppich WJ, Lappe M, Green M, Mangold K. Use of simulation to test systems and prepare staff for a new hospital transition. J Patient Saf. 2018;14(3):143–7.
13. Lapkin S, Fernandez R, Levett-Jones T, Bellchambers H. The effectiveness of using human patient simulation manikins in the teaching of clinical reasoning skills to undergraduate nursing students: a systematic review. JBI Libr Syst Rev. 2010;8(16):661–94.
14. Brewster DJ, Barrett JA, Gherardin E, O'Neill JA, Sage D, Hanlon G. Evaluating team-based inter-professional advanced life support training in intensive care-a prospective observational study. Anaesth Intensive Care. 2017;45(1):79–87.
15. Ventre KM, Barry JS, Davis D, Baiamonte VL, Wentworth AC, Petras M, et al. Using in situ simulation to evaluate operational readiness of a children's hospital-based obstetric unit. Simul Healthc. 2014;9:102–11.

16. Villamaria FJ, Pliego JF, Wehbe-Janket H, Coker N, Rajab MH, Sibbitt S, et al. Using simulation to orient code blue teams to a new hospital facility. Simul Healthc. 2008;3:209–16.
17. Gardner AK, Ahmed RA, George RL, Frey J. In situ simulation to assess workplace attitudes and effectiveness in a new facility. Simul Healthc. 2013;8(6):351–8.
18. Lamers K, Janisse L, Brown G, Butler C, Watson B. Collaborative hospital orientation: simulation as a teaching strategy. Nurs Leadersh (Tor Ont). 2013;26 Spec No 2013:61–9.
19. Gardner AK, Nepomnayshy D, Reickert C, Gee DW, Brydges R, Korndorffer JR, et al. The value proposition of simulation. Surgery. 2016;160:546–51.
20. Kohn LT, Corrigan JM, Donaldson MS, editors. To err is human: building a safer health system. Washington, D.C.: National Academies Press; 1999.
21. Brennan TA, Leape LL, Laird NM, Herbert L, Localio AR, Lawthers AG, et al. Incidence of adverse events and negligence in hospitalized patients. Results of the Harvard Medical Practice Study I. N Engl J Med. 1991;324:370–6.
22. Decker SI, Anderson M, Boese T, Epps C, McCarthy J, Motola I, et al. Standards of best practice: simulation standard VIII: simulation-enhanced interprofessional education (Sim-IPE). Clin Simul Nurs. 2015;11:293–7.
23. Gardner AK, DeMoya MA, Tinkoff GH, Brown KB, Garcia GD, Miller GT, et al. Using simulation for disaster preparedness. Surgery. 2016;160:565–70. https://doi.org/10.1016/j.surg.2016.03.027.
24. Guttman O, Gardner AK. Personal protective equipment and simulation: chemiluminescent glow sticks as a game changer? Jt Comm J Qual Patient Saf. 2015;41:234–5.
25. Kobayashi L, Shapiro MJ, Sucov A, Woolard R, Boss RM 3rd, Dunbar J, et al. Portable advanced medical simulation for new emergency department testing and orientation. Acad Emerg Med. 2006;13:691–5.
26. Sutton RM, Niles D, Meaney PA, Aplenc R, French B, Abella B, et al. Detecting breaches in defensive barriers using in situ simulation for obstetric emergencies. Qual Saf Healthc. 2010;19:i53–6.
27. Gardner AK, Ahmed RA. Transforming trauma teams through transactive memory: how simulation can enhance performance. Simul Gaming. 2014;45:356–70.
28. Gardner AK, Scott DJ. Important concepts for developing expert surgical teams using simulation. Surg Clin N Am. 2015;95:717–28.
29. Gardner AK, Kosemund M, Martinez J. Examining the feasibility and predictive validity of the SAGAT tool to assess situation awareness among medical trainees. Simul Healthc. 2017;12(1):249–52.
30. Gardner AK, Scott DJ, AbdelFattah KR. Do great teams think alike? An examination of team mental models and their impact on team performance. Surgery. 2017;161:1203–8.
31. Ross BK, Metzner J. Simulation for maintenance of certification. Surg Clin North Am. 2015;9594:893–905.
32. Chih-Hsien C, Wen-Hsin C, Chia-Chang C, Tsai MC, Tsai LM. Emergency medical technicians' disaster training by tabletop exercise. Am J Emerg Med. 2001;19(5):433–6.
33. Atack L, Parker K, Rocchi M, Maher J, Dryden T. The impact of an online interprofessional course in disaster management competency and attitude towards interprofessional learning. J Interprof Care. 2009;23(6):586–98.
34. Miller JL, Rambeck JH, Snyder A. Improving emergency preparedness system readiness through simulation and interprofessional education. Public Health Rep. 2014;129:129–35.
35. Livingston LL, West CA, Livingston JL, Landry KA, Watzak BC, Graham LL. Simulated Disaster Day: benefit from lessons learned through years of transformation from silos to interprofessional education. Simul Healthc. 2016;11(4):293–8.
36. Sorensen JL, Ostergaard D, LeBlanc V, Ottesen B, Konge L, Dieckmann P, et al. Design of simulation-based medical education and advantages and disadvantages of in situ versus off-site simulation. BMC Med Educ. 2017;17(1):20.
37. Patterson MD, Blike GT, Nadkarni VM. Advances in patient safety: new directions and alternative approaches. Rockville: Agency for Healthcare Research and Quality; 2008.

38. Couto TB, Kerrey BT, Taylor RG, Fitzgerald M, Geis GL. Teamwork skills in actual, in situ, and in-center pediatric emergencies: performance levels across settings and perceptions of comparative educational impact. Simul Healthc. 2015;10:76–84.
39. Sorensen JL, van der Vleuten C, Rosthoj S, Oestergaard D, Leblanc V, Johansen M, et al. Simulation-based multiprofessional obstetric anesthesia training conducted in situ versus off-site leads to similar individual and team outcomes: results from a randomized educational trial. BMJ Open. 2015;5:e008344.
40. Pessin J. The effect of similar and dissimilar conditions upon learning and relearning. J Exp Psychol. 1932;15:427–35.
41. Smith KK, Gilcreast D, Pierce K. Evaluation of staff's retention of ACLS and BLS skills. Resuscitation. 2008;78(1):59–65.
42. Yang CW, Yen ZS, McGowan JE, Chen HC, Chiang WC, Mancini ME, et al. A systematic review of retention of adult advanced life support knowledge and skills in healthcare providers. Resuscitation. 2012;83(9):1055–60.
43. Rudolph JW, Simon R, Rivard P, Dufresne RL, Raemer DB. Debriefing with good judgment: combining rigorous feedback with genuine inquiry. Anesthesiol Clin. 2007;25(2):361–76.
44. Husebø SE, Dieckmann P, Rystedt H, Søreide E, Friberg F. The relationship between facilitators' questions and the level of reflection in postsimulation debriefing. Simul Healthc. 2013;8(3):135–42.
45. Tannenbaum SI, Cerasoli CP. Do team and individual debriefs enhance performance? A meta-analysis. Hum Factors. 2013;55:231–45.
46. Ahmed R, Hughes PG. Simulation directors as improvement leaders. Phys Leadersh J 2017;4(1):44–7.
47. Bajaj K, Rivera-Chiauzzi EY, Lee C, Shepard C, Bernstein PS, Moore-Murray T, et al. Validating obstetric emergency checklists using simulation: a randomized controlled trial. Am J Perinatol. 2016;33(12):1182–90.
48. Arriaga AF, Bader AM, Wong JM, Lipsitz SR, Berry WR, Ziewacz JE, et al. Simulation-based trial of surgical-crisis checklists. N Engl J Med. 2013;368(3):246–53.
49. Ericsson KA. Acquisition and maintenance of medical expertise. Acad Med. 2015;90(11):1471–86.
50. Bingham AL, Sen S, Finn LA, Cawley MJ. Retention of advanced cardiac life support knowledge and skills following high-fidelity mannequin simulation training. Am J Pharm Educ. 2015;79(1):12.
51. Ackermann AD, Kenny G, Walker C. Simulator programs for new nurses'orientation: a retention strategy. J Nurses Staff Dev. 2007;23(3):136–9.
52. Bullough AS, Wagner S, Boland T, Waters TP, Kim K, Adams W. Obstetric team simulation program challenges. J Clin Anesth. 2016;35:564–70.

Considerations and Strategies for Assessing: Simulation-Based Training in Interprofessional Education

9

Kristen L. W. Webster, Amanda C. Tan, Nicholas Unger, and Elizabeth H. Lazzara

Introduction

Medical care is a complex and dynamic system that requires a diverse arsenal of relevant knowledge, skills, and attitudes. Medical education has made substantial strides to ensure that clinicians are fit to provide safe, high-quality care. One of the greatest progressions in achieving such care was the enactment of competency-based education requiring professionals to first show competency in a skill before moving on to the next skill (e.g., Accreditation Council for Graduate Medical Education [ACGME] and American Board of Medical Specialties six competency domains) [1]. Although identifying and establishing competencies is a crucial step to strengthening education, it is insufficient for learning. The crux of learning and developing efficient and effective health professionals is contingent upon comprehensive, rigorous, and robust assessment [2]. Understanding the need for such assessment, competency-based education is now used in every phase of the medical education curriculum – medical school application process [3], residency training [4, 5], and maintenance of certifications [6]. Regardless of the phase in medical education, all assessment has three overarching goals: (1) to serve as a basis for

K. L. W. Webster (✉)
Johns Hopkins Hospital, Department of Anesthesiology and Critical Care Medicine and Department of Surgery, Baltimore, MD, USA
e-mail: kwebster@jh.edu

A. C. Tan
Fuqua Center for Late-Life Depression, Emory University, Atlanta, GA, USA

N. Unger
Department of Research & Synthesis, BlackHägen Design, Dunedin, FL, USA

E. H. Lazzara
Department of Human Factors and Behavioral Neurobiology, Embry-Riddle Aeronautical University, Daytona Beach, FL, USA

J. T. Paige et al. (eds.), *Comprehensive Healthcare Simulation: InterProfessional Team Training and Simulation*, Comprehensive Healthcare Simulation,
https://doi.org/10.1007/978-3-030-28845-7_9

selecting applicants, (2) to enhance the competency of all learners and practitioners by motivating and encouraging learning, and (3) to protect patients by identifying incapable clinicians [7].

Many recognize the importance of assessment [8, 9]; however, effectively executing assessment efforts can be challenging as it is time- and resource-intensive with little clarity [9]. To elaborate, accurately determining learners' improvements requires that assessments be conducted longitudinally. Also, assessment often mandates that faculty serve the role of an evaluator. These duties often exist in conjunction with clinical productivity, patient care, and teaching requirements, compounding faculty's existing responsibilities [5]. In addition to these challenges, little guidance and lack of standardization make assessment difficult, leaving evaluators to question whether learners are competent and capable of safely practicing patient care independently [5]. The ability to develop assessment is made even more difficult as evaluators often have little familiarity with assessment and the psychometric properties of effective assessment [10], despite the fact that most practicing physicians are involved in assessing other health professionals, in some capacity [7].

Unquestionably, assessment is difficult when targeting individuals. It becomes even more daunting when considering multiple individuals with varied backgrounds and expertise who are learning in a collaborative manner as is the manifested in interprofessional education (IPE). IPE involves students learning from others who are outside of their own field with the goal of providing patient centered health through collaborative practice [11].

One mechanism to begin to ameliorate some of these challenges, while providing other added benefits, is simulation-based assessment for IPE. Simulations often have dedicated faculty with protected time, which ensures that faculty are not juggling competing responsibilities. Further, simulations often accommodate a limited number of learners simultaneously; therefore, the ratio of students to faculty is favorable and creates a potentially better learning environment [12]. Another benefit to simulation-based training is that simulation scenarios can be designed a priori and adjusted to fit multiple needs of learners.

Although simulation-based assessments can be a useful educational tool, it must be developed and implemented in a scientifically sound manner. With that in mind, the purpose of this chapter is twofold: (1) to discuss the considerations when leveraging simulation-based training assessments and (2) to describe the advantages and disadvantages of various assessment strategies. The following sections will expand upon these stated objectives.

Considerations for Assessment

Bearing in mind that the overall goal of any training program or simulation is knowledge, skill, or attitude acquisition, it is prudent that the program be adequately developed, implemented, and evaluated to improve or further the development of the educational experience [13]. Although available resources will often dictate the specifics and the parameters of the assessment [13], there are other considerations that must be taken seriously. The following section outlines some of the considerations to undertake when creating and implementing assessment within IPE simulation.

Objectives (Processes and Outcomes) Patient care is a complex and dynamic process of events. Consequently, measuring all facets of provider behavior within one simulation is not feasible. Therefore, assessments should focus on select outcomes and processes that are correlated to patient safety and/or provider performance. Outcomes essentially answer the question of what happened; meanwhile, processes answer the question of why it happened [14]. Outcomes are unquestionably important as they indicate if the objective was accomplished, but processes are arguably equally important as they offer insights into the specific directions to remediate performance [13]. The amalgamation of assessing processes and outcomes is necessary to ensure both the outcomes and the processes to accomplish those outcomes are desirable. For example, processes and outcomes can include but are not limited to situation awareness, communication, knowledge acquisition, and psychomotor skills [15–18], accuracy of recording vital signs [19], compression rates [20], patient identification behaviors and vital sign monitoring [21], or confidence and knowledge [22].

Levels (Individual and Team) IPE inherently entails multiple individuals being trained simultaneously [8], which creates an opportunity to conduct a multi-level evaluation (i.e., individuals and teams). Assessing *only* individuals or *only* teams can provide useful information; however, it can also provide an artificial depiction of the training and the proficiency of the learners [8, 23]. A more robust and comprehensive approach is to assess individuals *and* teams [8, 23]. Evaluating teams provides an understanding as to how the team performed collectively. Considering that patient care is always delivered by teams, such assessment can offer useful insights. Only assessing teams, though, does not discern which individuals need to be reinforced for their efforts and which individuals need guidance and remediation to improve the necessary knowledge, skills, or attitudes [24].

Criteria (Content and Focus) A scientifically sound assessment is contingent upon a multi-dimensional approach. Within the domain of IPE, many have utilized Kirkpatrick's typology of training evaluation [25]. Kirkpatrick's [26] approach offers four criteria: reactions, learning, behaviors, and results by which to evaluate training programs. Reactions answers the question of the extent to which trainees *liked* the training. Learning addresses the extent to which trainees acquired the requisite knowledge. Behaviors refer to the extent to which trainees exhibited the actions in the real-world environment. Finally, results focus on the "bottom line" of the organization. In other words, did the organization see tangible changes as a result of the training? Although much of the literature has focused on reactions and learning [27], we argue that more successful assessments include all four criteria because together they offer a more accurate representation of the training program itself as well as the learners. However, some behaviors and results cannot be assessed during simulation, but rather in follow-up assessments in the clinical arena. Because the evaluation of the training can be distinct from the evaluation of the learners, it is crucial to be especially comprehensive and draw distinction between the simulation and how individuals engage in the simulation. For example, an individual cannot be measured on their ability to adequately check a medication dose if no medication is needed during the simulation.

Data Type (Subjective and Objective) A multitude of data types (e.g. qualitative or quantitative) exist within simulation training and selecting the most appropriate data type to assess can be difficult. As addressed previously, one must carefully select processes and outcomes for measurement to ensure that the appropriate data is being captured in accordance with the determined goals. As such, the type of data available can assist in the selection of these items for measurement during training. Subjective qualitative measurement techniques (e.g., interviews and focus groups), typically entail textual or verbal information and have advantages and disadvantages. One of the biggest advantages is that such qualitative techniques offer rich, in-depth data that cannot be captured by quantitative measurement techniques. Additionally, qualitative techniques are particularly useful for dissecting complex phenomena (e.g., decision making, communication) or uncovering individual nuances or idiosyncrasies. Conversely, these qualitative techniques are especially resource intensive. In addition, qualitative techniques are time-intensive for both the interviewers as well as the interviewees. With regards to the interviewers, much time is needed to train individuals, conduct the interviews, and code and analyze the data. From the interviewees' perspective, it can be time consuming to answer questions with great detail [28]; as a result, such studies may experience attrition, as learners may not want to continue.

The counterpart to subjective data, objective data, involves numerical and quantifiable metrics (e.g., surveys and automated systems) obtained through quantitative techniques. As an advantage, the rigidity of objective data affords reliability, precision, and standardization. Moreover, objective data limits bias, negating human nature to have preferences toward certain individuals in the simulation. Finally, quantitative techniques can oftentimes be easier to collect as they are often embedded or pre-programmed within the simulators and computer/software systems. Although these are unquestionable benefits, there are disadvantages to quantitative techniques. The most noteworthy disadvantage is the assumption that these techniques are "true" assessments [29] as there is always some inherent error even in quantitative techniques. In fact, because of their inflexibility, quantitative techniques often offer limited understanding surrounding complex phenomena and processes. Collecting quantitative observation data can be cumbersome when engaging in real-time assessment. Therefore, it may be necessary to audio or video record simulations to be viewed and analyzed when convenient. Recorded simulations can be paused, replayed, and watched multiple times with different learners as subjects of investigation each time, providing a level of convenience not available during real-time observations.

Types of Assessment

Choosing the correct type of assessment for simulation can be a complex task. Both qualitative and quantitative strategies offer a myriad of options to conduct assessment. Qualitative strategies for IPE assessment include protocol analysis, critical incident technique, communication analysis, and concept mapping. These qualitative strategies, by definition, are more subjective in nature. As described previously, these qualitative strategies utilize interviews, focus groups, and observation techniques to create non-numeric sets of data. Quantitative strategies for IPE assessment include behaviorally anchored rating scales (BARS), behavioral observation scales (BOS), event-based measurement, structural knowledge assessment, self-report measures, and automated performance recording and measurement [9]. These strategies are objective in nature, meaning they utilize more survey-based and automated techniques to create numeric data sets. Now that the objectives, levels, criteria, and data type considerations of assessment have been discussed, we will address the varying qualitative and quantitative strategies for IPE simulation training, recognizing their positive and negative attributes.

Qualitative Methods

Protocol Analysis Also called "think-aloud" analysis, protocol analysis is a method in which verbal reports are obtained from an individual regarding a task [30]. The think-aloud process allows individuals to literally 'think out loud' and describe their steps in how they problem-solved a task [31]. The 'thoughts' verbalized by an individual are recorded, transcribed, coded, and analyzed to understand the individual's cognitive processes during the problem-solving task [30]. Shadbolt [32] and Bainbridge and Sanderson [33] categorized the different channels of protocol analysis into three types: on-line, off-line, and cognitive walkthrough. In on-line protocol analysis, the individual is asked to think out loud *during* the performance of the task. This ensures that the individual does not miss a step in the explanation of a process since (s)he is actively performing the task while speaking; however, elaborating on the processes throughout the task may impede performance. Off-line protocol analysis is said to be less distracting because the individual is explaining a task while watching/listening to a video and/or audio recording of him/herself performing the task [32]. If only an audio recording is available, the transcription of the recording may not play back in a manner that is easily understood. Without visual cues of the behaviors being explained, the individual must rely on verbal explanation and memory, possibly creating a confusing situation. Finally, cognitive walkthrough is defined as explaining how to perform a task out loud without physically performing, listening, or actively seeing it [33]. In cognitive walkthrough, the advantage is that the individual is not distracted by the performance of the task or trying to decipher a video or audio recording. On the other hand, the likelihood of missing or forgetting a step in the process becomes more prevalent since the task is not being actively watched or performed. Protocol analysis can be used within IPE simulations where groups need to complete a step-by-step process. For example, while healthcare professionals are working in a team setting, they can describe out loud what they are doing each step of the way, taking turns and ensuring that their words are being recorded in the consecutive order of events. This allows them to replay the process that each provider takes to complete the team-oriented task, and analyze it later for future enhancement purposes.

Critical Incident Technique Critical incident technique (CIT) is a "set of procedures for collecting direct observation of human behavior in such a way as to facilitate their potential usefulness in solving practical problems" [34]. Incidents are defined as critical when the observer can definitively distinguish the individual's intent(s) and action and can conceive the consequences of said action [9]. The advantage of CIT is that it is easily understood, assists in process development and safety, and can focus on sporadic yet dangerous events. One disadvantage of CIT is that it can be difficult to make comparisons longitudinally since the method inherently focuses on critical, infrequent, and potentially catastrophic events. Relatedly, the events are based upon memory, creating the potential for bias which can interfere with the details of events being recalled correctly (if at all) [9]. CIT is useful in IPE simulations as it provides examples of catastrophic events and gives the team an opportunity to discuss possible future solutions if said event occurs again. Each team member can provide input as to how they would personally solve the problem, and a collective solution can be identified through discussion.

Communication Analysis This form of analysis involves evaluating verbal discourse exchanged between two or more individuals. Within communication analysis, there is content analysis, which is defined as a qualitative research method that analyzes the manifest content involved in communication [35]. The conversation is coded and themes/words are identified [36]. An asset of communication analysis is that it dissects communication granularly, making it easier to identify successful team performance. In fact, some researchers argue it is the best technique for measuring team processes [9]. Such measurable team processes can include, but are not limited to, coordination, leadership, group consciousness, and shared vision [37]. The downside of communication analysis is that it only accounts for team analysis and does not account for each separate individual [9], which can present an inaccurate depiction of how the team functions collectively as a unit.

Concept Mapping Concept mapping is both an individual and team-based assessment that measures knowledge and maps how cognitive concepts, like steps in thought processes, are interrelated [9]. Concept mapping was developed to make connections between key concepts in individual and team-based assessment. By making these connections, individuals and teams can create a network of relationships between the concepts [38]. Particularly within team concept mapping, members participate in processes such as “brainstorming” and organization of ideas to provide meaning to their experience [39]. An asset of this technique is that it enables the measurement and analysis of concepts over time rendering it possible to determine how concepts have evolved [9]. A hindrance of concept mapping is that it can be difficult to develop if all the individuals on a team cannot come to consensus. For example, concept mapping in IPE healthcare simulations would be useful for each team member to present to one another how (s)he is interrelating ideas in his/her own mind as well as for the team as a unit to come up with a shared mental model on how to pursue a process. A surgeon, circulating nurse, and anesthesiologist each have a different priorities and processes when preparing a patient for surgery. Through concept mapping, they can identify ways to make the processes more streamlined by synthesizing their efforts effectively.

Quantitative Methods

Behaviorally Anchored Rating Scales Consisting of a Likert-type scale where numbers represent quality of performance, BARS, use narrative behavioral anchors [40] that can be developed through (but not limited to) data collected using CIT or task analysis [34]. BARS typically ask a question related to performance (e.g., “the employee practices safe tool-handling procedures” with answer options ranging from “(7) Strongly Agree” to “(1) Strongly Disagree,” with “(4)” being neutral). One benefit of a BARS is that it can provide a more accurate rating of an individual’s behavior and performance since the anchors are specific, observable behaviors that are developed by experts [9]. By using the experts to develop the anchors, the opportunity for observer bias greatly diminishes, and the scales become more job-oriented instead of trait-oriented [41]. Although the granularity of the anchors can be seen as advantageous, it can also be detrimental. To elaborate, the specificity of the anchors forces the observer to put behaviors into predetermined categories. These predetermined categories cause the observer to focus solely on how the individual is performing and does not take into account the results of the task itself [42]. This leads to two issues: (1) observers may have categorized a behavior differently on their own but were forced to pick a category they may not agree with, and (2) observers may see the individual performing a task “incorrectly” or simply in a different way and may categorize the individual’s behavior as defiant even though the individual may have completed the task in a more effective manner.

Behavioral Observation Scales BOS analyze "typical" performance [9]. BOS use the Likert-scale as a frequency counter of specific task- or team-oriented behaviors; that is, instead of the Likert-scale representing "unacceptable" to "excellent" it ranges from "never" to "always." An advantage of a BOS is that it is described as being user-friendly [43]. On the other hand, because a BOS is akin to frequency counts, it relies on human memory and is subject to recall bias. Certain steps can be taken to prevent and restrict these biases (e.g., reviewing and editing the desired BOS scale before administering it to ensure there is minimal errors) [35]. A BOS is useful specifically in IPE simulation-based training in the event that the goal of the team training is to identify who is performing what task and at what frequency. If the BOS is used by multiple observers, each observer can identify the tasks completed by each individual in the simulation. Assessing team members simultaneously provides an interprofessional team the ability to compare performance across disciplines and then discuss the differences in performance and provide constructive feedback for performance improvement.

Event-Based Measurement Event-based measurement techniques are traditionally checklists that record the presence or absence of specific, acceptable behaviors determined by experts a priori [44]. One of the most noteworthy perks of this technique is that observers experience little cognitive demand since behaviors are previously established and are presented chronologically [44]. For IPE simulation assessment, this is beneficial because the observers can evaluate a scenario swiftly. A drawback to this technique is that because domain experts develop the checklist prior to performance, the observers may overlook behaviors not included on the checklist. Excluding potentially relevant behaviors is important in a healthcare simulation because an overlooked event can end up resulting in a travesty if not properly addressed. Another hindrance is that event-based measurement is customized for a specific scenario, which makes development of an event based measurement protocol time consuming [18].

Structural Knowledge Assessment Structural knowledge assessment requires individuals to pair presented concepts together to create a map where similar concepts are more closely grouped than dissimilar concepts [9]. For example, in a healthcare simulation, someone like a nurse would present his/her knowledge in a concept map, and a program using an algorithm would assess the degree of similarity/dissimilarity to an expert's concept map on the same topic. An advantage of structural knowledge assessment is that it can investigate performance and knowledge longitudinally (i.e., throughout the duration of a simulation). Another advantage of this technique is that it can be used to guide decisions to improve future outcomes by analyzing individual's completed structure concept maps. By assessing the similarity to an expert's concept map, feedback is immediate and can be used to navigate the individual's idea more similarly towards the expert's idea. As a downside, structural knowledge assessment is the only method that does not assess the process level of analysis [9]. To put it simply, as described by Nau [45], when holding your cards in a card game, you are at the structural level. When you play a card, you are at the process level. Structural knowledge assessment puts together concepts but does not portray the process of how these concepts play out together. For IPE simulation assessment, this means that it can only portray a gross concept similarity between the individual's and expert's maps and does not analyze how those maps could be intertwined to possibly yield the same outcome.

Self-Report Measures Self-report measures (e.g., surveys or questionnaires) can evaluate people globally (team only), at the shared level (team members), and configurally (separate individuals) [46]. Once the evaluation method is determined (i.e., globally, shared, or configurally), they are assessed by aggregating one level to another level's attributes [9]. For example, most commonly the configural level is translated to the shared level, where many individuals are analyzed to understand the team-level attributes [47]. The upside of self-report measures is that they are easy to implement and are time- and cost-effective. Conversely, self-report measures have several disadvantages. Self-report measures are particularly susceptible to biases and validity issues, such as social desirability bias and response bias [48]. The self-report measure is useful in IPE simulation when assessing interpersonal skills (e.g., assessing conflict resolution among team members to provide better training for said concept).

Automated Performance Recording Automated performance recording and measurement involves the use of equipment to automatically record data, as the name suggests. Such equipment can include video cameras, audio recorders (for example, microphones attached to recorders), or a combination of both. Automated performance recording monitors communication and behavior in a two-step process. The first step involves the researcher observing each team member individually to determine if (s)he has the ability to perform the training objective. In the second step, the researcher observes the team as a whole to measure functionality of said training objective based upon team communication and team behaviors [49]. For example, if the training is targeting clinical skills, the observer would first analyze the team members individually to determine his/her understanding of his/her clinical skills, then the observer would analyze the team's clinical skills collectively. A benefit of using automated performance recordings is that a researcher or observer does not have to be present to record the events, making this technique minimally invasive. Moreover, relying on technology as opposed to a human observer limits the Hawthorne effect (i.e., the known effect that people change their behavior when being observed) [50]. On the other hand, automated technology makes it practically impossible to measure cognitions and attitudes, as the task is simply being observed and questions are not able to be asked to the individuals performing the task [9]. For a summary of all of the strategies along with their corresponding advantages and disadvantages, refer to Table 9.1.

Table 9.1 Assessment strategies for IPE simulation

Strategy	Description	Advantages and disadvantages
Qualitative		
Protocol analysis	Verbal thoughts are transcribed, coded, and analyzed to understand the individual's cognitive processes during the problem-solving task.	Advantage(s) – Steps are not skipped during the explanation process. Individuals are not distracted by the performance of the task.
		Disadvantage(s) – Elaborating on the processes throughout the task may impede performance. The individual may have difficulty remembering the process if not being acted out.
Critical incident technique	A set of procedures for collecting direct observation of human behavior in such a way as to facilitate their potential usefulness in solving practical problems	Advantage(s) – Easily understood, assists in process development/safety, and can focus on sporadic yet dangerous events. Allows each team member the opportunity to provide input as to how they, as the individual, would solve the problem.
		Disadvantage(s) – It can be difficult to make comparisons longitudinally since the method inherently focuses on critical, infrequent, and potentially catastrophic events. Events are based on memory, creating potential for bias which can interfere with the details of events being recalled incorrectly.
Communication analysis	Analysis of verbal discourse Contains communication and content analysis The conversation is coded and themes/words are identified	Advantage(s) – Dissects communication, measures team processes
		Disadvantage(s) – Only accounts for team analysis, not for separate individuals
Concept mapping	Both an individual and team-based assessment that measures knowledge and maps how cognitive concepts, like steps in thought processes, are interrelated	Advantage(s) – it enables the measurement and analysis of concepts over time, rendering it possible to determine how concepts have evolved. They can identify ways to make the processes more streamlined by synthesizing their efforts effectively
		Disadvantage(s) – it can be difficult to develop if all the individuals on a team cannot come to consensus
Quantitative		
Behaviorally anchored rating scales	A Likert-type scale where numbers represent quality of performance it uses narrative behavioral anchors that can be developed through (but not limited to) data collected using CIT or task analysis. It typically asks a question related to performance	Advantage(s) – it can provide a more accurate rating of an individual's behavior and performance since the anchors are specific, observable behaviors that are developed by experts. By using the experts to develop the anchors, the opportunity for observer bias greatly diminishes, and the scales become more job-oriented instead of trait-oriented
		Disadvantage(s) – the specificity of the anchors forces the observer to put behaviors into predetermined categories. These predetermined categories cause the observer to focus solely on how the individual is performing and does not take into account the results of the task itself.

Table 9.1 (continued)

Strategy	Description	Advantages and disadvantages
Quantitative		
Behavioral observation scales	Analyzes "typical" performance. Uses the Likert-scale as a frequency counter of specific task- or team-oriented behaviors; that is, instead of the Likert-scale representing "unacceptable" to "excellent" it ranges from "never" to "always"	Advantage(s) – user-friendly; If utilized by multiple observers, each observer can identify the tasks completed by each individual in the simulation. It enhances the ability to compare performance across disciplines and then discuss the differences in performance to provide constructive feedback for performance improvement Disadvantage(s) – relies on human memory and therefore is subject to recall bias
Event-based measuring	These techniques are traditionally checklists that record the presence or absence of specific, acceptable behaviors determined by experts a priori	Advantage(s) – Limited cognitive demand, swift evaluation of scenarios Disadvantage(s) – Previously created checklist allows observers to overlook behaviors not included. Development of the tool is time consuming because of customization requirements
Structural knowledge assessment	Individuals pair presented concepts together Similar items are more closely grouped together	Advantage(s) – Analyzes performance and knowledge longitudinally Disadvantage(s) – Does not assess the process level of analysis or portray the process of how these concepts play out together
Self-report measures	Self-report measures (e.g., surveys or questionnaires) can evaluate people globally (team only), at the shared level (team members), and configurally (separate individuals)	Advantage(s) – they are easy to implement and are time and cost effective. It is also useful when assessing interpersonal skills Disadvantage(s) – Self-report measures are particularly susceptible to biases, such as social desirability bias and response bias, as well as to validity issues
Automated performance recording	Automatically recorded data (video cameras, audio recorders)	Advantage(s) – An observer does not have to be present to record the events Disadvantage(s) – Automated technology makes it difficult to measure cognitions and attitudes

Conclusion

Simulation-based training is essential for strengthening the competencies of medical and other health care professionals; assessment is at the crux of enhancing knowledge, skills, and attitudes. We hope that by delineating the considerations for effective assessment as well as discussing specific measurement techniques along with their strengths and weaknesses, we have provided researchers, educators, and practitioners with some guidance to pursue IPE assessment within the context of simulation.

References

1. Swing SR. The ACGME outcome project: retrospective and prospective. Med Teach. 2007;29(7):648–54.
2. Tabish SA. Assessment methods in medical education. Int J Health Sci. 2010;2(2):3–7.
3. Eva KW, Reiter HI, Rosenfeld J, Norman GR. The ability of the multiple mini-interview to predict pre-clerkship performance in medical school. Acad Med. 2004;79:S40–2.
4. Nasca TJ, Philibert I, Brigham T, Flynn TC. The next GME accreditation system—rationale and benefits. N Engl J Med. 2012 Mar 15;366(11):1051–6.
5. Frey-Vogel AS, Scott-Vernaglia SE, Carter LP, Huang GC. Simulation for milestone assessment: use of a longitudinal curriculum for pediatric residents. Simul Healthc. 2016;11:286–92.
6. Batmangelich S, Adamowski S. Maintenance of certification in the United States: a progress report. J Contin Educ Health Prof. 2004;24:134–8.
7. Cox M, Irby DM. Assessment in medical education. N Engl J Med. 2007;356:387–96.
8. Rosen MA, Weaver SJ, Lazzara EH, Salas E, Wu T, Silvestri S, et al. Tools for evaluating team performance in simulation –based training. J Emerg Trauma Shock. 2010;3(4):353–9.
9. Salas E, Rosen MA, Held JD, Weissmuller JJ. Performance measurement in simulation-based training. Simul Gaming. 2009 June;40(3):328–76.
10. Reinert A. Assessment in medical education: a primer on methodology. News-Columbia University: College of Physicians and Surgeons. [Internet]. 2013 Sep 09. [cited 2017 Apr 10]. Available from: http://www.ps.columbia.edu/education/sites/default/files/student_life/Assessment%20in%20Medical%20Education%20-%20A%20Primer%20on%20Methodology%5B1%5D%20copy.pdf.
11. Centre for the Advancement of Interprofessional Education (CAIPE). Interprofessional education – a definition. London: CAIPE Bulletin 13; 1997. p. 19.
12. Quilici AP, Bicudo AM, Gianotto-Oliveira R, Timerman S, Gutierrez F, Abrão KC. Faculty perceptions of simulation programs in healthcare education. Int J Med Educ. 2015;6:166–71.
13. Patton M. Utilization-focused evaluation. Los Angeles/London/New Delhi/Singapore: Sage Publishing; 2008. p. 4.
14. Salas E, Benishek L, Coultas C, Dietz A, Grossman R, Lazzara E. Team training essentials: a research-based guide, vol. 1. New York: Routledge; 2015.
15. Levett-Jones T, Lapkin S. A systematic review of the effectiveness of simulation debriefing in health professional education. Nurs Educ Today. 2014;34(6):58–63.
16. Boet S, Bould MD, Bruppacher HR, Desjardins F, Chandra DB, Naik VN. Looking in the mirror: self-debriefing versus instructor debriefing for simulated crises. Crit Care Med. 2011;39(6):1377–81.
17. Savoldelli GL, Naik VN, Park J, Joo HS, Chow R, Hamstra SJ. Value of debriefing during simulated crisis management. Anesthesiology. 2006;105(2):279–85.
18. Welke TM, LeBlanc VR, Savoldelli GL, Joo HS, Chandra DB, Crabtree DB, et al. Personalized oral debriefing versus standardized multimedia instruction after patient crisis simulation. Anesth Analg. 2009;109(1):183–9.
19. Byrne A, Sellen A, Jones J, Aitkenhead A, Hussain S, Gilder F. Effect of videotape feedback on anaesthetists performance while managing simulated anaesthetic crises: a multicentre study. Anaesthesia. 2002;57:176–9.
20. Dine C, Gersh R, Leary M, Riegel B, Bellini L, Abella B. Improving cardiopulmonary resuscitation quality and resuscitation training by combining audiovisual feedback and debriefing. Crit Care Med. 2008;36:2817–22.
21. Grant JS, Moss J, Epps C, Watts P. Using video-facilitated feedback to improve student performance following high-fidelity simulation. Clin Simul Nurs. 2010;6:177–84.
22. Van Heukelom J, Begaz T, Treat R. Comparison of postsimulation debriefing versus in-simulation debriefing in medical simulation. Simul Healthc. 2010;5:91–7.
23. Grand JA, Pearce M, Rench TA, Chao GT, Fernandez R, Kozlowski SWJ. Going DEEP: Guidlenies for building simulation-based team assessments. BMJ Qual Saf. 2013;22(5):436–48.
24. Salas E, Cannon-Bowers J, Smith-Jentsch K. Principles and strategies for team training. In: International encyclopedia of ergonomics and human factors, vol. 2. Boca Raton: CRC Press; 2006.

25. Institute of Medicine. Conceptual framework for measuring the impact of IPE. Measuring the impact of interprofessional education on collaboration and outcomes. Washington, D.C.: The National Academies Press; 2015. p. 25–38.
26. Kirkpatrick DL. Evaluation of training. In: Craig RL, Bittle LR, editors. Training and development handbook. New York: McGraw-Hill; 1967. p. 87–112.
27. Thistlethwaite J, Kumar K, Moran M, Saunders R, Carr S. An exploratory review of prequalification interprofessional education evaluations. J Interprof Care. 2015;29(4):292–7.
28. Rimando M, Brace AM, Namageyo-Funa A, Parr TL, Sealy D, Davis TL. Data collections challenges and recommendations for early career researchers. Qual Rep. 2015;20(12):2025–36.
29. Vincenzi DA. Human factors in simulation and training. Boca Raton: CRC Press; 2009.
30. Azevedo R, Taub M, Mudrick N. Think-aloud protocol analysis. Thousand Oaks: Sage Publications Inc; 2015. p. 764–6.
31. Ericsson KA, Simon HA. Protocol analysis: verbal reports as data. Cambridge, MA: The MIT Press; 1993.
32. Shadbolt N. Eliciting expertise. In: Wilson JR, Corlett NE, editors. Evaluation of human work. Boca Raton: Taylor & Francis; 2005. p. 185–218.
33. Bainbridge L, Sanderson P. Verbal protocol analysis. In: Wilson JR, Corlett EN, editors. Evaluation of human work: a practical ergonomics methodology. 3rd ed. Boca Raton: Taylor & Francis; 2005. p. 159–84.
34. Flanagan JC. The critical incident technique. Psychol Bull. 1954;51:327–58.
35. Hassan E. Recall bias can be a threat to retrospective and prospective research designs. Int J Epidemiol. 2006;3(2):4.
36. Berelson B. Content analysis in communication research. New York: Free Press; 1952.
37. Nancarrow SA, Booth A, Ariss S, Smith T, Enderby P, Roots A. Ten principles of good interdisciplinary team work. Hum Resour Health. 2013;11(19):1–11.
38. Given LM, editor. The SAGE encyclopedia of qualitative research methods. 2nd ed. Thousand Oaks: Sage Publications; 2008. p. 108–9.
39. Trochim W. Concept mapping. In: Mathison S, editor. Encyclopedia of evaluation [Internet]. Thousand Oaks: Sage Publications; 2005. p. 73–4.
40. Martin-Raugh M, Tannenbaum RJ, Tocci CM, Reese C. Behaviorally anchored rating scales: an application for evaluating teaching practice. Teach Teach Educ. 2016;59:414–9.
41. Schwab DP, Heneman HG III, DeCotiis TA. Behaviorally anchored rating scales: a review of the literature. Pers Psychol. 1975;28:549–62.
42. Rarick CA, Baxter G. Behaviorally anchored rating scales (BARS): an effective performance appraisal approach. SAM Adv Manag J. 1986 Jan;51(1):36–9.
43. Wiersma U, Latham GP. The practicality of behavioral observation scales, behavioral expectation scales, and trait scales. Pers Psychol. 1986;39:619–28.
44. Fowlkes J, Dwyer DJ, Oser RL, Salas E. Event-based approach to training (EBAT). Int J Aviat Psychol. 1998;8(3):209–21.
45. Nau HR, editor. Perspectives on international relations. 2nd ed. Washington, D.C.: CQ Press; 2009.
46. Kozlowski SWJ, Klein KJ. A multilevel approach to theory and research in organizations: contextual, temporal, and emergent processes. In: Klein KJ and Kozlowski SWJ, editors. Multilevel theory, research, and methods in organizations: foundations, extensions, and new directions. San Francisco: Jossey-Bass; 2000. p. 3–90.
47. Driskell JE, Salas E. Collective behavior and team performance. Hum Factors. 1992;34:277–88.
48. DeVellis RF. Scale development: theory and applications. 2nd ed. Thousand Oaks: Sage Publications; 2003.
49. Brannick MT, Prince C. An overview of team performance measurement. In: Brannick MT, Salas E, Prince C, editors. Team performance assessment and measurement. Mahwah: Lawrence Erlbaum; 1997. p. 3–16.
50. Gillespie R. Manufacturing knowledge: a history of the Hawthorne experiments. Cambridge: Cambridge University Press; 1993.

Logistics in Simulation-Based Interprofessional Education

10

Stephen Charles and Mary L. Koehn

Introduction

Simulation and interprofessional education (IPE) have become key components of health professions education. Both are increasingly being required by accrediting bodies for multiple health professions [1–4]. Healthcare simulation, in its modern form, is a result of rapid advances in technology along with advances in aviation training, computer science, and health care education [5]. However, the purpose of simulation for healthcare education has always been to improve the quality of patient care. Each healthcare profession values its own professional identity formation and this independent formation tends to create silos of learners. By learning in silos, learners may develop stereotypes of other professions and may not be prepared to work in a healthcare team in the clinical environment to provide optimal patient care [6]. Simulation and IPE are effective teaching methodologies to break down silos, increase communication between professions, understand the scope of practice and roles of professions, and improve teamwork [7–9].

On the other hand, while many health professions educators value IPE, the implementation of such initiatives are complex and the logistics can create barriers. Thus, as IPE becomes more widely implemented in health professions education, it is critical that educators have the knowledge of how to optimize their resources to

S. Charles (✉)
Office of Medical Education, Brody School of Medicine, East Carolina University, Greenville, NC, USA
e-mail: Charless16@ecu.edu

M. L. Koehn
University of Kansas School of Medicine-Wichita, Wichita, KS, USA

J. T. Paige et al. (eds.), *Comprehensive Healthcare Simulation: InterProfessional Team Training and Simulation*, Comprehensive Healthcare Simulation,
https://doi.org/10.1007/978-3-030-28845-7_10

overcome these logistical barriers [10]. In this chapter, we will present recommendations that educators may use to develop and implement interprofessional simulation programming. The recommendations are based on current available empirical and theoretical literature as well as the authors' experiences over the past decade. This chapter will identify key components in creating an IPE simulation program and how to overcome barriers in the following stages: organizational planning, developing a curriculum, implementing simulation curricula and evaluating programming.

Organizational Planning

Committed Leadership

Planning an IPE simulation program begins with engaging and procuring upper level administrative support. Thibault [6] defines upper level administration as deans, associate deans for education, and/or their designee(s). These decision makers are key to providing the resources necessary to plan, implement, and evaluate an IPE simulation program. Although interprofessional simulation activities will most often start with innovative educators, it is imperative to seek administrative support. This is particularly important when working across the factions of siloed professional programs. Quality simulation activities can be costly and rarely can one discipline supply and sustain the resources needed for these activities. Furthermore, upper administration support provides "permission" for more flexibility in schedules or curriculum. The authors of this chapter found the upper level administration group formation relatively easy to start, but more challenging to update. However, formation of an administration group provides increased support for faculty networking, and thus, begins to break down the silos. Networking also helps to create a group of committed IPE simulation educators. If possible, plan for at least biannual meetings with the administration group to update it on progress, successes, and outcomes.

Committed Educators

Another key component in developing an IPE simulation program is to identify IPE champions. Champions are the educators who are willing to actively work to create interprofessional programming by communicating to and convincing others to participate in IPE [11]. Seek those who have the passion and the commitment to make the simulation program work and who are early adopters [12]. These champions will assist in maintaining sustainability of the IPE simulation program by (1) advocating for IPE simulation, (2) actively finding and procuring resources, (3) providing awareness of organizational/political changes, (4) recruiting faculty for simulation sessions, (5) and providing a detailed understanding of their own institutional needs and curriculum. Do not be concerned if, at first, all professions in the area are represented within an IPE; this may not happen. In fact, it is best to start small [13]. Do not be surprised if it feels uncomfortable and even risky for faculty to delve into working across professions. Remember that the goal is to establish a successful simulation IPE program. If the programming is successful, more professions will seek to be included [13].

Developing an IPE Simulation Curriculum

IPE simulation activities can be developed and packaged in many ways. Typically, these activities are referred to as the IPE simulation curriculum [13]. While there are many factors that need to be considered when developing a curriculum (such as learners, faculty, and goals of the curriculum) engagement of the IPE champions is essential. Engagement of the IPE champions ensures that all interested professions are represented and that all members are committed to a successful IPE program [7]. At the first meeting, take the time for educators to describe their institutional curriculum, schedules (some programs are on semesters, some on quarters, etc.), goals for IPE, and number of health professions learners in their programs, and even something personal about themselves. This sets the tone for a greater understanding of the professions and what Rudolph, et al., refers to as a safe container for learning [14]. A safe container is an environment where learners are challenged professionally and are held to high standards but are not humiliated or intimidated [14].

Learner Considerations

Although health professionals of all levels work together, for learning purposes, we highly recommend leveling professional learners according to clinical experience. The authors recommend using a theory, such as Benner's Novice to Expert as a framework for leveling [15]. Benner's model identifies five stages of clinical competence from novice, advanced beginner, competent, proficient, and expert. These stages describe the knowledge and skills acquired from education and experiences. The authors have provided a possible framework for leveling in Appendix 10.A. However, be flexible and use the framework as a guide and not a rule.

Faculty Considerations

Faculty who facilitate IPE simulations need to have the following background: knowledge of their own health profession's current professional practice issues, knowledge of best practices in simulation, and experience with IPE [16]. Yet, faculty often lack firsthand experience with interprofessional simulation [10]. Thus, IPE as a collaborative initiative provides an opportunity for faculty development [7,

17]. Although involved faculty may come with teaching experience and even simulation experience, they most likely have not personally experienced an interprofessional simulation. We suggest that the group of faculty members not only design an interprofessional simulation, but also put themselves into the activity itself – practice it, rehearse it, and learn from doing it.

Goal Setting

Setting goals for curricular programs are important [18, 19]. Although the initial activity may be a single interprofessional activity, it is important to discuss and work towards a longitudinal curriculum plan. These long-term goals are essential to setting the groundwork for unifying all professions and setting the requisite knowledge, skills, attitudes, and behavior outcomes. Until faculty are comfortable with IPE, it is easy to err in design by falling back into using familiar discipline specific skills, such as physical assessment skills, as the focus of the activities [17].

Practical advice includes using the Interprofessional Education Collaborative (IPEC) competencies [20] as the overall outcomes for the programming (see Table 10.1). These competencies were developed and supported by 15 different institutional organizations including the American Council of Academic Physical Therapy, Association of Schools of Allied Health Professions, and American Association of Colleges of Nursing. The competencies span four domains: Values/Ethics for Interprofessional Practice, Roles and Responsibilities, Interprofessional Communication, and Teams and Teamwork [20]. As interprofessional education is about the process of care, keeping the competencies in the forefront will help to remind the IPE planners of that goal.

Table 10.1 Interprofessional core competencies for collaborative practice

Interprofessional core competency	Definition
Values/Ethics for Interprofessional Practice	Work with individuals of other professions to maintain a climate of mutual respect and shared values
Roles/Responsibilities	Use the knowledge of one's own role and those of other professions to appropriately assess and address the health care needs of patients and to promote and advance the health of populations
Interprofessional communication	Communicate with patients, families, communities, and professionals in health and other fields in a responsive and responsible manner that supports a team approach to the promotion and maintenance of health and the prevention and treatment of disease
Teams and teamwork	Apply relationship-building values and the principles of team dynamics to perform effectively in different team roles to plan, deliver, and evaluate patient/population-centered care and population health programs and policies that are safe, timely, efficient, effective, and equitable

Data from: IPEC 2016 [20]

Designing Simulation Scenarios

Template Simulations scenarios include multiple components and sections such as objectives, scenario, equipment, etc. [21]. In order to ensure all components are included many IPE simulation curriculum designers will document the information on an interprofessional simulation template. The simulation template helps create a structured, consistent process for developing scenarios and helps to ensure that steps are not left out. A sample template is found in Appendix 10.B. This template has sections for addressing objectives, type of assessment, space, number of professions, numbers of learners, patient scenario, assigning responsibilities, creating scenario, equipment, faculty script, and props.

Objectives When designing a simulation IPE program begin with the end in mind. The stated objectives will drive the entire simulation session. Try to keep the number of objectives to no more than 3 to 4 per session. One tip is to use the IPEC Competencies as the main focus of the objectives [20]. Then, add an additional focused objective that is achievable by all participating professions, not just one profession [5]. To ensure the objectives are appropriate, scenario designers can use SMART (specific, measurable, achievable, relevant and timely) objectives [22]. For example, an achievable team objective may be: "By the end of this interprofessional simulation session, learners will be able to collaboratively develop a short term plan of care."

Scenario designers will need to be aware that, when developing objectives, different professions may at times be in conflict with one another. For example, a simulation could involve social work and medical learners addressing a Standardized Patient (SP) portraying a homeless veteran. Conflicting objectives could arise from medical learners addressing an open wound which could be sepsis and social workers addressing the homeless situation. The medical learners may want to stop the encounter and have the SP seek urgent help from an emergency department. Again, one suggestion to avoid conflicting objectives is to focus on objectives that all professions can achieve, not just one profession [5].

Scheduling Getting multiple professions to agree on a date and time to have even one IPE simulation session requires collaboration, navigation, and possibly even political maneuvering. Many health professions have different admission cycles (fall and/or spring), lengths of time to graduation, and course and clinical rotation requirements. Thus, upper level administration support may be valuable and helpful in navigating curricular schedules. Unless this is a large scale event, such as TeamSTEPPS® [23], we recommend including no more than 3–4 professions per activity. With more than 4 professions, it is hard to agree on objectives, scenario details, and balancing competing healthcare priorities. Ultimately, this may mean multiple dates of the same activity; however, from a logistics point of view, this is beneficial. Scheduling is much easier and the scenarios can be tailored to be more inclusive of and specific to the participating professions.

Scenario Creation Creating a new simulation scenario needs to be a collaborative effort with faculty from all of the participating professions. Throughout the scenario planning, revisit the objectives often to maintain focus and to ensure that the scenario is designed so that the learners can achieve them. From experience, ideally this planning is best done face-to-face. This allows more accurate interpretations of body language, undertone, and better supports the smooth flow of ideas. Without all professions represented, although not intentional, the planning team runs the risk of designing a scenario that does not meet the objectives of the profession not present. A further risk is that the one profession may perceive the activity as a waste of time and may even refuse to participate in the future.

We suggest an unfolding case scenario [24, 25] with three scenarios. This allows for a slightly larger overall group of learners who can be divided into three interprofessional teams. Experience suggests a maximum 6–7 learners per team. This allows for a total of 18–21 learners per simulation activity. Using an unfolding scenario allows for changes in the scenarios, yet keeps a case with the same background information, the same as a "real" patient. Add complexity with each unfolding scenario, but create a scenario where the patient will ultimately recover at the end. Using the leveling document as a guideline will help to create scenarios for the intended learners. Above all, develop a case that is relevant to the participating professions.

Simulation Modality The term "simulation" most often triggers the use of high-fidelity manikins; however, not all simulations are best served by their use. Consider all of the possibilities: standardized patients, high fidelity simulators, low fidelity simulators, partial task trainers, virtual reality, augmented reality, and gaming. Each of these modalities has its advantages and disadvantages, but to assist in which modality is best for the scenario return to the objectives. Using objectives to select the appropriate simulation modality is called modality matching [5]. Consider the expectations as well as the level of the learners. In addition, consider the resources and space available. For example, in the homeless veteran case previously mentioned, one of the objectives might be to engage other health professionals in shared patient centered problem solving. In order to have interprofessional patient-centered problem solving, partial task trainers are not appropriate. Although a high fidelity mannequin could be appropriate, the level of realism is not as much as a standardized patient. Thus, curriculum planners may decide to use standardized patients to portray the homeless veteran and his sister. The homeless veteran can then have mannerisms and physical appearances similar to that of a real patient. Furthermore, the homeless veteran can participate in debriefing and provide feedback about interpersonal communication skills, which a high fidelity mannequin cannot.

Space Space is a very important consideration for IPE simulation sessions. The physical space utilized must be conducive to the type of simulation modality and the number of learners participating. For example, consider what is needed: inpatient, outpatient, *in situ* setting, small group rooms, or a computer lab. A simulation lab space that can manage a scenario with 6–7 learners with additional space for the other 12–14 learners is ideal. If not available, consider other non-traditional spaces as a possibility. If the scenario does not require specific clinical equipment, this is feasible. For example, one of our initial interprofessional activities was set in an outpatient clinic setting. As no participating school had a large enough simulation lab for 21 learners, we used a large mega church in our area that had closed its doors. It had a large room, and, as the scenario required few props, it was ideal. The only props included a small table, two chairs, a white board, and a wheel chair. Although unintentional, this added the benefit of neutral ground and helped break down silos as we started the journey into IPE simulation. Later, one of the health professional institutions in our area remodeled space for a new simulation center which provided a large simulation lab room. However, by then, IPE was established and the group welcomed the "real lab". Thus, focus on the interprofessional learning and do not let space be a prohibiting factor.

Implementing an Initial Simulation Event

Plan adequate time for set-up of the environment and to ensure that any needed equipment is working. Plan to have the interprofessional faculty arrive early enough to huddle prior to the event. Depending on the degree that the group has worked together or if last-minute changes in faculty had to occur, start with introductions. Talk through the event; make sure all faculty members know their roles. Go through the timeline. See Appendix 10.C for an example overview for a 3-hour interprofessional activity.

Ask and seek clarification for any aspect of the event. Then, as the learners arrive, welcome them and engage with all learners; model interprofessional teamwork and communication.

Pre-briefing: Preparing the Learners

The importance of pre-briefing cannot be overemphasized. Learners often come to an interprofessional activity with multiple perceptions and experiences [26, 27]:

- Uncertainty of the expectations
- Pre-conceived biases about other professions
- Hierarchical biases and experiences
- Lack of confidence in their skills
- Positive or negative experiences with other professions

- Unfamiliarity with the physical environment, especially if the experience is using simulation as the learning modality

Any or all of these perceptions may contribute to anxiety and frustration with the impending interprofessional experience. A well-planned pre-briefing can help to alleviate much of the anxiety and allow for a more focused attention to the learning. Depending on the activity, some of the pre-briefing, such as objectives and reading assignments, can be given prior to the activity. However, fundamental elements contributing to a successful "pre-brief" for the activity are addressed here.

Start with Introductions

Consider having everyone, including the facilitators, sit in a circle or around a conference table. This creates an expectation of inclusion and participation of everyone; and it creates an atmosphere of non-hierarchy [28]. Thus, no one is "higher" or "lower" than anyone else and this should be explicitly stated. Take the time for relationship building as this contributes to trust and collaboration - important components of teamwork. Windover et al. [29] said it well: "Each time an emotional connection is made, it is equivalent to making a deposit in the emotion account with that person. Building up the emotion account is important to sustain a personal connection" (p. 9).Thus, consider having learners tell their name, profession, and at least one thing personal about themselves. For example, "share one of the best things happening in your life today" or "what is your favorite thing to do when you are not working". The point is to have them share something that initiates a personal connection with someone else in the room.

Role Identification IPEC Competency 2 is "Use the knowledge of one's own role and those of other professions to appropriately assess and address the health care need of patients, and to promote and advance the health professions" [20]. During introductions, it is helpful to have the learners explain their educational paths as well as what their professions do. This will help learners to articulate their own expertise, to hear the roles of others, and to recognize the similarities and the differences across their professions. As an example, the facilitator may say something like this:

> As we go around the circle, if you are the first person speaking from your profession, please tell the group about your program – the path to your degree/specialty. In addition, each of you, please tell the group something you do in your profession, i.e., name one thing that you do as a nurse, etc.

Learners having recognition of their profession and other health professions is a prerequisite for interprofessional collaboration to occur [30]. Learners gathering knowledge of other team members roles and responsibilities is defined as interpositional knowledge [31]. Interpositional knowledge has been documented to be correlated to team performance [32].

Overview of the Session

Provide a brief outline or overview of the day as this will help learners with mental organization and may alleviate some of the uncertainty. Details of the simulation are not needed at this point; just a brief overview of the timeframe and activities.

The Basic Assumption and Ground Rules

Following the expertise of Harvard's Center for Medical Simulation [33], it is important to share the "The Basic Assumption" each and every time in an interprofessional activity. The assumption is that every participating learner is "intelligent, capable and is trying to do their best to learn and improve" [14, p. 349]. The authors of this chapter follow this statement with the explanation that this is a safe, nurturing place for learning. Learners need to know that they can make suggestions and ask questions. They need to know that there are boundaries of confidentiality and privacy. Although interprofessional activities can be used for summative assessment, they are most suited for formative learning; let the learners know this. If they are focused on "the grade" they will be less likely to be relaxed and willing to experiment with teamwork.

Teamwork and Interprofessional Communication

Besides fostering the understanding of roles and responsibilities, the pre-brief is a time to clarify the teamwork and interprofessional communication competencies expected to be acquired by learners [20]. Making the competencies explicitly known helps give purposeful direction and focus for the session.

Although there is no one perfect way to initiate a discussion on teamwork, consider asking the learners for a definition or description of what teamwork means to them. One option is to discuss this as a whole group, or, alternatively, one can divide learners into sub-groups. All learners have either been on or know of a highly functioning team (and this does not have to be a healthcare team; a baseball team will have the same characteristics). The learners will be able to articulate the characteristics, but reviewing them here will highlight and bring to the forefront the learners' thinking for application in the activity. It is helpful to have the learners not only state a characteristic but to also provide an example of what those characteristics look like. Baker, Day, and Salas [34] have published a clearly articulated resource for effective team characteristics that may be helpful as a guide (see Table 10.2).

Table 10.2 Characteristics of effective teams

Team knowledge, skills, and attitudes	Characteristics of effective teams [35]
Team leadership	Have a clear common purpose Team member roles are clear but not overly rigid Involve the right people in decisions Conduct effective meetings Establish and revise team goals and plans Team members believe the leaders care about them Distribute and assign work thoughtfully
Backup behavior	Compensate for each other Manage conflict well-team members confront each other effectively Regularly provide feedback to each other, both individually and as a team ("debrief") "Deal" with poor performers Are self-correcting
Mutual performance monitoring	Effectively "span" boundaries with stakeholders outside the team Members understand each others' roles and how they fit together Examine and adjust the team's physical workplace Periodically diagnose team "effectiveness," including its results
Communication	Communicate often "enough"
Adaptability	Members anticipate each other Reallocate functions Recognize and adjust their strategy under stress Consciously integrate new team members
Shared mental models	Coordinate without the need to communicate overtly
Mutual trust	Trust other team members' "intentions"
Team orientation	Select team members who value teamwork Strongly believe in the team's collective ability to succeed

Reprinted with permission John Wiley and Sons [34]

Along with team characteristics, include a discussion on "who" makes up the team. Learners will generally always name all of the health professions. But, rarely do they include the patient and family as part of the team. Discuss the importance of active engagement of patient and family – what they add and why it is important to be inclusive [28].

Finally, any method that encourages communication among and across the professions contributes to relationship building; therefore, think of a collaborative approach to the topic. Avoid lecture but use interactive methods that will encourage learners to "…learn about, from and with each other to enable effective collaboration…" [36].

Objectives for the Session

Clearly articulate the objectives of the session. Consider providing the learners with pre-work or pre-handouts with details of the case or the problem to be solved. Then, they will be less focused on drug dosages, procedures, lab results, diagnoses, etc. If not provided, it is easier for the learners to default to "skills" as opposed to focusing on the interprofessional work.

Introduction to the Activity

Finalize the pre-brief with the directions or specific information related to the activity. The learners may have the background, but they need to know where to begin. Include any additional background information or materials they have not already received. Ask for any needed clarification. If the activity involves role play or simulation, introduce the learners to the physical environment. For example, if a manikin is being used, have the learners "meet" the "patient" in a normal state, let them practice finding pulses, etc. Make sure the learners know their roles and the roles of any embedded participants (such as "family member" in a scenario). Although the pre-brief can be of varying length, consider the extra time and added value that a well-planned pre-brief can contribute to the overall flow and learning of the actual activity.

Implementing the Event

If there has been interprofessional planning and an interprofessional "huddle" prior to the beginning of the event, implementing the activity should be smooth and enjoyable. Assign faculty roles such as: primary facilitator, time keeper, and technology facilitator. Encourage all faculty to engage in cross-monitoring the simulation activity.

Interprofessional Debriefing

As much has already been published on the value and the methods of the debriefing process itself [33, 37–41], this section focuses on the logistics of debriefing with the goal of helping learners work as an interprofessional team whether there is one or more debriefers [42], or no instructor debriefer [37]. Interprofessional debriefing is a complex and demanding activity [43]. Debriefing requires facilitator training and practice [44]. Just as learners come from mostly professional siloed training, so do the faculty. Second, there are elements that can either enrich or hinder interprofessional learning. For optimal results, consider the following:

- Co-debriefers [42] can model effective teamwork, they can complement each other's facilitating style, and they can help to cross-monitor reactions and engagement of the learners. On the other hand, unless trained and practiced, co-facilitating can be challenging. Be watchful that one facilitator does not dominate, interrupt, speak only to one professional group, or engage in open disagreement with the other facilitator.
- Start the debrief session by asking for reactions, first from the participating team, then the observers (if present). There are no right or wrong feelings but learners have the need to express them – either here or afterwards in out-of-session time.
- Balance debriefing of the therapeutic objectives and teamwork/communication objectives. While it is important that skills are optimally performed, the primary focus of the debriefing is what the learners have learned about working as a team and how they communicate with each other, the patient, and the family.
- Focus on digging deeper to discern mental models and decision making processes [45]. Ask questions about how the team made the decisions that they did. Be specific, i.e., "how did the team make the decision to use that particular treatment plan?"
- Avoid personal agendas and biases. These can come from either facilitators or learners. Personal agendas may lead a discussion away from the objectives of the session and do not contribute to interprofessional learning. An experienced facilitator will redirect the discussion and will explore biases that may arise. This is an opportune time for learning about roles and responsibilities of professions as well as the overlap in what professions do.
- Engage all of the learners in the conversation. This helps to develop mutual understanding and leads to better communication and patient outcomes [45]. Consider (if used) including the actor, staying in role, as part of the debriefing. Ask the "patient" for how the scenario went; were they included; was the family member included? However, there is a risk in including the actor, in role: the learners will want to revert to continuing to assess/question the "patient". A good facilitator keeps the learners focused on the "debrief" and not on gathering new information.
- Solicit feedback from the faculty as well as the learners. Be aware that faculty may easily fall into "teaching" or "lecture". A good facilitator will not let this happen but rather asks for input on their observations [46].

Overall, focused debriefing with experienced facilitators will create an environment of learning such that when the learners leave the activity, they will continue to reflect on the interprofessional experience. They will have gained new insights into how they can contribute to the team and improve the quality of healthcare to their patients and families.

Evaluating Programming

Learner Assessment

Learner assessment and program evaluation are imperative. It is necessary to determine whether to use formative or summative assessment. Formative assessments are designed to provide immediate feedback about how a learner can improve and does not typically involve grades. The summative assessment typically involves grades and involves a judgement of the student's capabilities. We realize that both formative and summative assessment methods have their benefits and uses. However, we prefer, when beginning IPE simulation programs, to use formative assessment. Summative assessment methods, especially if "high stakes" may increase the learners' anxiety and stress about IPE simulation [47]. On the other hand, formative assessment allows for genuine conversations between the multiple health professions learners. Thus, we clearly state this at the beginning: the goal is learning.

Program Evaluation

Program evaluation is a process to determine whether the design and implementation of a program were effective [19]. There are numerous models to help distinguish levels of effectiveness. One of the most popular models in the interprofessional literature is the Kirkpatrick's framework of four levels [48]. Level one is the learners' reaction to the program. Level two includes quantifiable measures that learning has taken place. Level three assesses whether the learners applied the behavior change to their job and level four describes results or outcomes due to the training program. The authors of this chapter find the reaction to be the easiest way to measure level one. We ask the learners at the end of the sessions to describe one or two words about how this experience made them feel. We have found that incorporating a few multiple choice questions or free response questions on a post survey or quiz after the program helps to measure if they did in fact meet objectives and if learning took place. Additionally, the authors have conducted focus groups to see if, in fact, the learners met the objectives of the simulation. Level three and level four are by far the most challenging to measure [19]. To see if the learners are implementing behavior change, direct observation must occur. One barrier is limited faculty time. One way to overcome this barrier is to adjust clinical/workplace evaluations so that preceptors/attendings can report on the observed behaviors. The final level is to identify outcomes in regards to improved quality, decreased costs, reduction in errors, etc. With the addition of the electronic health record, some of these measures can be tracked.

Conclusion

As the demand for IPE simulation programs increases, more faculty and staff are embarking on planning these complex programs. While planning these programs, many components can create barriers, but the authors have suggested several strategies to overcome these barriers. To begin organizing an IPE simulation program, the authors recommend having committed leadership and IPE champions. When developing IPE simulations, it is important to level the learners based upon clinical experience and to have all participating professions represented during face to face planning sessions. The authors recommend using an IPE simulation planning template and IPEC competencies to set goals for programming. In order to avoid competing goals, the authors recommend focusing objectives on all learners. not just one profession. Enlisting committed leadership to address scheduling issues will help balance the needs of all professions. The authors recommend having a well-planned pre-briefing session with time for introductions, role identification, The Basic Assumption and ground rules. In order to assure the maximum amount of learning, the authors recommend faculty training and practice in debriefing IPE simulation sessions. Finally, the authors recommended using Kirkpatrick's model of evaluation to assist and guide programmatic outcomes. With these strategies, IPE simulation programs can be established, refined, and sustained.

Appendix 10.A

Interprofessional Learner Leveling Guidelines

Level 1 learners are defined by the following:

- Novice stage with minimal experience in the situations in which they are expected to perform.
- Generally students at this level will be in the 1st year of their program.
- Learners may lack confidence to demonstrate safe practice and will likely require verbal and physical cues.

Level 2 learners are defined by the following:

- Efficient and skillful in parts of the practice area but are still developing the knowledge and skills.
- May require occasional supportive cues.
- Generally, they are students in the 2nd year of their program.

Level 3 learners are defined by the following:

- Verbalize and uses a plan that is based on considerable conscious, abstract, and analytic problem solving.
- Patient care is completed within a suitable time frame without supporting cues.
- Generally, students in advanced stages of their programs, i.e. residency, last practicum/rotation of physician assistant/nursing/social work/physical therapy, new graduate etc.

Level 4 learners are defined by the following:

- Generally, practitioners with a minimum of 6 months to 1 year clinical experience at the practitioner level

Appendix 10.B

HealthSim UNITED HealthSim UNITED **Scena rio Devel opme nt**

Scenario patient:		
Case Type:	**Date:**	**Location:**
Level: I II III IV		
Facilitator:		
Operator:		
Patient Voice:		
Family:		
Confederate:		
Debriefer:		

Template
Single Patient Scenario
Changing condition

Learners: **Set up:**			
Environment/Setting: **Objectives/Competencies:** 1) 2) 3) 4)			
Simulation Set-Up ___ **Manikin** ___ **Task-trainer** ___ **Simulated Patient**	**Equipment & Supplies**	**Moulage**	**Audio/Visual**

Patient Background

Introduction: Healthy Patient

Scene 1 – (Location of setting)		
Vital Signs: • HR • Rhythm • BP • RR • SaO2 % **Test results:**	**Allergies:**	**Medications Given:**
Relevant Medical & Social History:		
Family Present & Concerns:		
Other Relevant Patient Information & Concerns: **Starts:** **Change:**		

Scene 3 –		
Vital Signs: • HR • Rhythm • BP • RR • SaO2 **Test results:**	**Allergies:**	**Medications Given:**
Relevant Medical & Social History:		
Family Present & Concerns:		
Other Relevant Patient Information & Concerns:		

Appendix 10.C
Example: Interprofessional Activity: Tentative Timeline Morning Session for a 3-Scene Unfolding Simulation Activity

Time	Who/Item	Activity	Designated lead person
8:00 am	Faculty arrive	Set up learning environment for gathering/pre-briefing – chairs in circle (or tables/chairs) Set up sim lab Faculty huddle Introductions "Run thru" the scenario	
8:45–9:00 am	Students arrive	Students gather meeting/pre-briefing room Other faculty continue with finalizing set up	
9:00–9:30 am	Introduction to session	Where are we from? Introductions of learners/faculty (sit interspersed with learners) Overview/timeline Basic Assumption and Ground Rules Interprofessional Teamwork and Communication Objectives What are doing today? Introduction to the activity Teams formed – self-select or have the teams pre-selected and sitting together	
9:30 am		Break	
9:45–10:00 am	Team 1 Sim	Team 1 participates in the simulation All others form semi-circle at the back of the room	
10:00–10:20	Debriefing	Entire group in simulation lab – participating team starts Format: Description – How did it feel? Analysis – what worked? What didn't? What may be better? Application – What did I learn? What will I change in how I care for my patient? Does this transfer to the workplace?	
10:25–10:40	Team 2 Sim	Team 2 participates in the simulation All others form semi-circle at the back of the room	
10:40–11:00	Debriefing	Entire group in sim lab – as above	
11:05–11:20	Team 3 Sim	Team 3 participates in the simulation All others form semi-circle at the back of the room	
11:20–11:40	Final debriefing	Entire group in sim lab – as above	
11:45 – noon	Evaluation		

References

1. American Association of Colleges of Nursing. CCNE accreditation. 2017. Available from: http://www.aacn.nche.edu/ccne-accreditation.
2. Liaison Committee on Medical Education (LCME). Functions and structure of a medical school: LCME. 2016. Available from: http://lcme.org/publications/.
3. Accreditation Council for Pharmacy Education (ACPE). Accreditation standards and key elements for the professional program in pharmacy leading to the doctor of pharmacy degree Chicago. 2015. Available from: https://www.acpe-accredit.org/.
4. Verma S, Patterson M, Medves J. Core competencies for healthcare professionals: what medicine, nursing, occupational therapy, and physiotherapy share. J Allied Health. 2006;35(2):119–5.
5. Palaganas JC, Epps C, Raemer DB. A history of simulation-enhanced interprofessional education. J Interprof Care. 2014;28(2):110–5.
6. Thibault GE. Interprofessional education: an essential strategy to accomplish the future of nursing goals. J Nurs Educ. 2011;50(6):313–7.
7. Buring SE. Interprofessional education supplement: keys to successful implementation of interprofessional education: learning location, faculty development, and curricular themes. Am J Pharm Educ. 2009;4:1–11.
8. Kroboth P, Crismon LM, Daniels C, Hogue M, Reed L, Johnson L, et al. Getting to solutions in interprofessional education: report of the 2006-2007 professional affairs committee. Am J Pharm Educ. 2007;71(Suppl):S19.
9. Shoemaker MJ, Beasley J, Cooper M, Perkins R, Smith J, Swank C. A method for providing high-volume interprofessional simulation encounters in physical and occupational therapy education programs. J Allied Health. 2011;40(1):15E–21E.
10. Reeves S, Perrier L, Goldman J, Freeth D, Zwarenstein M. Interprofessional education: effects on professional practice and healthcare outcomes (update). Cochrane Database Syst Rev. 2013;3(3):CD002213.
11. Barker KK, Bosco C, Oandasan IF. Factors in implementing interprofessional education and collaborative practice initiatives: findings from key informant interviews. J Interprof Care. 2005;19(Suppl 1):166–76.
12. Rogers EM. Diffusions of innovations. New York: Free Press of Glencoe; 1962.
13. Freeth DS, Hammick M, Reeves S, Koppel I, Barr H. Effective interprofessional education: development, delivery, and evaluation. Hoboken: John Wiley & Sons; 2008.
14. Rudolph JW, Raemer DB, Simon R. Establishing a safe container for learning in simulation: the role of the presimulation briefing. Simul Healthc. 2014;9(6):339–49.
15. Benner P. From novice to expert: excellence and power in clinical nursing practice. Menlo Park: Addison-Wesley; 1984.
16. Reeves S, Goldman J, Oandasan I. Key factors in planning and implementing interprofessional education in health care settings. J Allied Health. 2007;36(4):231–5.
17. Pardue KT. A framework for the design, implementation, and evaluation of interprofessional education. Nurse Educ. 2015;40(1):10–5.
18. Dick W, Carey L, Carey JO. The systematic design of instruction. Boston: Pearson Higher Ed; 2014.
19. Caffarella R. Planning programs for adult learners: a practical guide for educators, trainers, and staff developers. San Francisco: Jossey-Bass; 2002.
20. Interprofessional Education Collaborative. Core competencies for interprofessional collaborative practice: 2016 update. Washington, DC: Interprofessional Education Collaborative; 2016.
21. Seropian MA. General concepts in full scale simulation: getting started. Anesth Analg. 2003;97(6):1695–705.

22. Tofade T, Khandoobhai A, Leadon K. Use of SMART learning objectives to introduce continuing professional development into the pharmacy curriculum. Am J Pharm Educ. 2012;76(4):68.
23. Agency for Healthcare Research and Quality. TeamSTEPPS 2.0. Rockville: Agency for Healthcare Research and Quality; 2016. Available from: http://www.ahrq.gov/teamstepps/instructor/index.html.
24. Carr KC. Using the unfolding case study in midwifery education. J Midwifery Womens Health. 2015;60(3):283–90.
25. Mills J, West C, Langtree T, Usher K, Henry R, Chamberlain-Salaun J, et al. 'Putting it together': unfolding case studies and high-fidelity simulation in the first-year of an undergraduate nursing curriculum. Nurse Educ Pract. 2014;14(1):12–7.
26. Boet S, Bould MD, Layat Burn C, Reeves S. Twelve tips for a successful interprofessional team-based high-fidelity simulation education session. Med Teach. 2014;36(10):853–7.
27. de Voest M, Meny L, VanLangen K, DeVuyst-Miller S, Salvati L, Bright D, et al. Four themes to enhanced interprofessional education integration: lessons learned from early implementation and curricular redesign. Inov Pharm. 2016;7(2):4.
28. Uhlig P, Raboin W. Field guide to collaborative care: implementing the future of health care. Overland Park: Oak Prairie Health Press; 2015.
29. Windover AK, Boissy A, Rice TW, Gilligan T, Velez VJ, Merlino J. The REDE model of healthcare communication: optimizing relationship as a therapeutic agent. J Patient Exp. 2014;1(1):8–13.
30. Henneman EA, Lee JL, Cohen JI. Collaboration: a concept analysis. J Adv Nurs. 1995;21(1):103–9.
31. Gum L, Greenhill J, Dix K. Clinical simulation in maternity (CSiM): interprofessional learning through simulation team training. Qual Saf Health Care. 2010;19(5):e19.
32. Cooke NJ, Cannon-Bowers JA, Kiekel PA, Rivera K, Stout RJ, Salas E. Improving teams' interpositional knowledge through cross training. Proc Hum Factors Ergon Soc Ann Meet. 2000;44(11):390–3.
33. Center for Medical Simulation. Debriefing as defined by CMS. 2016. Available from: https://harvardmedsim.org/resources-other.php.
34. Baker DP, Day R, Salas E. Teamwork as an essential component of high-reliability organizations. Health Serv Res. 2006;41(4p2):1576–98.
35. Salas E, Sims DE, Klein C. Cooperation at work. Encyclopedia of applied psychology. 2004;1: 497–505.
36. World Health Organization. The framework for action on interprofessional education and collaborative practice. Geneva; 2010. Report No.: WHO/HRH/HPN/10.3.
37. Boet S, Bould MD, Sharma B, Revees S, Naik VN, Triby E, et al. Within-team debriefing versus instructor-led debriefing for simulation-based education: a randomized controlled trial. Ann Surg. 2013;258(1):53–8.
38. Rudolph JW, Simon R, Rivard P, Dufresne RL, Raemer DB. Debriefing with good judgement: combining rigorous feedback with genuine inquiry. Anesthesiol Clin. 2007;25:361–76.
39. Sahakian GD, Alinier G, Savoldelli G, Oriot D, Jaffrelot M, Lecomte F. Setting conditions for productive debriefing. Simul Gaming. 2015;46(2):197–208.
40. University of Alberta. Debriefing using the advocacy-inquiry. n.d. Available from: http://www.hserc.ualberta.ca/en/TeachingandLearning/VIPER/EducatorResources/~/media/hserc/Documents/VIPER/Advocacy_Inquiry_Method.pdf.
41. Levett-Jones T, Lapkin S. A systematic review of the effectiveness of simulation debriefing in health professional education. Nurse Educ Today. 2014;34(6):e58–63.
42. Cheng A, Palaganas J, Eppich W, Rudolph J, Robinson T, Grant V. Co-debriefing for simulation-based education: a primer for facilitators. Simul Healthc. 2015;10(2):69–75.
43. Lindqvist SM, Reeves S. Facilitators' perceptions of delivering interprofessional education: a qualitative study. Med Teach. 2007;29(4):403–5.

44. Cheng A, Grant V, Dieckmann P, Arora S, Robinson T, Eppich W. Faculty development for simulation programs: five issues for the future of debriefing training. Simul Healthc. 2015;10(4):217–22.
45. Brown MR, Watts P. Primer on interprofessional simulation for clinical laboratory science programs: a practical guide to structure and terminology. Clin Lab Sci. 2016;29(4):241–6.
46. Willgerodt MA, Abu-Rish Blakeney E, Brock DM, Liner D, Murphy N, Zierler B. Interprofessional education and practice guide no. 4: developing and sustaining interprofessional education at an academic health center. J Interprof Care. 2015;29(5):421–5.
47. Lyndon MP, Strom JM, Alyami HM, Yu T-C, Wilson NC, Singh PP, et al. The relationship between academic assessment and psychological distress among medical students: a systematic review. Perspect Med Educ. 2014;3(6):405–18.
48. Bates R. A critical analysis of evaluation practice: the Kirkpatrick model and the principle of beneficence. Eval Program Plann. 2004;27(3):341–7.

Developing a State-of-the-Art Simulation-Based Education Center

11

Robert V. Rege

Introduction

The competency of physicians has classically been judged on their ability to make medical decisions, perform technical skills, and communicate with patients and co-workers [1]. These skills were obtained in clinical settings using an apprenticeship model where learners were assigned to faculty preceptors or to clinical teams. Students learned by observing and then performing tasks under supervision ("See one, do one"). As medical technology and the complexity of medical practice increases, the traditional medical school curriculum and structured residency program no longer suffices. For patient safety reasons, students should have an appropriate level of skill before they interact with patients. Simulation-based education is progressively filling voids in medical education by teaching prerequisite procedural and non-procedural skills in a safe simulated environment [1–3]. Proliferation of simulation across all medical disciplines and levels of instruction has now established simulation-based education as a pertinent tool to teach most of the skills and competencies required to be a healthcare provider or worker [2–6].

Although medical simulation began over 50 years ago, a surge in its use over the last two decades paralleled introduction of minimally invasive technology into medical practice. It is a logical and effective tool for teaching surgical skills using task-specific simulators, and skills acquired in the simulation laboratory transfer to the operating room [5, 7–9]. Surgical and gynecologic departments became early adopters of simulation-based education to teach laparoscopic skills, and the number of skills training facilities increased greatly in these departments. A need to prepare trainees to perform history and physical exams, to improve their communication

R. V. Rege (✉)
Distinguished Teaching Professor of Surgery, Associate Dean for Undergraduate Medical Education, University of Texas Southwestern Medical Center, Dallas, TX, USA
e-mail: Robert.rege@utsouthwestern.edu

J. T. Paige et al. (eds.), *Comprehensive Healthcare Simulation: InterProfessional Team Training and Simulation*, Comprehensive Healthcare Simulation,
https://doi.org/10.1007/978-3-030-28845-7_11

with patients, families, and colleagues, and to manage critical/emergent medical problems before encountering them clinically also fueled growth in simulation education [1, 3]. Methods of simulation ranging from clinical skills programs using objective structured clinical examination (OSCE), standardized patients, and high-fidelity mannequins to teach responses to life-threatening medical problems such as cardiac arrhythmias, shock, and cardiac arrest, and strategies to enhance team performance and improve patient safety like TeamSTEPPS® evolved to meet these latter needs [1, 10, 11]. While much of simulation education is directed at teaching patient-centered skills, simulation education can also address process-centered or environmental-centered skills [3]. Lane and colleagues define process-centered skills as those required for providers "to practice" in their local environment like information skills and teamwork. Environment-centered skills include business management, administrative, and leadership skills required to practice medicine. Finally, a demand to train all medical personnel in interprofessional teams expanded the breadth of learners who benefited from simulation-based training beyond physicians, including physician assistants, nurse practitioners, nurses, and availing healthcare workers. Today, simulation is commonplace at all levels of medical training and across all medical disciplines [1, 4, 12].

Simulation mimics real-world processes or procedures by approximating or modeling key features of a simple skill, complex tasks, or an entire procedure or process [1]. Simulation education utilizes scripted scenarios with role playing or standardized patients, animate or inanimate models, computer programs, or virtual reality environments [1–4]. Models range from simple box trainers to anatomical models and sophisticated high-fidelity mannequins. Simulation exposes trainees to new skills and allows repetitive practice of these skills in a safe environment. It is also capable of assessing individuals to certify that proficiency for a skill has been acquired.

The comprehensive menu of simulation activities required at teaching institutions can be quite expensive, taxing institutional resources. Faculty with specific skills and knowledge in simulation-based education, as well as staff trained to participate and assist in guiding simulation activities, are essential to the process. In addition, simulation centers require adequate space for simulation events and storage of equipment, sophisticated information technological support, and costly simulators to accommodate the needs of learners. To provide these services across a broad spectrum of learners, many institutions find it advantageous to centralize simulation activities [13]. This chapter outlines key points in establishing, developing, and maintaining a successful simulation center. In this context, the term "simulation-based center" denotes more than a facility providing simulation programs. Many successful simulation programs arise in a single department to meet the specific needs of trainees. Stand-alone facilities can and do provide excellent skills training and meet the mandatory needs of a well-defined group of trainees. On the other hand, a center concept is appropriate to efficiently teach multiple skills to a wide variety of learners, especially if training spans across the continuum of medical education.

The principles and examples presented in this chapter are based on literature directed toward managing state-of-the-art simulation centers. Experience of organizations such as the American College of Surgeons and the American Society of Anesthesiologists that set standards for medical simulation-based education exemplify this process [4, 12–18]. For example, the American College of Surgeons has assembled a consortium of over 90 accredited education institutes in the United States and worldwide that integrate simulation-based education with traditional medical education [14, 15]. These centers range considerably in size, mission, and types of simulation education offered, providing a myriad of models for institutions interested in building a simulation center. The criteria used by the American College of Surgeons to accredit education institutes [14, 15] and standards for simulation programs set by the American Society of Anesthesiologists [16] are excellent guides for institutions embarking on the establishment of a simulation center, and they will serve as touchpoints for this paper. Although not focused on in this chapter, the Society for Simulation in Healthcare [17] also has an accreditation process with standards which may also be of assistance.

Decision to Develop a Simulation Center

As the volume and complexity of simulation education grows within an institution, overlap of the needs of existing simulation programs and growth of programs across disciplines at an institution creates competition for resources and escalation of costs. At this point, an institution may opt to centralize resources into an institution-wide simulation center to achieve efficiencies in the use of space, personnel, and equipment while improving access to and quality of education provided. To be successful, the center must have a defined purpose, start-up investment funds, an adequate ongoing operating budget, high quality simulation curricula, and dedicated faculty and staff with simulation-education experience [13]. Too often, the development of a simulation center is propelled by a single infusion of start-up funds directed toward building of a facility and equipping it with the latest, most sophisticated simulators. Achieving the desired goals of a simulation center depends on more than a physical plant and hi-tech simulators. Rather, the pillars supporting a center-based concept are the desire to enlarge the number and diversity of learners at an institution, to improve the quality of simulation education for all learners, to achieve efficiencies in use of center space, personnel, and equipment, and ultimately to improve patient safety and patient outcomes (Fig. 11.1). Accomplishing these goals requires standardization and sharing of resources across providers from all pertinent disciplines at the institution [13].

The decision to establish a simulation center begins by assembling a core planning group (Fig. 11.1). Inclusion of key members from departments already using simulation-based education is essential because complete buy-in must be obtained from these individuals if the center is to share resources [13, 16, 18]. Established programs also provide needed expertise in simulation to advise the process. However, wide acceptance of the center concept by the entire institution requires individuals beyond this group. Funding, space, and management plans for the center benefit from the expertise and participation of business administration, facilities

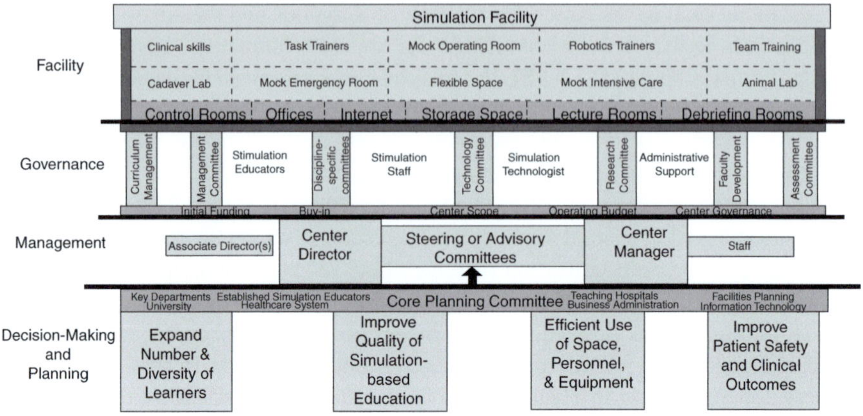

Fig. 11.1 The figure illustrates key components required to establish and maintain a comprehensive state-of-the-art simulation education center. The expansion of the number and quality of simulation education events, a need to achieve efficiencies in the use of resources, and a desire to improve patient safety and outcomes provides justification and are the foundation for development of a center simulation-education center. A successful center requires careful planning by stakeholders at the institution, dedicated management for the center, governance that ensure good business management, a robust curriculum development process, development of faculty and staff to provide simulation events, careful assessment of courses and learners, and scholarly activity. Simulation education facilities should be designed to support a variety of simulation-based curricula that meet the needs of multiple disciplines across the entire continuum of healthcare professional education

planning, and information technology resources in the institution. If the simulation center is to provide training to healthcare workers and continuing medical education, representatives from the healthcare system and hospitals, and from the continuing education office, are needed. The mission of the core planning group is to make a decision about proceeding with development of the simulation center. If the decision is to proceed, this group will also be responsible for developing a coherent plan for implementation of the center [13, 16, 18, 19].

A single formula for developing a state-of-the-art simulation center does not exist that meets the needs of every institution. Centers vary considerably in size, mission, funding mechanisms, and governance structure. However, choices about how to structure and operate a simulation center can be informed by the experience of others who have tackled similar problems. Examining, visiting, and partnering with established centers can be of great value. Considering important characteristics of state-of-the-art simulation centers can be quite helpful in the decision to establish a simulation center. Based on the accreditation processes for American College of Surgeons educational institutes [15] and the endorsement of the American Society of Anesthesiologists [16] for simulation programs, well-established simulation centers exhibit the following characteristics:

- Affiliation with a university or healthcare system.
- Oversight by a university/healthcare system administrator(s).

- Stable funding.
- Strong center leadership.
- Integration of the curricula across disciplines by talent, not by specialty training, department, or learner level.
- Well-defined governance.
- A clear process for curricular development that sets high quality standards for simulation programs at the center.

A series of questions one might contemplate in making a decision to develop a simulation center is provided in Table 11.1.

Scope of the Center

The institution must have a clear purpose for its simulation center, and the center mission must be well-defined and clearly articulated to institutional leadership, educators and staff in the center, and entities that provide or could potentially provide support for the center. Complete buy-in by all stakeholders should lead to a unified vision for the institution, establishment of a clear and effective governance structure, and seamless operation of the center on a daily basis. A needs assessment and gap analysis is the critical first step in determining a scope for the center. Identifying learner groups and assessing their needs is of utmost importance to determine center purpose and scope as well as decision-making about center size and configuration, types of simulation-education provided, equipment to be purchased, and the number and categories of personnel needed to manage the program. A simulation center focused on providing procedural skills will be sized and configured differently compared to a center teaching communication and/or teamwork skills. Additionally, a center focusing on pre-licensure healthcare students has different needs compared to one targeting practicing clinicians. The planning group must tailor the scope of the project to available funding, but should not compromise essential features of a center that correlate with long-term

Table 11.1 Considerations in making a decision to develop a simulation-based education center

Is your institution committed: To become a high quality simulation-based educational center? To improving the quality of simulation-based education at your institution?
Are simulation-based education programs expanding at your institution? Are resources adequate to accommodate growth for all stakeholders on campus?
Do you have adequate funding for the center? Will start-up funds create a facility that meets the needs of the institution? Is there sufficient ongoing funding for long-term operation of the facility?
Do you have buy-in from all stakeholders at your institution to build the governance required to manage the center?
Will a center: Expand the number of learners you can educate? Improve the quality of simulation-based education you are providing?

Table 11.2 Potential factors influencing design of a simulation center

Venue and location
General purpose space
Lecture rooms
Debriefing rooms
Exam rooms for clinical skills using standardized patients
Rooms for task-specific trainers
Specialty rooms
Mock patient exam rooms
Simulated specialty rooms (ED, OR, delivery rooms, etc.)
Animal facility
Cadaver laboratory
Size
Numbers of learners
Number and type of simulation events
Types of simulation-based education provided
Number and type of personnel
Support staff for facility
Simulation-based education coordinators
Simulator technologists
Infrastructure
Office space
Storage space
Lecture rooms
Debriefing rooms
Video-based control rooms
Internet and information technology support space

success. Table 11.2 outlines the factors that influence the size and configuration of a simulation center [15].

Financial Support

Start-up funding is essential to establish the simulation center. Initially, capital investments are required to build or renovate facilities, acquire supporting infrastructure, and procure simulation devices. In some cases, the initial investment may also support recruitment and salary for personnel for a defined period of time. Initial investments most often come from one-time capital investments derived from the university or healthcare system, or from philanthropic donations (Table 11.3). Philanthropic donations can also be used to establish endowments that will earn revenue to support the simulation center in the future.

An operating budget needs to be established and funds secured to operate the simulation center. Ongoing support of salaries, supplies, maintenance of the facility and equipment, licenses for users of software, and replacement of equipment and simulators comprise the major categories of expense for a simulation center. Many simulation centers also fund internal competitive development grants to aid faculty who wish to introduce new curricula. Stable, balanced operating budgets can be difficult to secure for the long-term. As a rule of thumb, center budgets should have a

Table 11.3 Potential sources of simulation center funding

Source	Initial	Ongoing
University support	Capital investments Facilities Infrastructure Recruitment	School assessments Medical Allied health Graduate school Nursing Department assessments
Health care system/teaching hospitals	Capital investments Facilities Infrastructure	Assessments Training healthcare workers Graduate medical education
User fees	N/A	Continuing professional development programs Testing/certification services
Competitive grants	N/A	Government Non-profit organization Industry
Industry	Simulation equipment	Simulation equipment Educational Grants Simulation supplies
Philanthropy	Capital investments Facilities Infrastructure Endowment	Capital investments Facilities Infrastructure Endowments

3-year financial plan in order to anticipate and meet needs of the center. This often requires guarantees of funding from primary stakeholders in the center to ensure continued operation during difficult times. Most simulation centers are creative in obtaining funding by utilizing several sources (Table 11.3). Usually, the institution, individual schools or programs within the institution, and advocates for specific groups of learners derive considerable benefit from simulation-based education and support these activities enthusiastically. For example, many universities underwrite a significant portion of the budget to provide essential and required curriculum for students matriculating in their programs. Likewise, healthcare systems and teaching hospitals allocate funds to the center to provide required skills training for its graduate medical education programs or for training of nurses, ancillary healthcare workers, and staff. Industry and philanthropic sources typically provide educational grants to support the center or to support individual simulation programs they value. It is important to remember that not all support is monetary; often industries, such as those that manufacture minimal invasive surgery equipment with a vested interest in ensuring that students are well-trained in their technologies, will provide in-kind support in the form of donated equipment or supplies. In-kind support has the potential to supplement capital investments and to reduce operating budgets. The value of these donations should be included as part of the budget and recognized by the institution. Simulation centers who do not report in-kind donations greatly undervalue their enterprise.

User fees for courses focusing on continuing professional development that include simulation activities generate revenue for the simulation center and some centers generate additional revenue by marketing their services to other institutions, medical societies, and industry. Establishment of the center as a testing center for programs is another possible way to generate support for simulation programs. For example, a simulation center receives fees for Fundamentals of Laparascopic Surgery Training, and for maintenance of Compliant Anesthesia Training. Finally, investigators who secure government and non-government grants generate financial support for the simulation center. The scholarly activity generated from such projects also exposes the center to new technology and prototype simulators keeping education programs on the forefront of simulation education. Funding formulas to determine assessments to different entities in the center can be derived based on numbers of learners, amount of time utilized by programs and the intensity of the programs presented within the center [13, 18, 19].

Monetary support is not the only means of building a sustainable budget. Institutions provide considerable internal support by protecting faculty and learner time for participation in simulation activities, providing existing educational offerings to build upon, and contributing by allowing access to existing amenities such as animal care facilities or cadaver laboratories. They also provide expertise from established educational support services and support systems like learning management or scheduling systems. The value of this type of support cannot be underestimated. Most simulation centers find they must make the center available for self-practice after hours. For example, the requirements for the Fundamentals of Laparoscopic Surgery certification require the learner to practice the skills to an expected level of proficiency before testing. Considering the busy schedule of medical trainees, this practice time is unlikely to occur during working hours and access to the simulation facility is required in the evenings and on weekends [13, 18, 19].

Leadership and Governance Structure

Once simulation center scope is determined and funding is secured, strong leadership is required to guide the institution through the process of establishing a state-of-the-art simulation center [13, 18]. A shared governance model with representation from each academic department and with oversight from the university, healthcare system, and teaching hospitals is invaluable. Administrative and business expertise already exists within the latter entities that can assist in establishment, and later in operation of the center, which can be facilitated by including institutional leadership in simulation center governance. This expertise needs to be tapped by the center. Although the planning group creates the implementation plan, specific leadership with expertise in managing a simulation center is required to execute the plan. A simulation center director and manager should be recruited and appointed early to help guide the process to fruition. The institution must ensure that these individuals have adequate dedicated administrative time with concomitant financial support to implement and manage the center [13, 18].

The director and manager are responsible for the actual implementation of the institution's simulation education center plan and for management of the center thereafter. Initially, they report to the planning group and to institutional leadership overseeing and supporting the project. Later, an advisory committee should replace the planning group (Fig. 11.1). Reporting lines within the center and to the larger entity from which it arises should be clearly defined in an organization chart.

Dedicated faculty educators and staff who are immersed in simulation-education are needed as programs within the center are implemented. They become stewards of the center's space and equipment, and are indispensable in designing and executing curricula on a daily basis. The center director and manager are responsible for recruiting faculty to teach at the center and assembling an administrative staff to support simulation programs. Faculty and staff candidates include personnel from existing programs at the institution, or may be individuals recruited to the simulation center based on results of the gap analysis. Large centers require associate directors to manage various aspects of the center such as curriculum development, curricular and learner assessment, faculty development, or simulation education research. Obviously, large centers with complex structures also require more complex governance. Smaller centers can manage by having faculty and staff assume more than one responsibility.

The specific goals and objectives and the size of a simulation center determine the number of committees and subcommittees a center establishes. At a minimum, a center requires an advisory committee and a curriculum management committee. The advisory committee replaces the core planning group who made the decision to proceed with center implementation. It sets center policy, establishes center priorities, and provides counsel to the director and the administrative team that manages the center on a daily basis. It also makes strategic decisions concerning changes in the centers mission and structure. In some centers, the advisory committee is replaced by a steering committee that makes high level strategic decisions while a management committee establishes center policy and counsels the director. Institutional leadership is usually included at the steering or advisory level.

A curriculum management committee establishes educational standards for the overall simulation center curriculum and applies them to individual courses. It reviews proposals for courses, prioritizes the proposed offerings, and decides what is actually taught at the simulation center. Prioritization is especially important when there is competition for space and time at the center by several groups. The curriculum management committee must assure that all proposed curricula meet both the goals and objectives of the simulation center and quality standards that have been set for courses. Commonly, simulation centers have a faculty development committee and a research committee [15]. Very large centers may have curricular subcommittees for different types of simulation education, for each of the key aspects of curriculum development, and/or for discipline-specific needs dealing with nuances of training in each field.

Some simulation education centers choose a distributed model of governance, especially when their centers include two or more simulation facilities at different sites. Separate facilities, whether on the same or different campuses, require some degree of autonomy to function on a daily basis and each facility develops local governance. However, they must report to an overarching management group that ensures uniformity and the quality of education provided at each individual site to be an integral part of the simulation center. The institutional oversight committee makes strategic plans for the entire program. This model can be quite effective, but it lacks some of the efficiencies of a single site, single governance model. On the other hand, it may be necessary to provide adequate simulation education to trainees who rotate between campuses or hospitals that are remote from the main teaching institution.

Simulation Center Curriculum

The simulation center curriculum is a plan for all of the learning activities at the simulation center. Each course of study will also develop a plan, or course curriculum, consistent with the center curriculum. Best educational practices necessitate that curriculum development follow several key steps. The center curriculum must start with an assessment of learner needs and gap analysis, but this may have been accomplished to some extent to make the decision to proceed with a center concept. If so, the assessment may need to be updated and refined to provide more granular data for specific course design. The curriculum should then establish educational goals and overall objectives, determine the most judicious and effective methodology to teach learners, select the optimal and most cost effective simulators and simulator environments to achieve the stated goals and objectives, and choose how the program and learners will be assessed to guarantee that goals and objective are met. Similar steps should be followed for each individual course curriculum.

The highest quality simulation-based education programs build on the expertise of all educators at the institution since course curricula usually must be designed to meet the learner needs from several disciplines. Integration of the course curricula across disciplines achieves this result by bringing all of the institution's pertinent expertise together to make decisions about best practices for both the learners and the institution. Integrated curricula leads to standardization of procedures, uniform protocols across the institution, better patient outcomes, and reduced healthcare costs. Achieving these outcomes enhances continuing support for the center. Finally, complex skills are acquired gradually by students as they progress from year to year in their educational program.

Integration of course curricula across each level of education brings together educators from pre-licensure programs through continuing professional development courses to decide what skills will be taught at each level of education. At each stage, skills training must benefit from the foundational skills taught during earlier phases of an individual's education, expanding the learner's level of expertise by acquisition of additional and more advanced skills as the person progresses toward graduation. At some point, the learner should have developed competency in a task expected of a physician or healthcare worker and should be tested to ensure competency. Fully integrating center curricula horizontally across disciplines and vertically over stages of education ensures that learners achieve the competencies they require to provide excellent patient care, and is essential in development of sophisticated simulation-based education.

Ultimately, the curriculum management committee has the responsibility for ensuring course quality and learner outcomes. The committee must monitor course evaluations and short- and long-term learner outcomes to guarantee that curricular goals and objectives are met. The principles of continuous quality improvement apply to curricular improvement and a data-driven quality improvement program is essential at a state-of-the-art simulation center.

Assessment of Courses and Learners

Determination of how courses and learners will be assessed is critical for a state-of-the-art simulation center. Objective data on the quality of simulation programs and documentation of learner outcomes will garner continued buy-in from stakeholders at the center, and funding decisions depend heavily on demonstrating the value of simulation education to the institution. In addition, in most incidences, quality data will drive the priority decisions placed before the curriculum management committee and ensure an effective curricular improvement program.

Each course must determine the parameters to follow to determine if the course has met its goals and objectives. The simulation center needs to decide how the data will be collected and stored. Some data will be in other institutional systems and connectivity/interoperability of educational databases with databases already in place at the institution, such as electronic medical records, might be an issue. These issues should be dealt with up front. For example, the increasing desire to demonstrate differences in patient outcomes that result from simulation-based education programs requires interface between educational and patient outcome databases. Planning information resource needs early avoids conflicts due to patient and student confidentiality, Institutional Review Board issues when publications result, and technical (interface) issues between information systems. State-of-the-art simulation centers often have center-dedicated information technologists, statisticians, and education assessment experts who help navigate through these problems. An assessment team helps gather data, analyzes it, and generates reports or dashboards on course and learner outcomes. An evaluation/assessment committee may also be included in center governance.

A nationally validated course, Fundamentals of Laparoscopic Surgery (FLS), arose from efforts to standardize laparoscopic skills training and led to the requirement that every surgical resident in the United States must pass an FLS test and demonstrate competency in laparoscopic skills before they are allowed to sit for board certification [20–22]. Other programs to teach and assess the fundamentals of endoscopy are on the horizon [22]. Courses such as Advanced Life Support (ACLS) and Advanced Trauma Life Support (ATLS) include simulation and are required for credentialing at most hospitals. The American Society of Anesthesiologists endorses programs using simulation for continuing professional development and maintenance of competency of practicing anesthesiologists [4, 16]. United States Medical Licensing Exam Step 2 Clinical Skills (USMLE Step 2 CS) is an OSCE-based exam that medical students must pass for licensure [23]. These examples illustrate the current use of simulation for high-stakes assessment of learners. The future likely will include an even larger and more important role for simulation in testing and certifying healthcare workers.

Scholarly Activity

Successful simulation centers participate in the design and assessment of novel curricula for simulation, develop new simulators, and perform studies which validate curricula. At a minimum, a center participates in scholarly activity by enrolling learners in multicenter investigative studies designed by others and shares information with their colleagues at peer institutions. Although not a prerequisite for providing quality curricula, centers participating in simulation research stay on the cutting edge as the field of simulation evolves and contribute to the evolution of simulation-based education. Participation and presentation of experiences and networking with colleagues at regional and national simulation conferences is helpful in staying well-informed of the latest advances in simulation education and builds the reputation of the simulation center, opening opportunities for further scholarly activity and research funding. If scholarly activity is a focus of the center, infrastructure will be required to support research efforts and a research committee would be appropriate in the governance structure of the center (Fig. 11.1).

Faculty Development

Simulation is an educational methodology that requires specific skills. The individuals who manage or teach at the simulation center require specific expertise in these methodologies to effectively educate learners using simulation techniques. Although content expertise is needed to run a simulation activity, being an excellent physician is not in itself sufficient to guarantee that a faculty member will be an effective teacher in the simulation center. Knowledge of simulation devices, training in running a simulation event, special skills in assessment of learners in simulation events, and the capability to debrief learners after a team-based event exemplify skills an educator may need to develop to facilitate a simulation event. Likewise, staff require special training in these areas and may require expertise in building, setting up, modifying, or maintaining simulation devices. Faculty development and staff training programs are essential for onboarding new faculty and staff, and ensure ongoing competence of staff and faculty. The cost of establishing a faculty development program and logistical problems with providing faculty the time to pursue these programs are frequently overlooked in the planning process. Development of faculty simulation skills is essential for success and must be a clear focus of a state-of-the-art simulation center. Its role in the center may dictate a faculty development committee (Fig. 11.1).

Faculty and staff development can be assured in several ways besides creation of specific center programs to teach simulation courses. Hiring individuals with specific expertise in simulation education sets a standard for others who teach at the center and provides experts to direct design of simulation courses and to train their colleagues at their institution. Alternately, faculty members might be sent to simulation education programs sponsored by other institutions, including programs to obtain advanced degrees in education with a simulation emphasis. Faculty who facilitate simulation events not only need simulation expertise to participate in courses, but they require orientation to the unique methodologies used to teach simulation events, training in their specific roles during simulation events, or instruction in techniques of assessing or debriefing learners. A program to educate and orient course facilitators is as important as having well-trained simulation-based educators at the center to lead curricular development and courses.

A shortage of individuals specifically trained with the unique skills required for simulation-based education and to manage a simulation center has led to the establishment of simulation education fellowships [23, 24]. The American College of Surgeons now accredits simulation education fellowships based in accredited educational institutes [23, 24]. Fellows learn theory of simulation education, develop expertise in providing simulation-based education and training, and perform simulation research. A goal of the program is to groom fellows to become future leaders of simulation centers.

Staff and standardized patients also require training in carrying out simulation scenarios or in guiding and coaching learners in simulation tasks. Most centers have programs to orient and train staff and standardized patients. Other staff members require orientation and training to specifically setup and manage simulation equipment. Although internal programs may suffice for much of this training, staff benefit from attendance at simulation conferences and courses outside the institution. In addition, complex equipment and the nuances of sophisticated software programs dictate that individuals have special training that can only be obtained at specific training courses or from the manufacturer. Planning for continued training and updating of staff is essential for optimal use of the sophisticated technology required for simulation education and needs to be considered in the center budget.

Conclusion

Development of state-of-the-art simulation based education centers can enlarge the number of learners at an institution and improve the quality of simulation education. To be successful, an institution should define its needs, secure adequate start-up funds, ensure ongoing financial support for program, and develop a clear governance structure that guarantees high quality simulation-based curricula. Top-notch centers also have robust faculty development and research programs. Simulation-based education centers may benefit from seeking accreditation for their center by one of the specialty societies that set standards for simulation-based education. These accreditation processes lead a center through the steps required to become a state-of-the-art simulation center.

References

1. Rosen KR. The history of medical simulation. J Crit Care. 2008;23:157–66.
2. Datta CR, Upadhyay BKK, Jaideep CN. Simulation and its role in medical education. MJAFI. 2012;68:167–72.
3. Lane JL, Slavin S, Ziv A. Simulation in medical education: a review. Simul Gaming. 2001;32(30):297–314.
4. Passiment M, Sacks H, Huang G. Medical simulation in medical education: results of an AAMC survey. 2011 Sept. Available from: https://www.aamc.org/download/259760/data.
5. Scott DJ, Pugh CA, Ritter EM, Jacobs LM, Pellegrini CA, Sachdeva AJ. New directions in simulation-based surgical education and training: validation and transfer of surgical skills, use of nonsurgeons as faculty, use of simulation to screen and select residents, and long-term follow-up of learners. Surgery. 2011;149:735–44.
6. Scott DJ, Dunnington GL. The new ACS/APDS skills curriculum: moving the learning curve out of the operating room. J Gastrointest Surg. 2008;12:213–21.
7. Scott DJ, Bergen PC, Rege RV, Laycock R, Tesfay ST, Valentine RJ, Euhus DM, Jeyarajah DR, Thompson WM, Jones DB. Laparoscopic training on bench models: better and more cost effective than operating room experience? J Am Coll Surg. 2000;191(3):272–83.
8. Hamilton EC, Scott DJ, Fleming JB, Rege RV, Laycock R, Bergen PC, Tesfay S, Jones DB. Comparison of video trainer and virtual reality training systems on acquisition of laparoscopic skills. Surg Endosc. 2002;16:406–11.
9. Seymour N, Gallagher A, Roman S, et al. Virtual reality training improves operating room performance: results of a randomized, double-blinded study. Ann Surg. 2002;236:458–64.
10. Harden R, Stevenson M, Downie WW, Wilson GM. Assessment of clinical competence using objective structured examination. Br Med J. 1975;1:447–51.
11. King HB, Battles J, Baker DP, Alonso A, Salas E, Webster J, Toomey L, Salisbury M. TeamSTEPPS™: team strategies and tools to enhance performance and patient safety. In: Henriksen K, Battles JB, Keyes MA, et al. editors. Advances in patient safety: new directions and alternative approaches, vol. 3, Performance and tools. Rockville: Agency for Healthcare Research and Quality (US); 2008. Available from: https://www.ncbi.nlm.nih.gov/books/NBK43686/.
12. Seymour NE, Cooper JB, Farley DR, Feaster SJ, Ross BK, Pellegrini CA, et al. Best practices in inter-professional education and training in surgery: experiences from the American College of Surgeons Accredited Education Institutes. Surgery. 2013;154:1–12.
13. Gardner AK, Lachapelle K, Posner CN, Sullivan ME, Sutherland D, Scott DJ, Sillin L, Sachdeva AK. Expanding simulation-based education through institutional-wide initiatives: a blueprint for success. Surgery. 2015;158:1403–7.
14. Sachdeva AK. Credentialing of surgical skills centers. Surgeon. 2011;9:S19–20.
15. American College of Surgeons Accredited Education Institutes. Available from: https://www.FACS.org/Education/accreditation/aei.
16. Steadman RH. The American Society of Anesthesiologists' national endorsement program for simulation centers. J Crit Care. 2008;28:203–6.
17. Society for Simulation in Healthcare Accreditation. Available from: https://www.SSIH.org/Accreditation.
18. Meier AH. Running a surgical education center: from small to large. Surg Clin N Am. 2010;90:491–504.
19. Dunkin BJ. Surgical simulation centers as educational homes for practicing surgeons. Surg Clin N Am. 2015;95:801–12.
20. Peter J, Fried GM, Sanstrom LL, et al. Development and validation of a comprehensive program of education an assessment of basic fundamentals of laparoscopic surgery. Surgery. 2004;135:21–7.
21. Ritter EM, Scott DJ. Design of a proficiency-based skills training curriculum for the fundamentals of laparoscopic surgery. Surg Innov. 2007;14(2):107–12.

22. America Board of Surgery Training and Certification; General Surgery. Available from: http://www.absurgery.org/default.jsp?certgsqe_training.
23. USMLE®. United States Medical Licensing Examination. Available from: http://www.USMLE.org/step2-CS/.
24. American College of Surgeons Accredited Education Institutes. Available from: https://www.FACS.org/Education/accreditation/aei/accredit.

Part III

Perspectives of Interprofessional Education

Interprofessional Simulation in Prelicensure Learners

12

John C. Luk, M. Kathryn Sanders, Veronica Young, Barbara L. Jones, and Kimberly M. Brown

Introduction

The impetus for integrating interprofessional education (IPE) into the curricula of prelicensure health professions' educational programs comes from the evolving understanding of the critical role that well-functioning teams play in the delivery of safe, high-quality healthcare [1]. The knowledge, skills and attitudes of each team member contribute to team function, and like other clinical skills, expert performance is driven by proper instruction, multiple opportunities to practice and receive feedback, and a clear mental representation of the desired performance [2].

Unlike most clinical skills taught within medical, nursing, pharmacy, social work and other healthcare programs, formal IPE training is a recent addition to health professions' curricula. Thus, the current generation of educators did not have uniform instruction on teamwork skills in their professional training, and there are fewer resources available to assist faculty in the initial implementation of IPE into existing curricula. Likewise, there is tremendous variability in the level of

J. C. Luk
Dell Medical School, The University of Texas at Austin, Austin, TX, USA

M. K. Sanders
School of Nursing, The University of Texas at Austin, Austin, TX, USA

V. Young
College of Pharmacy, The University of Texas at Austin, Austin, TX, USA

B. L. Jones
School of Social Work, The University of Texas at Austin, Austin, TX, USA

K. M. Brown (✉)
Dell Medical School, The University of Texas at Austin, Austin, TX, USA

Department of Surgery and Perioperative Care, Austin, TX, USA
e-mail: kimberly.brown@austin.utexas.edu

J. T. Paige et al. (eds.), *Comprehensive Healthcare Simulation: InterProfessional Team Training and Simulation*, Comprehensive Healthcare Simulation,
https://doi.org/10.1007/978-3-030-28845-7_12

teamwork skills demonstrated by healthcare teams in the current clinical environment; however, a better understanding of the importance of teamwork will foster penetration of IPE into existing cultural norms. The variability in teamwork skills presents challenges in the clinical learning environment, specifically in ensuring that students receive proper instruction and uniform opportunities to practice teamwork skills.

Simulation-based training offers an ideal instructional method for all core competencies of interprofessional collaborative practice, and is particularly beneficial in teaching teamwork skills. The use of simulation for IPE training provides a safe, standardized learning environment for students to engage in deliberate practice and obtain feedback. While teamwork skills are applied in the context of clinical patient care, they can be separated from activities that require specific clinical knowledge, allowing for more intentional focus on the development of teamwork skills to maximize the benefits afforded to each level of learner participating. Simulation as an active, experiential learning modality is ideal for fostering the development of professional identity and role identity that occurs within the team, and offers an opportunity for socialization into one's profession.

The use of interprofessional education (IPE) simulation-based training in prelicensure education programs promotes achievement of learning objectives related to clinical decision-making and exposes students to team based competencies. Prior to the integration of IPE simulation-based experiences into an existing cognitive framework, students must first be instructed on the fundamentals of teams and teamwork, key attributes of a team, how a team functions, and how the members on a team contribute to the effectiveness of the team.

This chapter focuses on the use of IPE simulation-based training as a means of initial instruction on the formation and function of a high-performing team for prelicensure learners. We provide a summary of the current literature and examples of our personal experiences in creating and delivering IPE simulation activities for prelicensure learners at The University of Texas at Austin (UT). As a part of an introductory IPE course for students in medicine, nursing, pharmacy and social work, simulation provided a portion of the instructional methods as well as the capstone experience through which learners acquired and practiced the foundational knowledge and skills necessary for interprofessional collaborative practice.

Logistics

Simulation has been well-integrated into prelicensure health professions education [3, 4], and has been employed in team training of health care practitioners [5]. IPE simulation represents the culmination of efforts that bring together curricula, faculty, facilities, staff, and, most importantly, learners from across health professions programs. Its effectiveness hinges on the proper and pragmatic alignment of prelicensure health professions programs at three logistical levels: the macro, meso, and micro [6–8]. These levels exist organizationally and temporally from inception to delivery of the IPE simulation and are represented in Fig. 12.1.

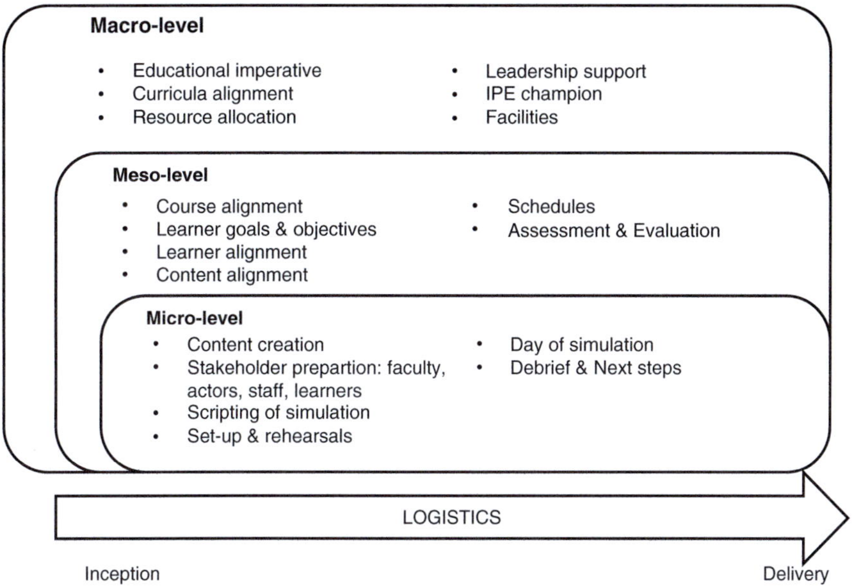

Fig. 12.1 Levels of prelicensure interprofessional simulation logistics

Table 12.1 IPE simulation champion key roles

Guide idea for interprofessional simulation into a curricular proposal and business plan
Solicit support from leaders and stakeholders
Communicate the opportunity widely
Work on all levels of logistics to deliver the simulation

Macro-level

Like many curricular innovations, IPE simulation starts as an idea that sparks a novel approach to better prepare health professions learners for interprofessional collaborative practice. The idea kindles initial enthusiasm and interest among stakeholders. Translating and guiding the idea from inception to implementation depends on a myriad of factors, starting with IPE champions [9]. These champions catalyze the synthesis of an IPE education proposal, of which simulation is a part (Table 12.1). Such synthesis starts with a working knowledge of IPE and the core competencies for interprofessional collaborative practice [10]. IPE simulation should also be mindfully coupled with contemporary prelicensure educational imperatives, objectives, and outcomes that drive curricular changes and accreditation. The creation of prelicensure IPE simulation tangibly focuses these areas into a demonstrable learning experience with measurable outcomes.

One of the early activities for IPE simulation champions is to compose a clear curricular proposal and strategic plan that delineates the justifications, organizational alignment, needed resources, and intended outcomes of the simulation-based

Table 12.2 Prelicensure interprofessional simulation stakeholders

Macro	Meso	Micro
IPE champions Institutional/Organizational leaders (e.g., Provost, Deans) Program/Curriculum leaders (e.g., Curriculum Deans, Department Chairs)	Course directors Course coordinators Simulation leader Standardized patient program leader Assessment & evaluation specialists Student leaders	Faculty Simulation staff Standardized patient program staff Standardized patients Students

Table 12.3 Resource considerations

Macro	Meso	Micro
Work effort of interprofessional educational leaders Prioritization & allocation of internal resources Pursuit of external funding Financial and service implications of faculty and staff participation Facilities	Work effort of interprofessional simulation planning stakeholders Work effort of faculty and staff involved in interprofessional simulation Operations	Simulation equipment Simulation technology Computer technology Video recording and archival Materials for training

activity for stakeholders. Champions must consider stakeholders' needs, interests, and benefits that provide both strategic and operational perspectives to IPE simulation planning and implementation. Consultation with stakeholders (Table 12.2) enables the champions to communicate the alignment of IPE simulation with the organization's vision and mission and to garner vital feedback for its development [11]. Senior leadership support of IPE simulation provides the crucial endorsement of its value and alignment with the organization's priorities, as well as paves the way for important and necessary decisions on resource allocation (Table 12.3).

At UT Austin, the IPE champions for health professions including nursing, social work, pharmacy, and medicine established collaboration prior to the recent inception of its medical school. The nascent collaboration yielded a pilot interprofessional course for advanced health professions learners, producing evidence of its feasibility, applicability, and scalability [12]. The subsequent creation of a medical school at UT refocused the effort on the opportunity for longitudinal integration for and across partnering programs, as charged by the deans of the partnering programs. The UT health IPE champions had formed an effective team based on mutual trust and shared accountability through early curricular and scholarly collaborations. As individually accomplished educational leaders and scholars, these champions brought together the necessary power and expertise to move the project from proposal to implementation at the university. For example, they leveraged their collective understanding of individual program curricula and learner outcomes to find common ground upon which to design IPE and IPE simulation-based activities.

Each champion brought to the team unique and complementary skill sets that enabled navigation through the political, educational, and logistical spheres of the university. The IPE champions periodically consulted with and reported on their planning to their deans as a group. This approach fostered collaborative discussions in real time. For example, as the interprofessional integration curriculum spanned four partnering programs, the IPE champions needed clarity on individual program contributions to the funding stream. Hosting quarterly meetings with the deans provided a ready forum to address this issue and resulted in an agreement to fund the curriculum proportionate to the number of students each program contributed to the experience. Likewise, the contribution of faculty effort followed the proportion of students from that program. One program's student population comprised about half of the first year interprofessional course student body, so this program also provided half of the funding support and half of the total faculty effort.

Meso-level

Prelicensure IPE simulation begins to come to life at this level through curriculum development. Simulation can be delivered as a stand-alone or integrated activity; however, there is a risk of isolation from the curricula and fading to an educationally unconnected activity when it is used as a stand-alone activity. Integrating IPE simulation into an existing or new curricula improves its sustainability and effectiveness as a meaningful learning experience and ensures that all students participate [13, 14]. Prelicensure health professions' educators might employ the "Backward Design" approach to IPE simulation, in which the outcomes and assessments provide the starting point for creating curricular experiences [15, 16]. If IPE simulation lies at the central focal point of the design process, centripetal consideration of its fit into curricula and intended outcomes, as illustrated in Fig. 12.2, enhances its meaningful integration into prelicensure curricula.

The path for successful prelicensure IPE simulation lies in a strategic approach to its challenges [17]. Scheduling of IPE experiences remains one of the biggest challenges and provides the first true test of IPE simulation champions seeking common ground on which to offer simulation. Curricular intricacies of IPE simulation scheduling include temporal placement in the academic calendar, sequencing among the

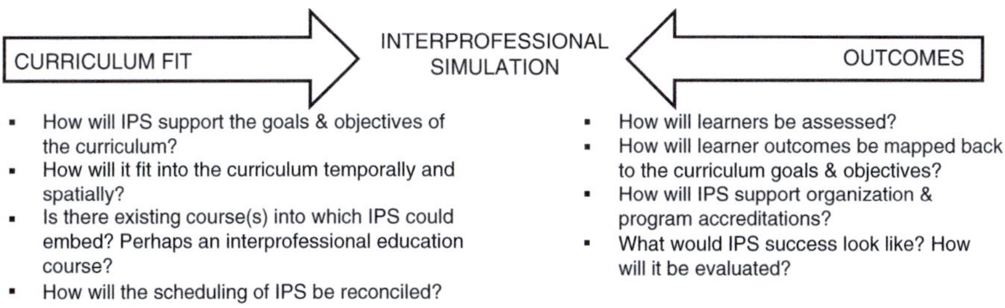

Fig. 12.2 Centripetal considerations for prelicensure curricular integration

curricular content, integration into existing or new courses, proximity to high-stake assessments (e.g., midterm and final course examinations), and spatial position among the other concurrent learning activities during the week. Other scheduling considerations include alignment of learners, their preparedness for IPE simulation, and the availability and readiness of faculty, staff, and facility to deliver the simulation.

Piloting an IPE simulation course or activity can be extremely helpful in identifying logistical challenges to full implementation; however, if the activity is not part of a curriculum, maintaining learner engagement can be a significant challenge. In addition, a pilot using volunteer students will yield a potentially unique experience due to a self-selected sub-group which may not be representative of the final student demographics [18].

At UT Austin, for the first year of the IPE curriculum across the partnering programs, the IPE champions searched for an optimal on-campus venue to host the IPE class, and learned that existing auditoria and meeting spaces on campus could not accommodate 330 individuals in team-based, experiential learning with a flipped-classroom approach. The champions devised a cohort approach to the first year of the IPE curriculum experience that delivered the learning experiences via three alternating cohorts of learners and faculty on the only day and time that partnering programs shared availability—Friday afternoons.

Micro-level

As planning moves closer to implementation, the focus of IPE simulation development shifts to the actual deliverable and its immediate enabling elements, described below. Ideally, IPE simulation planning on all three levels would move somewhat in parallel. The meso-level planning results inform the IPE simulation content. Development of IPE simulation content engages the collective interprofessional expertise of health professions educators, curriculum support staff, assessment and evaluation specialists, simulation and standardized patient program staff, technology specialists, and standardized patients. All contribute their talents in support of the learners' attainment of the experience outcomes through IPE simulation. The key micro-level stakeholders, who directly or indirectly interface with the learners in simulation, need training and preparation to effectively engage and assess learners as their roles dictate. Stakeholder preparation includes orientation to the IPE simulation learning objectives and outcomes, context and background, content, process, day-of-simulation scripting, simulation facility, and assessment instruments. Curriculum and IPE leaders also need to incorporate flexibility, remediation, and/or redundancy in IPE simulation to accommodate unexpected faculty, staff, and learner issues (e.g., absence due to illness or family emergencies). The desired learner outcomes determine the level of transparency of IPE simulation content and process provided to the learners, as illustrated in Fig. 12.3 and Table 12.4 [19, 20]. For all stakeholders immediately proximate to the IPE simulation, clear instructions minimize miscommunications and maximize intentions and expectations. Learner

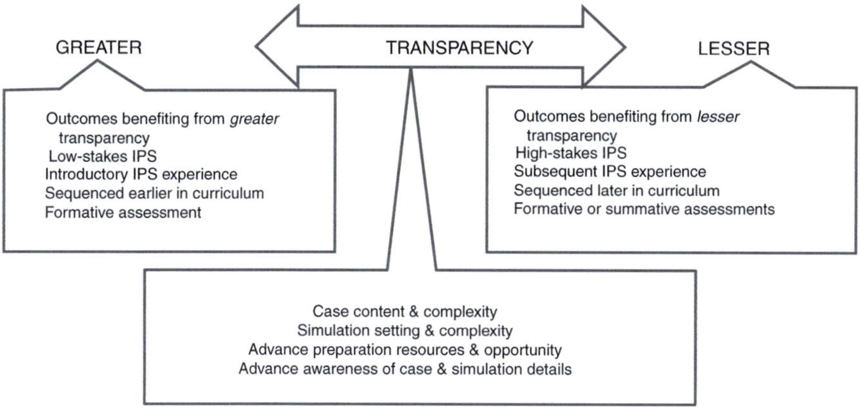

Fig. 12.3 IPS transparency to prelicensure learners

Table 12.4 Prelicensure outcomes for interprofessional simulation [19, 20]

	Knowledge	Skills	Attitudes
Interprofessional identity	Unique & overlapping roles & responsibilities Effective teamwork strategies	Collaboration Shared leadership Conflict resolution Team communication TeamSTEPPS®	Mutual respect & trust Shared accountability
Professional identity	Discipline-specific knowledge Patient safety Quality improvement	Critical reasoning Diagnostic Treatment planning Patient/client communication	Professionalism Ethics Leadership Humanism

instructions include IPE simulation goals and general details (e.g., duration), advance preparation details, recommended attire, permitted and prohibited items in IPE simulation, assessment approach, grading rubric, and security. Faculty instructions further expand on learner instructions to include guiding IPE simulation notes, copies of actual assessments, debriefing guides and details on viewing IPE simulation (e.g., live, recorded).

At UT Austin, IPE faculty champions committed to delivering simulation-based activities during the established class day and time confirmed reservation of simulation space well before the commencement of the first-year IPE course. As a part of the IPE simulation creation, IPE champions worked closely with the simulation staff to map out the simulation space, including envisioning team placement and flow through the simulation for optimal experience and video recording. Establishing redundancies and reserves on which to tap in case of unexpected faculty or standardized patient absences ensured minimal disruption of the simulation experience. IPE champions were available, in person and by mobile communication, to faculty members, learners, and staff for last minute or unanticipated issues. For example,

Table 12.5 Logistics lessons learned – UT Austin Health IPE simulation

Macro	Meso	Micro
Advance planning crucial to success Involve stakeholders early in development Clarify of simulation intent & learning outcomes drives simulation development Align learners & learning outcomes to optimize simulation outcomes Layering different levels of learners enhances simulation experience	Simulation must incorporate perspectives of partnering professions Simulation must be relevance to learners Applicability must be immediate & obvious to learners Plan contingencies for absences and/or remediation by offering more than one simulation date	Simulation debriefing imperative for learning & reinforcement of practice relevance Whenever possible, pilot simulation to obtain feedback from participants, identify barriers to implementation & meeting learning outcomes Clear communicate expectations, rules of engagement, instructions, & outcomes to learners & faculty

faculty member or student getting lost *en route* to simulation required real-time follow-up by IPE champions.

The IPE faculty champions developed unified standards of IPE simulation expectations, assessments, and learner experiences to provide a common platform for learner and faculty content engagement. They proactively collaborated with select faculty members with simulation experience to adapt an existing simulation activity into an IPE simulation-based activity using standardized patients. Simulation staff helped to organize the technical operation, including the standardized patient scripts, while faculty members with specific clinical expertise created the IPE simulation educational content and assessment. The IPE champions navigated both tracks of IPE simulation development. To afford sufficient complexity and to buffer against unpredictable team interactions with the standardized patients, IPE simulation champions collaborated with simulation staff to develop a richer patient script for the standardized patients. Learners and faculty members did not have access to the standardized patient script. Lessons learned from the UT Austin IPE are outlined in Table 12.5.

The desired learner outcomes inform the apposite complexity and necessary technology resource-level of IPE simulation. Lower complexity and lower technology-resourced IPE simulation can more easily integrate into the classroom and enhance instruction through experiential learning. Higher complexity and/or higher technology-resourced IPE simulation may not be necessary for achieving learning objectives among learners early in training; however, these elements offer more consequential clinical training for interprofessional teams comprising advanced learners. IPE simulation video recording provides additional post-IPE simulation learning opportunities and assurances of educational quality and outcomes. Video recording requires participant disclosure and consent. In addition, the frame composition and image capture in video recordings should focus on the learners for optimal educational impact.

Operational and educational IPE simulation debriefing by stakeholders provides important formative and summative lessons for process improvement and relevance for prelicensure learners, respectively. Programmatic evaluation of the IPE simulation and its effectiveness brings full circle the integration of IPE simulation in prelicensure health professions' educational programs.

At UT Austin, the IPE simulation followed the same process assessment and evaluation that applied to the in-class sessions. The IPE simulation assessment mirrored the in-class team assessment, minimizing learner anxiety with its use in IPE simulation and maximizing translation of in-class team experiences into IPE simulation. Similar to class session evaluations, IPE simulation evaluation flowed from direct observations by IPE champions and from feedback from course faculty, learners, and staff.

Curriculum Development

The complexities of integrating IPE into the curriculum of prelicensure health professions' educational programs and leveraging simulation as a component of the curricula require careful consideration of multiple aspects related to curriculum development. The following discussion explores the important components necessary for success, using the macro-meso-micro conceptual framework (Fig. 12.4).

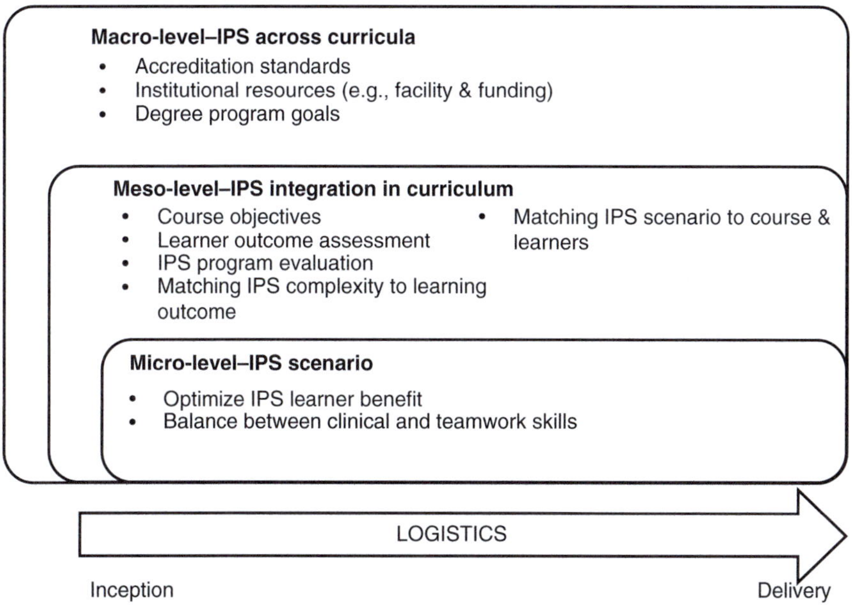

Fig. 12.4 Levels of prelicensure interprofessional simulation curricular considerations

Macro-level

Curricular elements in prelicensure health professions training are influenced by multiple factors at the macro level. Specific requirements for training in IPE-related competencies are found in the accreditation standards for most health professions programs. Discipline specific requirements are contained in the Essentials for Baccalaureate Education for Professional Nursing Practice (American Association of Colleges of Nursing, 2008), which emphasizes IPE as an integral element across nursing curricula [21]. The Liaison Committee for Medical Education Standard 7.9 states that "faculty of a medical school ensure that the core curriculum of the medical education program prepared medical students to function collaboratively on health care teams that include health professionals from other disciplines as they provide coordinated services to patients. These curricular experiences include practitioners and/or students from the other health professions." [22, p. 11] Similarly, Standard 11 of the Accreditation Council for Pharmacy Education states that "the curriculum prepares all students to provide entry-level, patient centered care in a variety of practice settings as a contributing member of an interprofessional team. In the aggregate, team exposure includes prescribers as well as other healthcare professionals." [23, p. 7] Similar standards exist for interprofessional or interdisciplinary collaboration for most health professions schools. At the macro level, IPE must also align with the program outcomes or objectives for each specific discipline.

Institutional, physical or financial resources required to conduct IPE simulation-based learning activities should be considered at this level, with an understanding that simulation does not necessarily require a high-stakes, high-fidelity simulation occurring in a high-technology environment. There are instructional methods using low fidelity simulation which can be equally effective in meeting curricular learning objectives in a resource-constrained environment.

Meso-level

At the meso level, implementation of an IPE curriculum begins with creating or evaluating the learning objectives for the course, and considering the overall objectives for the curriculum. Learning objectives require input and agreement from all professions represented in the learning, for alignment of the course objectives to individual discipline program outcomes. A method for assessing learner outcomes occurs at this level, specifically providing a method for evaluating simulation as part of the learning.

Using the definition of simulation put forth by Abdulmohsen of "an artificial representation of real world process to achieve education goals through experiential learning," [24, p. 35] simulation provides a mechanism through which students in an interprofessional curriculum course are able to practice and eventually demonstrate competency in the application of concepts and skills to practice. Simulation in an IPE curriculum occurs in many forms, from low-fidelity, low-stakes tabletop

Table 12.6 IPE curricular considerations for prelicensure participation

IPS curricular consideration	IPS approach
Maximal learner participation	Specific opportunities or roles for each level profession Utilize official class dates/times for simulation in lieu of class Offer multiple rounds of simulation
Variable health professions representation and/or availability	Nimble scenario development with flexible roles Flexible team member composition

discussions over a case presentation to high-fidelity, high-stakes, simulation activities. Development of scenarios requires an awareness that IPE learning must be maximized for all participants, with specific opportunities for each profession to meaningfully contribute to the success of the encounter. One of the main determinants of a scenario's ability to engage all learners is the level of clinical knowledge or experience required. Finding a scenario with enough clinical relevance to be interesting but not too much that learners cannot function in the roles required is the sweet spot of IPE simulation in early clinical training. Scenarios should also be nimble enough to allow for flexibility in the composition of participants, given that all professions may not be equally represented for every simulation. Scenarios written to allow role flexibility will have greater adaptability to variations in delivery, as illustrated in (Table 12.6).

At UT Austin, IPE champions sequenced the summative IPE simulation late in the year-long course to allow time for learners to form functioning interprofessional teams and to build simulation with more clinically-oriented content sequenced in the latter half of the course. The simulation was crafted to focus more on the team-centered attributes of interprofessional collaborative practice (e.g., mutual respect) and less on the clinical expertise and clinical decision-making process of the team. To make the clinical setting more contextual to the IPE simulation and to better prepare learners to engage, learners were provided the case information in advance along with clear team instructions, expectations and the IPE simulation assessment tool. The IPE simulation case stemmed from the IPE course module that immediately preceded the IPE simulation. This provided learners with some content awareness and preparation, utilizing in-class experiences and time to prepare for the IPE simulation. Faculty members received the same in-class preparation as students. They also received an advance preparation packet that included the student IPE simulation information bundle along with faculty IPE simulation instructions, expectations, and debriefing guidelines. Essentially, the IPE simulation-based activity became an extension of one module of the course.

Micro-level

The broader course outcomes drive the decisions around IPE simulation scenario transparency to learners and faculty. For example, faculty using IPE simulation in a capstone course may choose to provide learners with only a list of possible scenarios they may encounter. However, if the IPE simulation is sequenced within an introductory IPE course, the learners will need more details about what is expected to happen throughout the simulation. The level of clinical knowledge of each learner group must be considered in the sophistication of decision-making required in each scenario. For the early learner, a "clinical hook" assures sufficient engagement for all participants without over-emphasizing profession-specific skills. This allows emphasis to be placed upon demonstration of teamwork, professionalism, and communication rather than on clinical decision-making. The content and skills complexity for a given scenario may be tailored to the learners' progress in training.

Preparing Faculty and Students for Success

Macro-level

Preparation of faculty at the macro level starts with the development of IPE and IPE simulation champions. Formal training on the Interprofessional Education Collaborate (IPEC) core competencies and an IPE team consisting of equal representation of champions from all professions creates a cohesive core faculty who serve as leaders for their respective schools or divisions. The next consideration at the macro level is the appropriate population of students and faculty for the activity. Students are selected based on availability, their fit within the course culture and objectives, or flexibility within the program's curriculum to accommodate the IPE course. Discrepancies may emerge at this point regarding level of time available, cost versus benefit, and perception of the need for IPE activities, by administrators of different programs. Administrators and IPE champions must respond to potential resistance to the complexity of planning IPE, which may become apparent at this stage. Faculty selection requires consideration of availability during the course's activities and for training, funding mechanisms for faculty time and effort, as well as the school or program's mechanism for establishing expectations for faculty involvement in teaching. Heavy clinical requirements, inflexible schedules, and lack of incentives for teaching, can be significant barriers that the senior leadership champion within a school or program needs to address. Discrepancies in work load effort and other teaching commitments among the professions can manifest in unequal representation of all professional departments, and efforts should be made to minimize this impact on the learning activities.

Beyond logistical availability of faculty for the course, considerations to include in faculty selection are the faculty's understanding of their individual responsibility to interprofessional collaboration, time commitment to the learning activities of the course, and experience in education and simulation [25]. Faculty engaged in IPE simulation may not be comfortable with the learning modality; therefore, mentoring by colleagues from their own or other health professions who are comfortable with this modality and/or technology is important [26]. Implementation of IPE simulation within the greater framework of IPE requires attention to the inclusion or development of simulation experts to achieve the best outcomes for the learners. To sustain simulation in health professions curricula, structured faculty development is required [27]. Planning the faculty composition to allow a mix of content experts, committed to interprofessional learning, and simulation experts requires intentionality on the part of the collaborating professional schools. It may be necessary to balance simulation experts from one profession with IPE experts from another to assure appropriate delivery of the learning activity.

Meso-level

Faculty development in IPE begins in the meso level. IPE champions from each profession with extensive training in IPE and IPE simulation serve as the trainers for the remainder of the course faculty. All faculty involved in the course will require training over the Core Competencies for Interprofessional Collaborative Practice [28]. At UT, faculty development began with formal IPE course faculty training and continued through classroom experiences. IPE course faculty members participated in role-playing and tabletop simulation exercises as observers or patients. Learner preparation for IPE simulation paralleled that of their faculty members. Be extending content previously covered in the classroom and table top exercises, the IPE simulation represents a natural extension of the classroom experiences, requiring little additional formal preparation outside of the usual briefing prior to IPE simulation.

Micro-level

Faculty preparation on the day of an IPE simulation activity may include updates or instructions on the scenario, expectations, faculty role, assessment rubrics or other IPE simulation elements, depending on how much of this was done ahead of time. If the IPE simulation occurs in a formal simulation center, faculty may require orientation to the physical environment, instruction on controls, monitoring equipment, and where the faculty is positioned during the simulation. At UT, since the IPE course integrated simulation, faculty development occurred concurrently with the IPE course faculty development. The efforts of macro and meso levels of IPE simulation preparation greatly reduced the need for intensive faculty and student preparation on the day of the event and enabled IPE champions to focus on the event execution logistics, such as brief orientation to faculty's use of simulation monitoring equipment.

Evaluations and Outcomes

There is no consistent conceptual model in which the impact of IPE or IPE simulation can be described, due to variations in taxonomy, terminology, and educational structures reported in the literature [1]. We present consideration of the impact and outcomes of IPE simulation training using Kirkpatrick's model, which we have mapped onto the macro-meso-micro conceptual framework in Fig. 12.5. The majority of

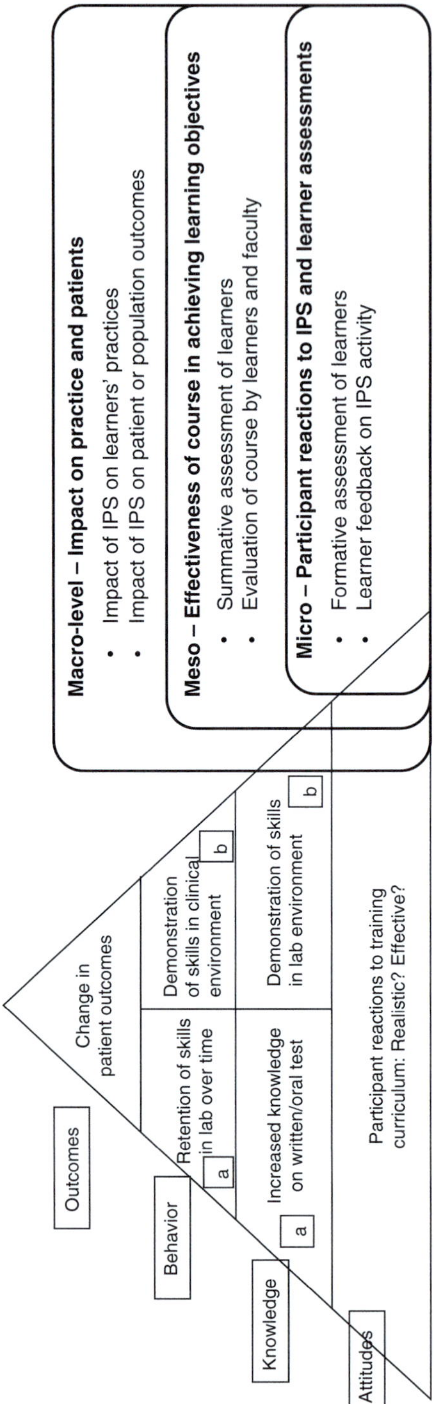

Fig. 12.5 Evaluation and outcomes

studies on learner and program outcomes in IPE simulation report Kirkpatrick's level 1 outcomes, highlighting significant gaps in evidence linking IPE and IPE simulation to patient outcomes. Despite these gaps, the importance of IPE in developing necessary collaborative practice skills in healthcare professionals is strongly supported by thought leaders in governmental, regulatory and education roles [1]. This learning starts in the prelicensure training programs, and should be considered alongside clinical skills as part of all healthcare professions' lifelong learning.

Macro-level

Outcomes at the macro level include evaluating the impact of IPE simulation on processes within a healthcare system, patient or population outcomes, corresponding to Kirkpatrick's level 4; however, the data supporting this impact are derived from training practicing providers and teams. Challenges to demonstrating the relationship between prelicensure IPE simulation and patient outcomes include the variable durations between the training and graduates' opportunity to independently influence patient care, and the fact that graduates will practice in multiple different settings, introducing confounding variables in each graduate's ultimate practice context.

Meso-level

At the meso level, summative assessment requires consideration of each professions' grading system, such that comparable grading criteria can be established for all students in the course. At UT, all partnering programs graded the course as pass/fail. Applying a uniform IPE simulation assessment allowed individual programs to extract necessary data to inform grading of their learners. For programs requiring letter grades, the IPE course was embedded as a component of another course in the curriculum, such that other activities in the parent course served as criteria for achieving a given letter grade.

Evaluation of the course's effectiveness in achieving its learning outcomes is an understood component of the curriculum development cycle, and considers learner performance in the course, learner and faculty evaluation of the course, and ideally a measure of impact through follow-up of the learners as they progress in their clinical experience. One of the early findings of our course is that the IPE simulation has removed barriers to communication and collaboration as the students enter or re-enter the clinical environment and interact with members of the professions participating in the course.

Micro-level

Studies on the impact of IPE simulation with prelicensure learners most commonly focus on students' reactions to the training, their changes in self-efficacy or attitudes regarding interprofessional learning or practice, corresponding to Kirkpatrick's Level 1 [29]. There are a variety of instruments that have been developed to assess learners' attitudes towards simulation, with varying levels of validity evidence in the prelicensure IPE simulation context. The Readiness for Interprofessional Learning Scale (RIPLS) is one of the most commonly used tools but we discontinued its use, like other centers, due to concerns over the nature of the items which encourage socially desirable answers and may not truly measure readiness for IPCP [30–32]. The Interprofessional Attitudes Scale (IPAS) is another validated instrument designed to assess students' attitudes towards IPE, with sub-scales designed to align with IPEC competency domains which we do currently administer in our program [33]. Participants' reactions to an IPE simulation activity can be collected through written feedback or debriefing; these micro-level evaluations do not require instruments with validity evidence, although the questions asked of participants should be thoughtfully crafted to generate useful information.

Also at the micro level, but corresponding to Kirkpatrick's level 2 is assessment of the students' performance, as individuals, and as a team. The instruments used in this level may be checklist or global rating tool specific to the clinical context, but there are also assessment tools for interprofessional teamwork skills that have varying levels of validity evidence in the prelicensure IPE simulation context, such as the Communication and Teamwork Skills assessment and the Teamwork Mini-Clinical Evaluation Exercise (T-MEX) [34, 35]. Of note, the T-MEX is designed for use in the clinical environment, but could be applied in the simulated environment.

One example of assessing learner outcomes at Kirkpatrick's level 2 is work by Paige et al., who demonstrated improvement in teamwork skills and team performance in fourth-year medical students, senior nursing students and nurse-anesthesia students following IPE simulation [36]. In this high-fidelity context, learners who have more sophisticated clinical knowledge and have already engaged in professional identity formation experiences are able to apply clinical skills and interprofessional competencies in the IPE simulation. In considering learner assessment, students should receive regular formative feedback on individual and team performance from peers and faculty facilitators. The process of peer feedback serves a dual purpose – on one hand, students provide a unique perspective in formative feedback to other team members as active participants in the IPE simulation scenario and its preparations; on the other hand, students are practicing the life-long skill of soliciting and receiving feedback from team members.

Faculty participation in debriefing sessions after each training activity provides feedback on the effectiveness of the simulation in achieving intended learning outcomes and on other aspects such as logistics. Student feedback on the simulation activity is ideally solicited at the end of each activity, to maximize recall, with attention to "survey fatigue," which can ultimately degrade the quality of feedback received.

Student feedback to faculty presents an opportunity for faculty to role model a flattened hierarchy in the educational setting through feedback agility. This is an important faculty development topic, as IPE simulation can uncover unconscious bias in faculty as well as students. Traditionally, student feedback occurs at the completion of a course or clerkship, but if a faculty's words or actions are received as offensive by a student, whether directed at the student, his or her profession, or a course faculty in the student's profession, the student may need a more timely resolution of his or her concern. Receiving feedback from students around unconscious bias is not easy for faculty, and focused effort should be directed at coaching faculty through this process before and during the course.

Conclusion

The use of simulation-based activities as a component of IPE is a powerful instructional method allowing for initial acquisition and deliberate practice of skills of IPEC Core Competencies for Interprofessional Collaborative Practice for prelicensure learners. The foundation for success lies in senior leadership buy-in and support in each partnering program and committed champions from each profession who function themselves as a high-performing, collaborative team. IPE simulation for development of teamwork skills can be employed early in the curriculum of a training program to allow focus on teamwork specifically, with enough clinical content to engage but not distract learners. Using a longitudinal approach rather than bringing early learners together for a single training activity allows meaningful team dynamics to develop through repeated opportunities to practice with the same team. However, more advanced learners do derive benefits from opportunities to practice applying clinical knowledge and skills in IPE simulation, even as standalone experiences.

The complexities of IPE simulation planning require extensive preparations and intentional consideration of multiple layers of logistics, curriculum development, faculty and student preparations by the IPE champions; the UT lessons learned in these areas are summarized in Table 12.5. Evaluation of outcomes is a unique challenge for prelicensure learners, given that they work under instructional supervision for a period of time before independent practice. As additional research emerges, the gaps between prelicensure IPE simulation and patient outcomes may be filled.

References

1. Institute of Medicine. Measuring the impact of interprofessional education on collaborative practice and patient outcomes. Washington, D.C.: The National Academies Press. 2015. [cited 2017 Apr 14]. Available from: https://www.nap.edu/read/21726/chapter/1.
2. Ericsson EA. Acquisition and maintenance of medical expertise: a perspective from the expert-performance approach with deliberate practice. Acad Med. 2015;90(11):1471–86.
3. Nehring WM. U.S. boards of nursing and the use of high-fidelity patient simulators in nursing education. J Prof Nurs. 2008;24(1):109–17.
4. Ryall T, Judd BK, Gordon CJ. Simulation-based assessments in health professional education: a systematic review. J Multidisp Healthc. 2006;9:69–82.
5. Robertson JM, Dias RD, Yule S, Smink DS. Operative room team training with simulation: a systematic review. J Laparoendosc Adv Surg Tech A. 2017;

6. Marcus W. Applying a framework to healthcare simulation: micro, meso and macro levels. In: Nestel D, Kelly M, Jolly B, Watson M, editors. Healthcare simulation education: evidence, theory, and practice. 1st ed. Oxford: Wiley; 2017. p. 29–34.
7. Craddock D, O'Halloran C, McPherson K, Hean S, Hammick M. A top-down approach impedes the use of theory? Interprofessional educational leaders' approaches to curriculum development and the use of learning theory. J Interprof Care. 2013;27(1):65–72.
8. Kahaleh AA, Danielson J, Franson KL, Nuffer WA, Umland EM. An interprofessional education panel on development, implementation, and assessment strategies. Am J Pharm Educ. 2015;79(6):78.
9. Speakman E, Tagliareni E, Sherburne A, Sicks S. Guide to effective Interprofessional education experiences in nursing education. Washington, D.C.: National League for Nursing; 2016. [cited 2017 Mar 26]. Available from: http://www.nln.org/docs/default-source/default-document-library/ipe-toolkit-krk-012716.pdf?sfvrsn=6.
10. Interprofessional Education Collaborative. Core competencies for interprofessional collaborative practice: 2016 update. Washington (DC): Interprofessional Education Collaborative. 2016. [cited 2017 Mar 26]. Available from: https://ipecollaborative.org/uploads/IPEC-2016-Updated-Core-Competencies-Report__final_release_.PDF.
11. MacKenzie DE, Doucet S, Nasser S, Godden-Webster AL, Andrews C, Kephart G. Collaboration behind-the-scenes: key to effective interprofessional education. J Interprof Care. 2014;28(4):381–3.
12. Jones BL, Luk JC, Phillips F. Transformative teams: co-teaching social work and medical students in interprofessional practice. Paper. Interprofessional and Transdisciplinary Practice Track. Council on Social Work Education 58th annual meeting. Washington, D.C. 2012.
13. Masters K. Journey toward integration of simulation in a baccalaureate nursing curriculum. J Nurs Educ. 2014;53(2):102–4.
14. Motola LA, Devine HS, Chun HS, Sullivan JE, Issenberg SB. Simulation in healthcare education: a best evidence practical guide. AMEE Guide No. 82. Med Teach. 2013;35(10):e1511–30.
15. Emory J. Understanding backward design to strengthen curricular models. Nurse Educ. 2014;39(3):122–5.
16. Daugherty KK. Backward course design: making the end the beginning. Am J Pharm Educ. 2006;70(6):135.
17. Goldman E, Schroth WS. Perspective: deconstructing integration: a framework for the rational application of integration as a guiding curricular strategy. Acad Med. 2012;87(6):729–34.
18. van Teijlingen E, Hundley V. The importance of pilot studies. Nurs Stand. 2002;16(40):33–6.
19. Holden MD, Buck E, Luk J, Ambriz F, Boisaubin EV, Clark MA, Mihalic AP, Sadler JZ, Sapire K, Spike J, Vince A, Dalrymple JL. Professional identity formation: creating a longitudinal framework through TIME. Acad Med. 2015;90(6):761–7.
20. Kirkpatrick DL, Kirkpatrick JL. Evaluating training programs. 3rd ed. San Francisco: Berrett-Koehler Publishers, Inc.; 2006.
21. American Association of College of Nursing. The essentials of baccalaureate education for professional nursing practice. Washington, D.C.: American Association of College of Nursing; 2008.
22. Liaison Committee on Medical Education. Functions and structure of a medical school: Standards for accreditation of medical education programs leading to the MD degree [Internet]. Association of American Medical Colleges and the American Medical Association, March 2017 [cited March 30, 2017]. Available from lcme.org.
23. Accreditation Council for Pharmacy Education. Accreditation standard and key elements for the professional program in pharmacy leading to the Doctor of Pharmacy degree [Internet]. Chicago: Accreditation Council for Pharmacy Education 2015 [cited March 30, 2017]. Available from ACPE.
24. Al-Elq AH. Simulation-based medical teaching and learning. J Fam Community Med 17.1 (2010): 35–40. PMC. Web. 26 Mar 2017.
25. Eddie M, Hamilton C, Hammett O, Hyde P, Pryde K, Sykes K. Operationalizing a new emergency department: the role of simulation. In: Nestel D, Kelly M, Jolly B, Watson M, editors.

Simulation education: evidence, theory and practice. West Sussex, UK: John Wiley & Sons, Ltd; 2018. p. 205–8.
26. Robertson J, Bandali K. Bridging the gap: enhancing interprofessional education using simulation. J Interprof Care. 2008;22(5):499–508.
27. Peterson, DT, Watts, P, Epps, CA, White ML. Simulation faculty development: a tired approach. SimulHealthc. 2017. Available from: https://doi.org/10.1097/SIH.0000000000000225. Accessed 11 April 2017.
28. Interprofessional Education Collaborative. Core competencies for interprofessional collaborative practice: 2016 update. Washington, D.C.: Interprofessional Education Collaborative 2016 [cited 2017 Apr 11]. Available from https://ipecollaborative.org/uploads/IPEC-2016-Updated-Core-Competencies-Report__final_release_.PDF.
29. Wang R, Shi N, Bai J, Zheng Y, Zhao Y. Implementation and evaluation of an interprofessional simulation-based education program for undergraduate nursing students in operating room nursing education: a randomized controlled trial. BMC Med Educ. 2015;15:115.
30. Curran VR, Sharpe D, Forristall J, Flynn K. Attitudes of health sciences students towards interprofessional teamwork and education. Learn Health Soc Care. 2008;7(3):146–56.
31. Parsell G, Bligh J. The development of a questionnaire to assess the readiness of health care students for interprofessional learning (RIPLS). Med Educ. 1999;33(2):95–100.
32. McFadyen AK, Webster V, Strachan K, Figgins E, Brown H, McKechnie J. The Readiness for Interprofessional Learning Scale: a possible more stable sub-scale model for the original version of RIPLS. J Interprof Care. 2005;19(6):595–603.
33. Norris J, Carpenter JG, Eaton J, Guo JW, Lassche M, Pett MA, Blumenthal DK. The development and validation of the interprofessional attitudes scale: assessing the interprofessional attitudes of students in the health professions. Acad Med. 2015;90(10):1394–400.
34. Frankel A, Gardner R, Maynard L, Kelly A. Using the communication and teamwork skills (CATS) assessment to measure health care team performance. Jt Comm J Qual Patient Saf. 2007;33(9):549–58.
35. Olupeliyawa AM, O'Sullivan AJ, Hughes C, Balasooriya CD. The Teamwork Mini-Clinical Evaluation Exercise (T-MEX): a workplace-based assessment focusing on collaborative competencies in health care. Acad Med. 2014;89(2):359–65.
36. Paige JT, Garbee DD, Kozmenko V, Yu Q, Kozmenko L, Yang T, Bonanno L, Swartz W. Getting a head start: high-fidelity, simulation-based operating room team training of interprofessional students. J Am Coll Surg. 2014;218(1):140–9.

Simulation-Based Training for Post-graduate Interprofessional Learners

13

Jannet Lee-Jayaram, Benjamin W. Berg, and Susan Steinemann

Introduction: The IPE Imperative

In 2002, the Committee on the Health Professions Education Summit was convened, involving leaders across multiple disciplines to discuss and develop strategies for restructuring healthcare education. This led to the 2003 Institute of Medicine (IOM) report: "Health Professions Education: A Bridge to Quality," which elaborated five core competencies expected of all health providers: Provide patient-centered care, employ evidence-based practice, apply quality improvement, utilize informatics and work in interdisciplinary teams [1]. The committee's recommendations for incorporating these competencies were directed mainly at national oversight organizations responsible for educational institution and professional association accreditation and certification. These included recommendations to overhaul training programs, certification requirements, and maintenance of certification requirements to demonstrate these competencies.

At the time of the IOM report, the Accreditation Committee for Graduate Medical Education (ACGME) had defined and incorporated requirements for six core resident competencies, regardless of specialty. The interprofessional education (IPE) paradigm directly addresses ACGME core competencies including: Interpersonal and Communication Skills (IV.A.5.d), Systems-based Practice (IV.A.5.f), Formative

J. Lee-Jayaram · B. W. Berg
SimTiki Simulation Center, John A Burns School of Medicine, University of Hawaii at Manoa, Honolulu, HI, USA

S. Steinemann (✉)
Department of Surgery, John A Burns School of Medicine, University of Hawaii at Manoa, Honolulu, HI, USA
e-mail: steine@hawaii.edu

J. T. Paige et al. (eds.), *Comprehensive Healthcare Simulation: InterProfessional Team Training and Simulation*, Comprehensive Healthcare Simulation,
https://doi.org/10.1007/978-3-030-28845-7_13

Evaluation (V.A.2), Transitions of Care (handoffs) (VI.B.3) and Teamwork (VI.F) [2]. Residencies must document resident competency in communicating effectively with other health professionals, working effectively as a member or leader of a health care team, and working in interprofessional teams to enhance patient safety and improve patient care quality. The ACGME requires that programs provide residents opportunities to work in interprofessional teams and ensure resident competency in handover communication. Residencies must provide formative feedback on progress of the competencies. Specific instructions as to how to demonstrate these interprofessional competencies were left up to each individual specialty.

The ACGME Milestones Project began in 2012 to define specialty-specific developmental outcomes for the six common core competencies. While the taxonomy and specifics vary between specialties, all the milestones include requirements for working and communicating in an interprofessional team. Surgery milestones for interpersonal skills and communication competencies fall under the practice domain of coordination of care [3]. Diagnostic Radiology milestones specify communication with the health care team in written and verbal domains, with various recommended methods of evaluation, including simulation and objective structured clinical examinations (OSCE) [4]. Methods for evaluation and formative assessment in these competencies vary by individual residencies and many have used simulation for this purpose.

Experience and Practical Considerations

There are a number of clinical environments that require interprofessional teamwork and many published reports of the successful use of simulation for IPE. A representative sample is discussed below and summarized in Table 13.1. Published experiences are diverse and describe clinical construct, methods of simulation, and educational focus, i.e. resident education versus inclusion of residents as a member of the team. Outcomes measured range from Kirkpatrick level 1 outcomes for learner reactions to level 4 outcomes for changes to the system [5].

Simulation-based IPE level 4 outcomes have been demonstrated in emergency trauma care. Capella et al. compared real trauma resuscitations before and after an IPE simulation including surgery residents, surgery attending physicians and nurses, and found improvements in the teamwork scores and in the clinical care of the patients in the emergency department (ED) [6]. Following IPE intervention, trauma patients had shorter times to computed tomography (CT) scan (26.4–22.1 minutes, $p = 0.005$), to endotracheal intubation (10.1–6.6 minutes, p-0.49) and to the operating room (OR) (130.1–94.5 minutes, $p = 0.021$). IPE consisted of a 2-hour didactic lecture for the residents, followed by 2 hours of simulation incorporating three high-fidelity simulation scenarios with interprofessional video co-debriefing by a PhD educator, surgery attending and trauma nurse. Participation in the training was high; 100% of the surgery residents and attendings completed the teamwork training and 80% of the ED nurses participated.

Table 13.1 Published reports of the successful use of simulation for IPE

Year	Author	Clinical team	Target learners	Simulator	Curriculum	Debriefing	Kirkpatrick level outcome
2010	Capella	Trauma resuscitation	Trauma team w/ Surg residents	HPS	TeamSTEPPS	Video, team	4
2011	Steinemann	Trauma resuscitation	Trauma team w/ Surg residents	HPS	Novel, based on Pittsburgh	Video, team	4
2010	Nishisaki	PICU	ICU team w/ Ped & EM residents	HPS	Novel	Team	3
2016	Wong	ED	EM residents and nurses	HPS	TeamSTEPPS + Novel	Team	2
2008	Falcone	Ped trauma resuscitation	Trauma team w/ Surg, Ped, EM residents	HPS	Novel	Video, team	2
2011	Sweeney	Inpatient Ped code	Ped residents and nurses	Not described	Novel	Team	1, 2
2013	Patterson	Ped ED	ED team w/ Ped residents	Not described	Novel	Team	1, 2, 4
2012	Salam	Inpatient ward	IM residents & nurses	SP	Novel	Video, team	2

Similarly, Steinemann et al. conducted in-situ (in the ED) trauma resuscitation simulations for interprofessional trauma team members. All surgical residents and trauma surgeons completed training, participation rates were 72–95% among the other trauma team members (ED physicians, nurses and technicians, respiratory therapists, and critical care nurses) [7]. The intervention consisted of a pre-course web presentation on teamwork, a 30-minute pre-simulation didactic lecture and 2.5 hours with 3 high-fidelity manikin in-situ trauma simulations each followed by a physician-facilitated debriefing. Kirkpatrick level 4 outcomes were evaluated in real trauma resuscitations before and after IPE showing improvements in the percentage of tasks completed and reported (34% with ≤1 unreported task pre-training, 60% post-training) and decreased mean resuscitation time in the ED (32 versus 26 minutes, $p < 0.05$).

IPE simulation with trauma team training involving residents can lead to system changes that positively improve the care of patients during trauma resuscitations [6, 7]. Pucher et al. demonstrated that regardless of injury severity score (ISS), improved teamwork has been correlated to decreased delays in interprofessional and interdisciplinary care of injured patients [8]. In a prospective observational study of trauma calls at an urban level I trauma center, teamwork performance was measured, and times to disposition, completion of assessment care processes, delays, errors and ISS were recorded. Cases with low teamwork scores had a greater time to disposition (24 versus 20 minutes, $p = 0.046$) and regression analysis revealed that teamwork was the only factor associated with delays (OR 0.24; 95% CI 0.06–0.95). Thus, the application of IPE training with residents to improve teamwork appears to yield tangible improvements in patient care.

Integrating labor- and time-intensive IPE requires coordination of training cycles with the annual influx of novice residents and optimization of recurrent training for other staff. Variable participation rates between professions highlight organizational limitations to comprehensive IPE initiatives in the clinical realm. Optimal interprofessional participation requires institutional buy-in and participation mandates. Application of IPE incorporating residents is a high yield target for evidence-based application of IPE to yield educational outcomes and tangible improvements in patient care.

To address feasibility issues of interprofessional simulation, Nishisaki et al. used a type of shorter, more focused training dubbed "Just-in-Time-Training" for airway intubation in a pediatric intensive care unit (PICU) [9, 10]. This randomized IPE intervention trial enrolled 78 emergency medicine and pediatric residents, 122 PICU nurses and 65 respiratory therapists. Immediately prior to shift change, participants completed a 20-minute high-fidelity manikin-based infant respiratory distress scenario followed by debriefing. Level 3 outcomes were evaluated for all patient intubations in the PICU during the study, comparing trained residents with non-trained residents and pre/post-intervention intubation metrics. Post-intervention, resident attempted intubations increased (pre- 20.9% to post-intervention 35.4%, $p = 0.002$). Overall success of intubation demonstrated a non-significant improvement (pre- 57.5% to post-intervention 75%, $p = 0.19$), as did first-attempt intubation success (pre- 50% to post-intervention 62.5%, $p = 0.44$). There was no increase in tracheal intubation adverse events (pre- 22% to post-intervention 19.9%, $p = 0.62$) [9]. It was speculated that the interprofessional training improved competency in the non-laryngoscopist team members, thereby preventing increased tracheal intubation adverse events. Teams randomized to the training intervention were ad-hoc interprofessional teams and were never the intact teams performing patient intubations due to scheduling complexity, which is an inherent challenge for all IPE. It is unusual that co-trained IPE participants will deliver care as an intact patient care team, especially for in-hospital crisis response teams. However, objectives and results of IPE carry through and lead to improved outcomes. This study also demonstrated that IPE simulation can be provided in shorter doses, diminishing the burdensome time commitment for training outside of regular duty hours.

Integrated instructional designs with longer, more formal didactics and simulations combined with brief "just-in-time" continuity simulations is one approach to creating sustainable, durable training and impact. In an adult emergency department, Wong et al. required all emergency medicine residents and staff nurses to participate in a 3-hour team training, consisting of a 30-minute didactic and two high-fidelity medical emergency simulations, followed by physician and nurse educator co-debriefing [11]. Thereafter, abridged versions of the same scenarios were conducted bi-weekly in-situ in the ED and a monthly staff newsletter reemphasizing teamwork principles was distributed. Individual attitudes toward teamwork and the perception of patient safety culture in the hospital showed improvement, except in the area of management support of patient safety. Pre- and post- surveys on attitudes towards teamwork were only slightly improved in the teamwork constructs of team structure (6.4%, $p < 0.0001$), leadership (2.8%, $p = 0.029$), situation monitoring (4%, $p = 0.014$), and mutual support (4%, $p = 0.003$). This result is similar to other studies in which most participants report positive attitudes toward IPE prior to the intervention and make marginal gains after the training [12–14].

Interprofessional simulations can serve as an evaluation method for teamwork and communication educational interventions. At a children's hospital trauma center, during a 1-year study period, Falcone et al. emphasized team function and communication in all trauma educational activities, both for residents and trauma core nursing teams [15]. Activities included lectures, conferences, video review, web-based curriculum, and a monthly 2-hour high-fidelity simulation session on two pediatric trauma scenarios. There were 160 participants from surgery and pediatric residencies, emergency medicine and critical care fellowships, surgery and emergency medicine attendings, trauma core nurses, paramedics and respiratory therapists. Only the trauma core nurses attended more than one session throughout the year. The scenarios were scored and the mean percentage of appropriately completed tasks were compared between scenarios scored early in the year and scenarios scored later in the year. The mean percentage of appropriately completed tasks improved from 65% to 75% ($p < 0.05$). Two, possibly overlapping, mechanisms to explain the improvements were proposed: the effect of the new teamwork and communication emphasis in trauma education and the effect of the trauma core nurses' participation in multiple simulation sessions.

IPE simulations have addressed not only the ACGME core competencies of interpersonal/communication skills and system-based practice, but also competencies of patient care, medical knowledge, practice-based learning/improvement, and professionalism. In a pediatric residency, Sweeney et al. had senior residents, under faculty guidance, create, coordinate and facilitate inpatient mock codes for inpatient residents and nurses [16]. Goals were established for both the resident educators and resident participants. Nursing leadership incorporated goals for the nursing participants and the hospital's code committee established goals addressing hospital quality improvement parameters. During a two week night float rotation, a resident educator created and implemented a 15–20 minute interprofessional mock code, followed by a 40–45 minute debriefing on resuscitation and crisis resource management. Following the team debriefing, a faculty supervisor debriefed the resident educator, focusing on leadership and teaching. Pre- and post-mock code surveys were collected from the resident educators and resident participants. Nursing participants completed a post-mock code survey. All of the residents involved in the mock code perceived the curriculum as useful for the care of patients and for collaborative teamwork and benefitted from inclusion of a robust educational component to a service-heavy night float rotation. The required interprofessional collaboration with nurses and the code committee to plan the curriculum led to improved communication and working professional relationships. Using IPE simulation to fulfill an expanded range of core competencies through learner-specific tiered learning objectives is a technique to optimize learning in an already overloaded resident curriculum.

IPE simulation including residents has been applied to identify latent safety threats in work environments. In a children's emergency department, Patterson et al. conducted 20-minute in-situ simulations one to two times per week, with debriefing focused on identifying latent safety threats and teamwork issues [17]. The simulations were based on problematic real cases (e.g. near misses, poor teamwork), seasonally relevant syndromes (drownings in the summer, hypothermia in the winter), and medical and traumatic emergencies. All staff members that would normally respond to these emergencies were required to participate in the simulations. A standardized debriefing checklist was used to guide reflection and discussion of teamwork skills, and then to identify threats and solutions, in the areas of medications, resources, and equipment. Threats such as missing critical medications and airway equipment, and inadequate staffing were identified based on findings during the simulations. In this high-volume ED, 90 interprofessional simulations were completed in 1 year, becoming a valued, regular activity. Culture and language changed in that ED; the Nurse Documenter was renamed as the Nurse Leader, explicitly incorporating a model of shared leadership in the culture of the department. Decay of knowledge and skills over time is problematic, emphasizing that regular interventions, such as this one, are key to effect pervasive change. When IPE simulation is regularized (e.g. not a special occurrence), its ability to mold culture and attitudes in daily healthcare practice has been best demonstrated.

Determining the best location to conduct team training can be a concern for educators. While logistics and other factors are more easily controlled in a classroom setting, in-situ simulation presents learners with a high fidelity environment that is extremely relevant to daily clinical practice. Challenges inherent to in-situ training include the impact on actual patient care, space constraints, and patient safety when training equipment is introduced in the patient care areas. In-situ benefits include enhanced realism and, perhaps more importantly, the ease of congregating individuals from different disciplines and departments. From an educational standpoint, while learners may prefer the in-situ setting, learning outcomes are equivalent whether in the classroom or in-situ setting, as long as IPE simulation is an expected and regular part of the curriculum [18].

IPE for high-acuity teams frequently employs simulation-based education, however communication and team skills may be better taught with standardized patients (SP). Salam et al. reported that internal medicine residents and novice nurses practiced and improved verbal and non-verbal skills, both with an SP and between team members, during a team observed structured clinical exam (TOSCE) evaluation of a patient with alcohol withdrawal symptoms [19]. SP's were undergraduate healthcare students trained by observing real patients with alcohol withdrawal, adhering to a script which realistically portrayed the disease. Both learner groups reported improved confidence in their ability to identify withdrawal symptoms (44% pre-, 94% post-encounter), communicate with the team (55% pre-, 81% post-encounter), and adhere to their institution's post-intervention protocol (41% pre-, 72% post-encounter). Bays et al. demonstrated that internal medicine residents, fellows, and nurse practitioner students also improved their skills in delivering bad news during an IPE simulation with multiple actors representing the patient and family [20]. Participants initially communicated a serious diagnosis, and in subsequent simulations informed family members of a patient death. Coded behaviors outlined for communicating bad news and showing empathy were evaluated pre- and post- intervention. Participants demonstrated significant improvement in 8 of the 11 coded behaviors ($p < 0.001$). Matching the simulation modality (e.g. manikin scenario, SP interaction, etc.) to well-defined objectives and subject matter of the IPE intervention is required for optimal training outcomes.

Virtual reality platforms are an evolving IPE format that may circumvent many of the challenges inherent in conducting live simulation exercises. Research comparing virtual reality to more conventional methods is lacking, but exploratory work has demonstrated feasibility and the concept is gaining traction [21, 22].

IPE Challenges

In 2014, the accrediting bodies for the six founding associations of the Interprofessional Education Collaborative (IPEC) came together to form the Health Professions Accreditors Collaborative (HPAC). HPAC released a press statement that IPE competencies are fundamental and integral to the accreditation standards for educational programs accredited by these agencies. Subsequently, medical schools responding to the Liaison Committee on Medical Education (LCME) questionnaire, reported increasing mandatory IPE, primarily in the classroom/seminar setting, ranging from 44% in the 2007–2008 academic year to 92% in the 2014–2015 academic year [23]. However, there are no requirements regarding the amount, type, objectives, and professions included in IPE during undergraduate education, so it is likely that students will arrive at residency programs with varying degrees of preparation for and attitudes toward IPE.

In addition to knowledge gaps about professional roles and responsibilities, residents may harbor personal bias against IPE. van Schaik et al. interviewed pediatric residents after an IPE mock code simulation with nurses; residents reported anxiety at having to perform in front of nurses, questioned the value of the interprofessional debriefing, and expressed inability for complete honesty during debriefings due to the need to maintain interprofessional working relationships [24]. Many residents expressed that debriefing separately would have been valuable, with reference to a power differential, and would have valued the opportunity to reflect on different aspects of the simulation specific to each profession's scope of practice. Such concerns can be addressed by "phased-domain" debriefing, in which intact team debriefing (Phase 1) is followed by break-outs into domain specific groups (Phase 2) for reflection and discussion of discipline or profession specific topics [25]. Despite the ACGME requirement for IPE, residents may have different priorities for their education, likely focused on rapid assimilation of medical knowledge and technical skills, rather than teamwork. Paradoxically, Lagan et al. reported that orthopedic surgery residents who worked in interprofessional groups during a standardized patient simulation had more negative attitudes toward interpersonal skills and communication than those who worked in resident-only groups [26]. Residents in the interprofessional group reported less willingness to improve their communication skills (post-pre difference −7.44, $p = 0.049$) and less improvement in professional satisfaction in effective communication when compared to the resident-only group (post-pre difference resident-only 7.11, interprofessional 1.89, $p = 0.047$). In this intervention, interprofessional participation appeared to detract from the experience. While individuals may presume they are team players and open-minded, questioning the value of IPE likely comes from a place of bias. For example, when van Schaik et al. asked residents and nurses to rate usefulness of written feedback after interprofessional, in-situ simulated pediatric emergencies, they perceived feedback from their own profession as more valuable, even when similar feedback was provided by individuals from the other profession [27]. In the same study, when the professional source of feedback was not identified, subjects attributed feedback they perceived to be useful to a facilitator from their own profession. Therefore, it is not only IPE content which creates bias but the tendency for individuals to identify with and more highly value input communicated by members of their own professional domain. This finding may support design of IPE debriefing which includes multi-professional facilitators.

The level and profession of learners are factors affecting IPE attitudes. Varying resident levels within a specialty, different specialties, medical students, nursing students, paramedics, pharmacists, advanced- and mid-level non-physician practitioners and other health care providers comprise the interprofessional environment, and no two institutions have the exact same interprofessional mix. For IPE, an optimal combination of learner professions and levels has not been empirically established, and depending on individual perspective, the valuation of IPE may vary. Stefanidis et al. highlighted this issue when surgical residents and senior nursing students rated their experience after a team-training simulation and expressed vastly different opinions [28]. Surgical residents' rating of educational value of the sessions was lower than nursing student ratings. Residents preferred practicing nurses as partners for this type of training, citing that lack of nursing student knowledge impeded flow of the scenarios. Nursing students similarly preferred residents to medical students as partners for this type of training. These conflicting learner assessments regarding the optimal interprofessional representation (e.g. level of learner) for IPE highlight the need for additional IPE curriculum development work. Future research should frame how to address the issue of priorities that pose interprofessional conflicts. Which professional priorities should be asserted? How should priorities be "balanced"? Non-physician providers work with multiple physician specialties and physicians at varying levels of training, during which the importance of IPE is thus manifest.

Experienced non-physician providers work collaboratively with medical trainees and frequently contribute to "360-degree" evaluation feedback regarding residents. A working knowledge of residents' background, training and responsibilities in the evaluation domain(s) is required for accurate feedback. This working knowledge is presumed. However, when Schlitzkus et al. surveyed surgical nurses on their understanding of surgical residents' educational goals, scope of practice and lifestyles, many misconceptions were revealed [29]. Some incorrect beliefs that nurses held about residents included: residents paid tuition, residents did not hold a medical license, residents devoted more time to studying than patient care, residents were not legally physicians, residents did not have significant debt, and residents were paid more than they actually were. These types of perceptions are not necessarily apparent prior to conducting IPE, yet may strongly influence how professionals interact and respond to each other in the educational and patient care environment. Sensitive misconceptions like these may not be revealed during large group debriefings as social constraints prevent professionals from discussing these types of topics.

This knowledge gap of professional responsibilities continues even with teams comprised of experienced healthcare providers. When Steinemann et al. surveyed trauma surgeons and nurses from a single institution about role responsibilities during trauma resuscitation prior to team-training simulations, they reported discordant perceptions for responsibilities of tasks [30]. The groups differed significantly in their perception of responsibility for 71% of the trauma resuscitation tasks, both groups assigning more responsibility to their respective profession. Incorporating understanding of roles in multiple interprofessional domains early in training may be a way to remedy relevant knowledge gaps that can persist many years into an individual's practice.

ACGME residency training hour restrictions were introduced in 2003 and revised in 2011 in an attempt to promote resident education while ensuring both patient and resident safety. Restrictions include maximum number of hours worked per week, amount of time off between duty hours, and the maximum length of continuous duty hours. Although the effect of these restrictions has had variable impact on different specialties, surgical specialties have been impacted the most due to the long working hours associated with that specialty [31]. Given that the need for direct patient care time and development of skills exists in the face of restricted work hours, programs struggle to find sufficient time in the curriculum to devote to IPE. Time in the simulation lab or in-situ clinical arenas may be preferentially dedicated to improving technical or medical decision-making skills. Programs may be loath to prioritize resource-intensive time for "soft" skills such as interpersonal skills, communication or professionalism.

Resources

MedEdPORTAL Publications [https://www.mededportal.org/] is a program of the AAMC providing open access health professions education curricula which have been classroom tested and are disseminated for implementation [32]. A collection of IPE resources is available and has been assembled in conjunction with IPEC, the American Psychological Association, Physician Assistant Education Association and the American Physical Therapy Association. These resources include cases, assessment tools, multimedia presentations, tutorials, faculty guides, references, and even simulator programming. This collection represents ready-to-use, peer-reviewed, established curriculum, and is recommended as an excellent initial resource for educators tasked with implementing IPE in their institution.

The Agency for Healthcare Quality and Research and the Department of Defense have developed TeamSTEPPS® 2.0, an evidence-based, free educational program to improve teamwork, collaboration and communication [33]. TeamSTEPPS® 2.0 is widely regarded as a standard-setting curriculum. Resources include lecture slides, workshop tools, instructor development guides, and measurement tools. Measurement tools include scales to evaluate learners' perceptions and attitudes toward teamwork (TeamSTEPPS® Teamwork Attitudes Questionnaire T-TAQ) and measure observed team performance. T-TAQ measures attitudes in domains of team structure, leadership, communication, situation monitoring and mutual support. Wong et al. used T-TAQ to measure the impact of simulated emergency patient training for emergency medicine residents and emergency nurses; they found improved scores in four of five teamwork domains [11] Statistically significant improvement in scores for team structure (6.4%, $p < 0.0001$), leadership (2.8%, $p = 0.029$), situation monitoring (4%, $p = 0.014$), and mutual support (4%, $p = 0.003$) were demonstrated; however baseline scores for each section were already above 4 on a scale of 5.

The American College of Surgeons (ACS), in collaboration with the Association for Surgical Education (ASE) and Association of Program Directors in Surgery (APDS), has developed simulation-based team training curricula for residents [www.facs.org/education/program] [34]. The ACS/APDS/ASE Resident Prep Curriculum and the ACS/APDS Surgery Resident Skills Curriculum contain interprofessional team-based scenarios including mock pages, transitions of care, and trauma resuscitation that can be adapted for IPE use by surgical, anesthesiology or emergency medicine programs.

Tools for measuring learners' perceptions, readiness or attitudes towards IPE have been translated into various languages. The Interdisciplinary Education Perception Scale (IEPS) was designed to measure student perceptions relative to their professions and other allied health disciplines [35]. IEPS measures attitudes considered important to the interprofessional setting including one's own professional competency and autonomy (self-efficacy), the need for professional cooperation, perception of current cooperation across professions, and valuation of contributions and resource-sharing from other professions. Mendel used IEPS to demonstrate statistically significant improved attitudes after IPE cardiopulmonary bypass simulations including nurse anesthetist students and perfusionist students [12]. However, the baseline characteristics of the students revealed high pre-simulation scores, and it is unclear how small improvements on the scale correspond to real life behaviors or attitudes. Thresholds of meaningful changes and effect size in IPE program outcomes remain largely unstudied.

The Readiness for Interprofessional Learning Scale (RIPLS) was designed to evaluate student readiness for shared learning by measuring attitudes and perceptions in teamwork and collaboration, professional identity and professional roles [36]. Rossler and Kimble used RIPLS to evaluate the effect of a high-fidelity human patient simulation for nursing, administration, respiratory therapy and physical therapy students [37] In the domain of negative professional identity, which included items such as "I don't want to waste my time learning with other healthcare students," physical therapy students maintained low post-IPE scores. These learners did not assess group learning as valuable to their profession and the authors posit that the simulation itself may not have been well suited to this profession. RIPLS may thus be a useful tool for program evaluation, to determine the correct fit of the simulation for each learner's profession. Studies with nursing students, social work students and medical students have shown improved RIPLS post-simulation intervention scores [13, 38].

A profession-specific scale called the Jefferson Scale of Attitudes Toward Physician-Nurse Collaboration (JSATPNC) was developed to assess attitudes towards collaboration in four domains; shared education and collaborative relationships; caring as opposed to curing, nurse autonomy, and physician authority [39]. Garber et al. reported significant interprofessional differences in the total JSATPNC for practicing nurses, physicians and residents in a single health system [40]. Nurse scores reflected a more positive attitude toward collaboration than physician/resident scores (52.3 versus 50.88, $p = 0.014$). Salam et al. reported nurse and resident JSATPNC attitudes after a standardized patient acute pain management experience [14]. Participants were very supportive of IPE before the intervention (73.7% strongly agreed), and after the intervention there was a shift toward even stronger support (83.9% strongly agreed, $p = 0.078$). The view that the nurse should be viewed as a collaborator and colleague with the physician also significantly increased after the intervention (82.5–92.9%, $p = 0.04$).

The use of scales such as the JSATPNC to determine the impact of a simulated intervention may not be as meaningful when the pre-intervention scores are already high. However, other applications include use for institutional needs assessment surveys, evaluation of the differential impact of programs between professions, and to serve as debriefing or content guides following educational activities.

American College of Surgeons (ACS) developed a program in 2005 for regional support to establish a consortium of Accredited Educational Institutes (AEI). Accreditation is conferred to programs that meet rigorous standards for simulation-based surgical education at two levels, depending on the learners served, curriculum offered, and availability of technology and resources [41]. These regional centers are intended to provide surgical education support for medical students, residents, attendings and other surgical healthcare providers to meet or maintain certification requirements, and accomplish competency requirements and surgical milestones. A complete list of accredited centers and the process for applying for accreditation is available on the ACS website [https://www.facs.org/education/accreditation/aei] [42]. Training programs or providers in institutions without a rigorous simulation-based curriculum for training, directors or individuals can seek training in one of the consortium AEIs.

Quantifying the Impact

Knowledge, skills and attitudes gained from IPE are most commonly measured and reported in domains of interpersonal skills, communication skills and professionalism. Assessment of residents' progress in these ACGME competencies may be a measurable and reportable metric of the activity and quality of the institution's IPE program. The 360-degree evaluation process, eliciting feedback not only from faculty, but from peers, students, patients and other non-physician healthcare staff, is ideally suited for this type of assessment. Ogunyemi et al. reported on the feedback gained from nurses regarding obstetrics/gynecology residents' rapport with patients, interaction with staff, and professionalism [43]. There was strong internal correlation between the nurses' evaluations but weaker correlation with the faculty's evaluations. These results suggest that the feedback was unique and would not have been illuminated without this type of evaluation.

360-degree evaluations are utilized at the ACGME program level as a contribution to individual resident specialty-specific Milestones. The ACGME six common core competencies are supplemented by specialty-specific sub-competencies, varying from 10 to 43 sub-competencies. Milestone achievement criteria are determined at the specialty program level. Seeking a tool to track milestone data, some programs have used radar plots as a visual representation of resident competencies to track individual milestone progress, to inform evaluation decisions, to guide learning needs, and to facilitate feedback. Radar plots are a method of displaying multiple quantitative variables on axes originating from the same point, with angles of the axes being equal. Data points between the axes can be connected resulting in the shape of a radar or spider web. Harrington et al. used radar plots in a surgical residency as a summative assessment of a resident's progress through the 16 surgical milestones [44]. Individual areas of weakness were identified by a concavity in the radar plot and did not require extensive training for faculty comprehension, interpretation, or use. Radar plots were used by the program's clinical competency committee to guide discussions on a resident's progress, leading to increased efficiency in identification of focus areas for remediation. Related milestones such as professionalism and interpersonal/communication skills were plotted in axes next to each other to determine if a pervasive problem exists in that area. The radar plots could also be used as a formative assessment of a resident's progress through the milestones by tracking the effect of IPE or identifying areas that could be remediated by further IPE.

An institutional method of determining the impact of and the need for IPE is assessment of the safety climate, reflecting frontline healthcare providers' perceptions and attitudes toward patient safety related factors. A frequently used safety climate measurement tool is the validated Safety Attitudes Questionnaire, which includes inquiry in six domains of safety culture: (1) teamwork climate, (2) job satisfaction, (3) perceptions of management, (4) safety climate, (5) working conditions and (6) stress recognition [45]. The instrument includes items regarding collaboration with other professionals, communication and teamwork – items addressed during IPE activities. The Safety Attitudes Questionnaire can be used to identify IPE focus areas for improvement/intervention and to subsequently assess effectiveness of a tailored intervention, at a unit, department, institutional, or organizational level.

The ACGME monitoring process for accredited programs requires resident/fellow and faculty participation in annual surveys to provide an early-warning system for program non-compliance with accreditation standards. Specific content areas for both residents/fellows and faculty include teamwork and patient safety [46]. Trainees are expected to learn to work effectively in interprofessional teams as a condition of program accreditation. The ACGME measures and assesses program compliance with this mandate, regardless of explicit program IPE curricular content, or skill/knowledge acquisition by other methods such as clinical experience.

Conclusion

IPE simulation has been used as an effective teaching tool to improve attitudes, knowledge, skill and, in some studies, patient care outcomes. Simulation-based IPE comes in many forms, including high-fidelity human patient simulators, standardized patients, and virtual reality. IPE can be delivered using a variety of educational constructs: team-based, hospital in-situ, simulation centers, traditional courses, or recurring and "just in time" learning. Logistical, methodological, and attitudinal challenges exist for implementation of IPE, yet there are significant existing support resources for program development of IPE. Evaluating and quantifying the impact of IPE endeavors can enhance participation and sustain support for this critical piece of graduate medical education.

References

1. IOM. Health Professions Education: a bridge to quality. In: Greiner AC, Knebel E, editors. Institute of Medicine Committee on the Health Professions Education Summit. Washington, D.C.; 2003.
2. ACGME. ACGME Common Program Requirements, A.C.f.G.M. Education, editor. 2016 rev.
3. ACGME and ABS. The General Surgery Milestone Project, American Council for Graduate Medical Education and American Board of Surgery, editors. 2015.
4. ACGME and ABR. The Diagnostic Radiology Milestone Project, American Council for Graduate Medical Education and American Board of Radiology, editors. 2015.
5. Kirkpatrick DI. Evaluating training programs: the four levels. 2nd ed. San Francisco: Berrett-Koehler; 1998.
6. Capella J, et al. Teamwork training improves the clinical care of trauma patients. J Surg Educ. 2010;47(6):439–43.
7. Steinemann S, et al. In situ, multidisciplinary, simulation-based teamwork training improves early trauma care. J Surg Educ. 2011;68(3):472–7.
8. Pucher PH, et al. Nontechnical skills performance and care processes in the management of the acute trauma patient. Surgery. 2014;155:902–9.
9. Nishisaki A, et al. Effect of just-in-time simulation training on tracheal intubation procedure safety in the pediatric intensive care unit. Anesthesiology. 2010;113:214–23.
10. Nishisaki A, et al. Evaluation of multidisciplinary simulation training on clinical performance and team behavior during tracheal intubation procedures in a pediatric intensive care unit. Pediatr Crit Care Med. 2011;12(4):406–14.

11. Wong AH-W, et al. Making an "attitude adjustment" using a simulation-enhanced interprofessional education strategy to improve attitudes toward teamwork and communication. Simul Healthc. 2016;11:117–25.
12. Mendel S. Interdisciplinary simulation using the cardiopulmonary bypass simulator. J Extra Corpor Technol. 2014;46:300–4.
13. Miller A, et al. Can a single brief intervention improve participants' readiness for interprofessional learning? J Interprof Care. 2013;27(6):532–3.
14. Salam T, Saylor JL, Cowperthwait AL. Attitudes of nurse and physician trainees towards an interprofessional simulated education experience on pain assessment and management. J Interprof Care. 2015;29(3):276–8.
15. Falcone RA, et al. Multidisciplinary pediatric trauma team training using high fidelity trauma simulation. J Pediatr Surg. 2008;43:1065–71.
16. Sweeney A, et al. Senior pediatric residents as teachers for an innovative multidsciplinary mock code curriculum. J Grad Med Educ. 2011;3(3):446.
17. Patterson MD, et al. In situ simulation: detection of safety threats and teamwork training in a high risk emergency department. BMJ Qual Saf. 2013;22:468–77.
18. Couto TB, et al. Team skills in actual, in situ, and in-center pediatric emergencies: performance levels across settings and perceptions of comparative educational impact. Simul Healthc. 2015;10:76–84.
19. Salam T, Collins M, Baker A-M. All the world's a stage: integrating theater and medicine for interprofessional team building in physician and nurse residency programs. Ochsner J. 2012;12:359–62.
20. Bays AM, et al. Interprofessional communication skills training for serious illness, evaluation of a small-group, simulated patient intervention. J Palliat Med. 2014;17(2):159–66.
21. Caylor S, et al. The use of virtual simulation and a modified teamSTEPPS training for multiprofessional education. Clin Simul Nurs. 2015;11(3):163–71.
22. McGrath JL, et al. Using virtual reality simulation environments to assess competence of emergency medicine learners. Acad Emerg Med. 2018;25:186–95.
23. AAMC. Curriculum inventory and reports. 2016 [cited 2017 March 20]. Available from: http://www.aamc.org/initiatives/cir/.
24. van Schaik SM, Plant J, O'Brien B. Challenges of interprofessional team training: a qualitative analysis of residents' perceptions. Educ Health. 2015;28(1):52–7.
25. Phrampus PE, O'Donnell JM. Debriefing using a structured and supported approach. In: Levine AI, et al., editors. The comprehensive textbook of healthcare simulation. New York: Springer Science & Business Media; 2013. p. 73–84.
26. Lagan C, et al. Evaluation of an interprofessional clinician-patient communication workshop utilizing standardized patient methodology. J Surg Educ. 2013;70(1):95–103.
27. van Schaik SM, et al. Does source matter? Nurses' and physicians' perceptions of interprofessional feedback. Med Educ. 2016;50(2):181–8.
28. Stefanidis D, et al. Are nursing students appropriate partners for interdisciplinary training of surgery residents. J Surg Educ. 2015;72(5):823–8.
29. Schlitzkus LL, et al. What do surgical nurses know about surgical residents. J Surg Educ. 2009;66(6):383–91.
30. Steinemann S, et al. Role confusion and self-assessment in interprofessional trauma teams. Am J Surg. 2016;211:482–8.
31. ACGME. ACGME Task Force on Quality Care and Professionalism, Philibert I and Amis S, editors. Chicago; 2011.
32. Interprofessional Education Collection. MedEdPORTAL Publications [cited 2017 March 17]. Available from: http://www.mededportal.org/collections/ipe/.
33. AHRQ. TeamSTEPPS(R) 2.0. 2016. Available from: http://www.ahrq.gov/teamstepps/instructor/index.html.
34. American College of Surgeons Educational Programs. [cited 2017 March 20]. Available from: http://www.facs.org/education/program.

35. Luecht RM, et al. Assessing professional perceptions: design and validation of an interdisciplinary education perception scale. J Allied Health. 1990;19(2):181–91.
36. Parsell G, Bligh J. The development of a questionnaire to assess the readiness of health care students for interprofessional learning (RIPLS). Med Educ. 1999;33(2):95–100.
37. Rossler KL, Kimble LP. Capturing readiness to learn and collaboration as exposured with an interprofessional simulation scenario: a mixed-methods research study. Nurse Educ Today. 2016;36:348–53.
38. Murphy JI, Nimmagadda J. Partnering to provide simulated learning to address Interprofessional Education Collaborative core competencies. J Interprof Care. 2015;29(3):258–9.
39. Hojat M, et al. Psychometric properties of an attitude scale measuring physician-nurse collaboration. Eval Health Prof. 1999;22(2):208–20.
40. Garber JS, et al. Attitudes towards collaboration and servant leadership among nurses, physicians and residents. J Interprof Care. 2009;23(4):331–40.
41. Sachdeva AK, Pellegrini CA, Johnson KA. Support for simulation-based surgical education through American College of Surgeons – Accredited Education Institutes. World J Surg. 2008;32:196–207.
42. American College of Surgeons Accredited Education Institutes. [cited 2017 March 20]. Available from: https://www.facs.org/education/accreditation/aei.
43. Ogunyemi D, et al. From the eye of the nurses: 360-degree evaluation of residents. J Contin Educ Health Prof. 2009;29(2):105–10.
44. Harrington DT, et al. What shape is your resident in? Using a radar plot to guide a milestone clinical competency discussion. J Surg Educ. 2015;72(6):e294–8.
45. Sexton JB, et al. The safety attitudes questionnaire: psychometric properties, benchmarking data, and emerging research. BMC Health Serv Res. 2006;6:44.
46. ACGME. Resident/Fellow and Faculty Surveys [cited 2017 March 17]. Data Collection Systems. Available from: http://www.acgme.org/Data-Collection-Systems/Resident-Fellow-and-Faculty-Surveys.

Simulation-Based Training for Interprofessional Teams of Practicing Clinicians

14

Jamie M. Robertson, Suzanne B. Klainer, Dorothy M. Bradley, Steven Yule, and Douglas S. Smink

Introduction

Team training fosters communication skills and teamwork, thereby improving patient safety in a variety of healthcare settings [1]. In the operating room (OR), communication breakdowns have been identified as a leading cause of intraoperative error [2–4]. Analysis of closed-claims data from malpractice insurers have shown that communication issues are associated with malpractice claims against both surgeons and anesthesiologists [3]. More importantly, the majority of the injuries and errors that occur as a result of communication breakdowns are considered preventable.

J. M. Robertson
STRATUS Center for Medical Simulation, Brigham and Women's Hospital, Boston, MA, USA

S. B. Klainer
Brigham and Women's Hospital, Department of Anesthesia, Harvard Medical School, Boston, MA, USA

D. M. Bradley
Center for Nursing Excellence, Brigham and Women's Hospital, Boston, MA, USA

S. Yule
Brigham & Women's Hospital/Harvard Medical School, STRATUS Center for Medical Simulation, Boston, MA, USA

D. S. Smink (✉)
Department of Surgery, Harvard Medical School, Boston, MA, USA

Center for Surgery and Public Health, Brigham and Women's Hospital, Boston, MA, USA
e-mail: dsmink@bwh.harvard.edu

J. T. Paige et al. (eds.), *Comprehensive Healthcare Simulation: InterProfessional Team Training and Simulation*, Comprehensive Healthcare Simulation,
https://doi.org/10.1007/978-3-030-28845-7_14

Interprofessional education (IPE) in communication and teamwork for residents has been employed in the OR setting, with teams of surgical and anesthesia trainees working together or teams of surgical trainees and nurses working together [5, 6]. Less frequently, full teams that include attending surgeons, anesthesiologists and nursing staff, have trained together in formal programs [7].

There are numerous barriers to providing simulation-based training to attending physicians together in an interprofessional setting. First, securing time away from clinical activities for multiple professional groups at the same time is difficult. There is a high opportunity cost for individuals to be out of the OR and clinic for any significant period of time due to the loss of revenue. Second, time scheduled for out-of-OR activities is typically taken up by faculty meetings, teaching, continuing education courses and other administrative responsibilities. Third, arranging schedules to allow all participants to be away from clinical requirements at the same time requires a great deal of planning, support, and administrative effort in order to achieve the program goals. Finally, simulation centers often do not have the money or expertise that is necessary to run programs at this level. Space limitations, technical resources, and staffing are all considerations for the level of fidelity necessary to engage learners from all disciplines in the simulation.

At Brigham and Women's Hospital in Boston, Massachusetts, we have been running an interprofessional team training program for full OR teams since 2011. Sponsored by The Risk Management Foundation of the Harvard Medical Institutions Incorporated (CRICO/RMF), the malpractice insurer of the Harvard-affiliated hospitals, these team-training sessions have provided training in closed-loop and directed communication, leadership and followership, and speaking-up regarding patient safety concerns to teams of attending surgeons, attending anesthesiologists, and practicing OR nurses and surgical technicians. This chapter will cover the process and strategies used in the planning and implemention of our interprofessional OR team training program.

Planning

Bringing together diverse professions and disciplines to participate in a half-day course on communication and teamwork is a daunting task. It is both labor- and cost-intensive to take time away from clinical practice to engage in continuing education. Despite this, the importance of providing training for teams that work together in a high-stakes environment similar to their actual practice is well established [8]. In 2010, CRICO/RMF, the malpractice insurer of the Harvard-affiliated hospitals, began the process of developing a simulation-based team training course to train OR teams within the Harvard system.

CRICO/RMF met with surgery and simulation leaders in Boston to discuss the feasibility of conducting simulation-based OR team training with full OR teams, including attending surgeons, attending anesthesiologists and OR nurses [9]. As a result, four test sites (Brigham and Women's Hospital, Beth Israel Deaconess Medical Center, Boston Children's Hospital and Massachusetts General Hospital) were chosen to participate in an eighteen-month pilot study to determine whether full OR team training was feasible.

The pilot study successfully trained 221 individuals from the four participating hospitals. Each hospital implemented their own version of the OR team training with simulation program, utilizing simulation and faculty resources within their institution. While each program was unique, they all included key elements within the learning objectives and simulation scenarios. The objectives of the course were to utilize the safe surgical checklist, speak up about patient safety concerns in the OR and to use closed-loop communication. The details of the scenarios in the program were ultimately left up to the faculty but were required to include one case that occurred in an out-of-OR environment, such as the pre- or post-operative care unit, and a case that involved significant blood loss.

Participant responses on the course evaluations overwhelmingly indicated that the course was both valuable and beneficial. In addition, the simulation teams demonstrated that they were able to create a high-fidelity environment for all of the participants, with 94% reporting that they found the scenarios realistic and 93% reporting that the scenarios prompted realistic responses.

After successful completion of the pilot program, CRICO/RMF created a grant to help fund a full team-training program for 3 years. The Harvard-affiliated hospitals, including Brigham and Women's Hospital, received funding for OR team training with simulation. In March 2014, our team at Brigham and Women's Hospital began training full OR teams using high-fidelity simulation. In preparation, we assembled the faculty expertise, institutional support and simulation collateral necessary to run a successful program.

In the 3 years since then, the program has changed and expanded. Though the course objectives and teaching points remain the same, the course and simulation training sessions have matured as the simulation center has grown and expanded its expertise. We have developed higher fidelity surgical training models, allowing our operations team to better control the rate of blood loss during simulated surgery. Additionally, we have iteratively added equipment and medications commonly requested by the teams during the scenarios. We have also adjusted the order in which the scenarios are presented to the participants. Originally, we had participants complete the out-of-OR scenario first. After several iterations, we instead chose to complete one of the OR scenarios first, offering participants an opportunity to work in a typical work environment as they adjust to the simulation setting.

Logistics

Participant Recruitment

Support from department chairs and division chiefs, as well as other key members of departments, has been key to the success of our program. The endorsement by these high-level members of the institution encourages participation and also ensures that participants take their engagement in the course seriously. Presentations during faculty meetings and grand rounds events, in addition to other means of encouragement have greatly contributed to participation in the program. Most department chairs and division chiefs have taken the course themselves and personally recommended it to the rest of their staff. In addition to these methods, we hear from participants that they specifically signed up for the course because colleagues who had participated in the course recommended and endorsed it. As planning begins for training for a new surgical specialty, leaders of that department are contacted. The course director meets with the division chief and any other key leadership figures to discuss the program, answer questions, and encourage participation.

Each session of our OR team training course includes a full OR team of two attending surgeons, two attending anesthesiologists, and two members of the OR nursing staff. After dates are arranged with the simulation center, emails are sent to the scheduling offices of each surgical department. Typically, emails listing the available dates are sent out to the members of the department and they are asked to sign-up for an available timeslot.

Anesthesiologists have a long history of simulation-based education. This type of training is an expectation of all attending anesthesiologists at Brigham and Women's Hospital and mandated by CRICO in order to obtain medical malpractice insurance at a reduced rate. Our anesthesiologists are divided into "pods" and routinely work with the same sub-specialty services. Whenever possible we attempt to schedule the anesthesiologist with surgeons, nurses and scrub technologists from the pod where they routinely work. However, when an anesthesiologist requires training to stay current with their CRICO requirements, they may be scheduled with a service with which they work less frequently. The Anesthesiology Scheduling Office, who makes the daily operating room schedule, does all scheduling for the anesthesiologists. Anesthesiologists are emailed available dates when they are due for training and have been eager to participate in the simulation training.

OR nurses and surgical technicians who attend the course receive relief from that portion of their shift for the day. As the nursing staff is key to the success of this program, we have worked closely with the OR nurse educators and nurse managers to identify staff to attend and ensure that the program is beneficial for their staff and educators. Nurses and OR techs are scheduled a month in advance to accommodate OR staffing. The nurses and OR techs are chosen, in most circumstances, by specialty area.

Participant Benefits

CRICO/RMF provides incentives to attendees in the form of malpractice insurance refunds. For surgeons who participant in the course, they receive 10% off their malpractice insurance rate for the year. Surgeons at our institution are not mandated to attend the course, but the rebate does provide incentive for the surgeon and their department. In the initial planning stages, we predicted that two-thirds of eligible surgeons would register for the course. So far, we have been successful in getting roughly 90% of eligible surgeons to attend, with nearly 100% participation from certain surgical divisions.

Anesthesiologists who participate in the course also receive a malpractice insurance discount for attending; however, at our institution the anesthesia department pays the malpractice insurance for providers in the department. As such, the anesthesia department mandates that all attending anesthesiologists attend simulation-based courses in order to receive the discount. Most anesthesiologists choose this course as they appreciate the interprofessional team approach, which is absent from most other qualifying courses.

Both surgeons and anesthesiologists receive 4.5 Category I Continuing Medical Education (CME) credits, which are designated as Risk Management. Nursing participants receive 4.5 Continuing Education credits from our institution for attending the course. Nurses attend during their normal paid work hours and are given leave from the OR for the duration of the course.

A total of 64 OR teams, consisting of 112 attending surgeons, 119 attending anesthesiologists, 122 OR nurses/scrub technicians, have attended the course since March 2014. As scheduled cases, sick leave, vacations and other events occasionally keep the course from scheduling a full team of individuals, we sometimes substitute residents or fellows into the course in order to ensure that course runs properly. During this time, five senior surgical residents participated in the course in place of an attending surgeon. While the course is designed for attending physicians to learn from and with one another, cancelling a course limits the number of sessions we are able to run each year and potentially means that others who originally signed up for that date will no longer be able to participate. We have found that senior residents and fellows are able to fully participate in the course and engage in the debriefings. We occasionally encounter hierarchical issues when trainees and attendings participate in training together. While the course is not an evaluation of performance for any team member, trainees may be concerned that their performance during the simulation and comments on institutional practice and culture in the debriefing will be used outside of the course. To counter this issue, we always discuss confidentiality at the beginning and end of the course, stressing that performance in the simulation center is not discussed outside of the simulation center. In our experience, the course is valuable experience for all involved, including trainees.

Scenario Design

One of the key features of our team training program is that there are very few prescribed features of the program. Each institution brings a range of knowledge, experience and resources to the project, in addition to a unique population of physicians with distinct needs. As a result, each of the affiliated institutions has had the ability to create a program that best fits the strengths and expertise of the faculty and simulation center.

Learning Objectives and Case Requirements

For our program, CRICO identified three major learning objectives: (1) consistent use of closed loop communication for communicating important information and requests to the team; (2) speaking up with new or changing information related to concerns for patient safety; and (3) proper and consistent use of the WHO Safe Surgery Checklist. In addition, at least one scenario needed to be an event outside of the operating room and one scenario needed to involve hemorrhage.

The initial scenarios were developed by an interprofessional team that included a surgeon, OR nurse, simulation operations specialists, anesthesiologist, and medical education expert. The combined expertise in simulation technology, clinical medicine, technical skills, role assignments and clarity for each team member, educational principles and evidence-based practice allowed for robust scenarios designed to achieve the learning objectives. In development of the initial scenarios, a key concern was to ensure that each one included elements to challenge and engage all member of the OR team as equally as possible. As such, no scenario is simply an "anesthesia problem" or a "surgery problem". It was important to include multiple opportunities for participants to demonstrate and practice each of the learning objectives for the session. Each scenario includes multiple areas where members of various teams need to communicate critical pieces of information in a timely fashion. In addition, there are multiple opportunities for various individuals to speak up about potential patient safety issues that have been built into the scenarios.

Scenarios

Two of the three cases included in the course are conducted in the OR. For each of these cases, participants receive a specialty-specific (surgeon, anesthesiologist, or nurse perspective) handout to read prior to the start of the case. These handouts include basic information on the patient, including chief complaint, history and physical exam, pre-operative lab results and a plan for the surgery. Each specialty also receives some unique pieces of information that is specific to their role and which they might normally have more knowledge of than other team members in the clinical environment. For example, the anesthesia handout includes information about the airway exam and any history of a difficult airway that is not included in the surgery or nursing handouts.

The first OR case is designed to be a tumor resection that results in massive blood loss during the case. The learning objectives of the case are as follows: (1) Describe the correct use of the surgical safety checklist, (2) demonstrate speaking up about new information during a case, and (3) provide examples of good closed-loop communication. The participants enter the room after the patient has been prepped, draped and induced. They are told that they have a few minutes to orient themselves to the room and the equipment and that they should begin the case by going through the surgery portion of the Safe Surgery Checklist. Once they complete the checklist, the surgery begins. A model made of gelatin, IV tubing, a simulated tumor and fake blood is used to create surgical fidelity during the case [10]. There are several pieces of information about the patient that must be effectively communicated during the case. For example, the nursing staff read prior to the scenario that the patient reported a penicillin allergy to a nurse at the last minute. This is in contrast to the printed records and other handouts that reported that the patient had no known drug allergies. During the case, one of the units of blood that is sent into the case when requested is actually labeled for the wrong patient. The scenario concludes when either the team is able to stop the bleeding or when the participants are in a holding pattern waiting for additional support from another service.

The second case occurs in the post-anesthesia care unit (PACU). The specific learning objectives for this case are as follows: (1) speaking up about new and changing clinical events, (2) use closed-loop and directed communication in a critical situation, and (3) explain the role of a leader in a critical situation. Unlike the OR cases, the participants do not receive handouts or have time to prepare before the start of this case. Instead, a non-clinical team-based activity is interrupted by a faculty member who informs the team that one of their patients in the PACU is having difficulty breathing and needs help. In most cases, this scenario involves a post-surgery patient that develops a pulmonary embolism (PE) and goes into a pulseless electrical activity (PEA) arrest. As the team treats the patient with cardiopulmonary resuscitation (CPR) and medications, the patient's rhythm converts to ventricular fibrillation. After appropriate CPR and defibrillation, the patient recovers.

The third case (and second OR scenario) begins prior to the anesthesia huddle that occurs prior to intubation and induction. The learning objectives for the case are as follows: (1) discuss patient care concerns collaboratively in an interprofessional team, (2) display use of closed-loop communication during a crisis, and (3) speak up about potentially unsafe patient care situations. In this case, the participants meet an awake patient who is able to answer basic questions and confirm information. The patient is undergoing surgery on a specific side of his or her body, but the surgeons' prior knowledge of the side is opposite to what the other team members read. In addition, the patient is site marked on the incorrect side. The team must agree on the appropriate course of action, after talking to the patient, looking at the available imaging and consulting the patient chart and consent forms. No matter what the participants decide, the next phase of the scenario involves the patient suffering from an allergic reaction to one of the pre-medications given prior to the start of the scenario. The patient suffers airway compromise, and the team is forced to begin the difficult airway algorithm. In most cases, the result is that the surgeons must perform an emergent cricothyroidotomy. Once the patient's airway is restored, the team must decide whether or not to continue with the procedure or cancel the case and send the patient to one of the hospital units.

Specialty Adjustments

As we have progressed through various surgical specialties, we have modified the above scenarios in order to meet the needs of the new group. In each case, we try and retain the overall structure of the scenarios in order to continue to include the elements that have been tried, tested and reviewed over the course of numerous trainings. However, each specialty has required multiple tweaks to the cases in order to allow the surgeons to perform simulated operations that would be within their practice parameters. For example, where general surgeons were asked to perform an inguinal hernia repair, thoracic surgeons were asked to perform wedge resection of a lung mass.

Though many of the elements of the scenarios remain consistent within each of the specialties, careful attention is paid to ensure that we maintain fidelity for each of the scenarios as they are changed. As a result, careful review of the equipment found in both the anesthesia cart as well as on the surgical instrument table in the real ORs is done to ensure the simulated environment closely approximates the real thing. Special trays of medications are created to provide the medications that would typically be present in these cases, as well as items that we anticipate may be requested throughout the surgery. Though it is impossible for the simulation center to obtain and stock all of the specialized surgical equipment that each surgeon might request during the surgery, we try to have at least the standard equipment prepared and ready to go.

As cases are developed for new surgical specialties, our simulation center performs two "dry runs" to practice the scenarios. The first dry run is a tabletop activity where faculty and operations staff go through each of the pieces and ensure that information is consistent throughout the curriculum, participant handouts, operation notes, and patient chart. This provides the chance for everyone to ask questions and ensure that there is a shared mental model about the flow of the scenarios. The second dry run is done with the rooms and manikins prepped as they would be on the day of the course. Faculty members stand in for participants during the run through and go through all of the actions that are expected to occur during the session. This is the last chance to identify items or information that are out of place or missing.

After the final dry run, all of the materials, including scenario and debriefing handouts for faculty members and participant handouts are finalized. Faculty guides are created with scenario write-ups, schedules and note pages to be used during the actual course.

Materials and Handouts

Paper copies of the patient chart are constructed with all of the standard forms and surgeon office notes that might be available for the case. Though much of the information contained in the chart is irrelevant and not reviewed by the participants, the availability of the records creates a certain level of fidelity as well as a rich patient background that they are able to draw upon during the case. Information about past surgical history, medication, history of present illness, living situation, social history, family medical history and preferred language are all included in the background information.

To accommodate differences in the composition of teams that work in the OR together we sometimes have to make additional adjustments in order to ensure the simulated experience is as close to the real OR as possible. For example, when we run the course for the cardiac surgery teams at our institutions, a full team included eight individuals due to the addition of a perfusionist and a physician assistant (PA). In order to continue to create an environment that was as close to the real OR as possible, we adjusted the composition and roles of the team in order to allow for them to train with the people they work with on a daily basis.

Faculty

We believe that having a faculty representative of the simulation participants is essential for conducting an OR team training curriculum. Just as we find that it is important for the participants to come together to learn from clinicians from different specialties and professions, we feel that our faculty greatly benefit from having a diverse range of background and experiences. Our faculty include an attending surgeon, attending anesthesiologists, OR nurse educators, simulation-based education experts and an organizational psychologist. Many, but not all, of our faculty members have an administrative function at the simulation center outside of teaching.

At any time, there are typically between five and seven members of our faculty who rotate facilitating sessions of the course, allowing for conferences, vacations, sick days and other competing priorities. This allows for us to staff each session with three to four faculty members. Faculty rotate roles throughout the session, providing didactic content, directing operations staff, serving as confederates, and debriefing the scenarios. As faculty members leave the institution for various reasons, efforts are made to replace them with a similarly qualified individual from the institution.

Faculty Roles

Faculty members take responsibility for course design, scenario development, didactic teaching, running scenarios and debriefing as part of their role in the course. Typically, each session is conducted with three to four faculty members present, allowing for faculty to rotate roles throughout the course. If multiple course sessions are envisaged, it makes sense to have a larger faculty than required, provide common training for the faculty, and then select specific faculty for each course. This reduces the burden on individual members and allows flexibility for multiple courses to be run at the same standard, with a different blend of faculty members.

On average, three to four members of our faculty participate in each session. One faculty member takes the lead on running the simulation scenario, including directing the simulation technicians in physiologic changes and other operational aspects of the scenario and answering the phone to talk to participants as the OR desk or blood bank. Two of the faculty members are focused on observing the actions and communication in the scenario and preparing for the debriefing. Occasionally, faculty members are needed to serve in embedded simulated participant roles ("confederates") during the scenarios. Participants are not scored or graded on any rubric system, but faculty observers take notes during the scenario on behaviors related to the learning objectives of the case. These notes are used in the debriefing to guide the discussion.

Selecting faculty for a particular course that reflects the variety of professional backgrounds of participants (e.g. surgeons, anesthesiologists, nurses, perfusionists) allows for a deeper and more credible learning experience than single discipline faculty (e,g, all surgeons). It has the added benefit of allowing expert knowledge to augment non-technical skills during debrief. Clinical knowledge is not sufficient, however, and having expertise in psychology, education, and research represented in the faculty team is also important to ensure that learning objectives are met. This also allows the simulation scenarios to be designed in a way that optimizes the physical and psychological fidelity of the scenarios in a way that maximizes that training potential.

Faculty Training

Prior to becoming course faculty, individuals must complete a training process. Studies have shown that debriefing is a key element to the success of team communication courses, as well as other simulation-based training courses [11–13]. As a requirement to join our faculty for this course, faculty members must complete a course in scenario debriefing from an appropriate educational provider. Potential faculty members also observe several courses in order to gain an understanding of the way the course works, participant reactions and debriefing styles of the other faculty members. If a course is also focused on formative assessment of non-technical skills of team members using tools like the NOTSS (Non-technical Skills for Surgeons) [14], then specific faculty development advice is available [15].

Once faculty members have completed a debriefing course, they are slowly introduced to the course through a series of guided debriefing experiences. In most cases, faculty start by debriefing pre-determined portions of the course under the mentorship of a senior faculty member. Feedback is provided via the Debriefing Assessment for Simulation in Healthcare (DASH) form [16]. The DASH scores debriefers on six element that have been shown to correspond to high-quality simulation-based learning experiences. The elements are setting the stage for an engaging learning experience, maintaining an engaging context for learning, structuring the debriefing in an organized way, provoking in-depth discussions that led participants to reflect on their performance, identifying what participants did well or poorly and why, and helping participants see how to improve or how to sustain good performance. Scores for each element range from 1 (extremely ineffective/detrimental) to 7 (extremely effective/outstanding). Feedback is provided to faculty both in quantitative scores and qualitative comments with constructive recommendations for improvement.

Session Logistics

The course begins with a brief introductory set of slides that include an introduction to the day, background on communication breakdowns and medical errors, course objectives and ground roles for simulation. Finally, participants engage in a non-clinical activity to prompt discussions of teamwork and role-clarity in the OR environment. A sample timeline is included in Table 14.1.

As many of the participants have not previously participated in a simulation course, we devote 10 minutes prior to the start of the simulations for introducing the participants to the simulation space, manikins, and supplies available at the center. A simulation specialist carefully explains the process of obtaining vital signs, listening for heart and respiratory sounds and performing procedures on the manikin. We also emphasize the process for calling consults and other phone numbers from the room and using the basic available supplies. The participants are encouraged to spend several minutes examining the manikin to gain comfort with the simulated environment. The tour ends in the OR when the participants are divided into professional groups for a more specific introduction to the equipment that they will be using. Specifically, the surgeons are introduced to the available surgical instruments as well as the surgical field and the process for making an incision in the model. Anesthesiologists are given basic instruction for use of the anesthesia machine in the room, as well as time to ensure that the anesthesia cart is stocked appropriately. Nursing staff are provided with information on making phone calls, obtaining equipment and working various machines around the OR.

Each of the three cases takes roughly 20 minutes and is followed by a 40 minute debriefing led by two of the faculty members. There is an additional set of slides covering closed-loop communication and speaking-up that are taught between the end of the first debriefing and the start of the second case. Along with these slides, participants engage in a teambuilding activity meant to help stimulate continued discussion.

Once all three cases and debriefings have concluded, participants are asked to go around the room and identify one learning point that they will take away from the session and back to their OR. This point can be related to the course objectives or to any other part of the course that the participant found useful. Finally, before they

Table 14.1 Sample Course Agenda

7:00 AM	Arrival and Breakfast
7:10 AM	Introductions and Course Overview
7:40 AM	Tour of Simulation Lab
8:00 AM	Scenario 1
8:20 AM	Debrief Scenario 1
9:00 AM	Break
9:20 AM	Didactic: Communication and Speaking-Up
9:40 AM	Scenario 2
10:00 AM	Debrief Scenario 2
10:40 AM	Break
11:00 AM	Scenario 3
11:20 AM	Debrief Scenario 3
11:50 AM	Wrap-Up

leave participants must complete an anonymous course evaluation. This is required in order to provide them with CME credit and the malpractice insurance discount. The evaluation asks 26 Likert-type questions about general impressions, quality of simulation scenarios, quality of debriefing, learning outcomes from the session, and whether the course improved their ability to function as a team. There are also sections for qualitative comments and suggestions for the course.

Conclusion

Our OR Team Training Program has been successful in engaging surgeons, anesthesiologists, OR nurses, and scrub technologists over the past 3 years. One of the major keys to our success is the creation of an interprofessional faculty to design and implement the course. Our group is composed of surgeons, anesthesiologists, nurses and educators, who lend credibility to the training program for the attendees from their field, serve as advocates for the program in their department, and provide valuable insight during the planning stages. The careful planning and design of the simulations themselves is time- and resource-intensive, but essential to creating a high quality program that is engaging, educational and well-received. Frequent comments from participants about the realism of the scenario and their ability to see beyond the manikins demonstrate the importance of the planning stages. While there are numerous logistical difficulties in bringing together groups from around the hospital, including timing, money and training priorities, we have found that incentives help diminish some of these issues. Though we are able to provide malpractice insurance discounts to those who attend, incentives can also be provided through departmental leadership and continuing education hours. In summary, our team training program has continued to develop and expand over the last 3 years as a result of careful planning, hospital engagement and faculty commitment. This program has created a beneficial training tool for the staff, departments and hospital.

The course focuses on high-priority patient safety concerns for the hospital. By providing OR teams the opportunity to discuss in-depth the teamwork, communication and leadership skills that have been shown to lower errors in the operating room, this course seeks to create a culture within our institution that values the non-technical skills that lead to safer patient care. Like any skill, the use of directed and closed-loop communication, proper setting of expectations around patient care, and use of the safe surgery checklist require ongoing training and preparation [1, 14]. This simulation session provides an opportunity for reflective practice to key members of OR teams at our institutions. Participants are encouraged to continue practicing skills from the course during their daily clinical practice.

References

1. Burke CS, Salas E, Wilson-Donnelly K, Priest H. How to turn a team of experts into an expert medical team: guidance from the aviation and military communities. Qual Saf Health Care. 2004;13(Suppl 1):i96–104. https://doi.org/10.1136/qhc.13.suppl_1.i96.

2. Rogers SOJ, Gawande AA, Kwaan M, et al. Analysis of surgical errors in closed malpractice claims at 4 liability insurers. Surgery. 2006;140(1):25–33. https://doi.org/10.1016/j.surg.2006.01.008.
3. Griffen FD, Stephens LS, Alexander JB, et al. Violations of behavioral practices revealed in closed claims reviews. Ann Surg. 2008;248(3):468–74. https://doi.org/10.1097/SLA.0b013e318185e196.
4. Gawande AA, Zinner MJ, Studdert DM, Brennan TA. Analysis of errors reported by surgeons at three teaching hospitals. Surgery. 2003;133(6):614–21. https://doi.org/10.1067/msy.2003.169.
5. Tan SB, Pena G, Altree M, Maddern GJ. Multidisciplinary team simulation for the operating theatre: a review of the literature. ANZ J Surg. 2014;84(7–8):515–22. https://doi.org/10.1111/ans.12478.
6. Cumin D, Boyd MJ, Webster CS, Weller JM. A systematic review of simulation for multidisciplinary team training in operating rooms. Simul Healthc. 2013;8(3):171–9. https://doi.org/10.1097/SIH.0b013e31827e2f4c.
7. Robertson JM, Dias RD, Yule S, Smink DS. Operating room team training with simulation: a systematic review. J Laparoendosc Adv Surg Tech A. 2017;27(5):475–80. https://doi.org/10.1089/lap.2017.0043.
8. Kohn LT, Corrigan JM, Donaldson MS, editors. To Err Is Human: Building a Safer Health System. Washington, D.C.: National Academies Press; 2000. https://doi.org/10.17226/9728.
9. Arriaga AF, Gawande AA, Raemer DB, et al. Pilot testing of a model for insurer-driven, large-scale multicenter simulation training for operating room teams. Ann Surg. 2014;259(3):403–10. https://doi.org/10.1097/SLA.0000000000000342.
10. Berry W, Raemer D. The tumor: a simulator for open surgery. Simul Healthc. 2006;1(2):115.
11. Rudolph JW, Simon R, Dufresne RL, Raemer DB. There's no such thing as "nonjudgmental" debriefing: a theory and method for debriefing with good judgment. Simul Healthc. 2006;1(1):49–55.
12. Rudolph JW, Simon R, Rivard P, Dufresne RL, Raemer DB. Debriefing with good judgment: combining rigorous feedback with genuine inquiry. Anesthesiol Clin. 2007;25(2):361–76. https://doi.org/10.1016/j.anclin.2007.03.007.
13. Rudolph JW, Simon R, Raemer DB, Eppich WJ. Debriefing as formative assessment: closing performance gaps in medical education. Acad Emerg Med. 2008;15(11):1010–6. https://doi.org/10.1111/j.1553-2712.2008.00248.x.
14. Yule S, Flin R, Maran N, Rowley D, Youngson G, Paterson-Brown S. Surgeons' non-technical skills in the operating room: reliability testing of the NOTSS behavior rating system. World J Surg. 2008;32(4):548–56. https://doi.org/10.1007/s00268-007-9320-z.
15. Hull L, Arora S, Symons NRA, et al. Training faculty in nontechnical skill assessment: national guidelines on program requirements. Ann Surg. 2013;258(2):370–5. https://doi.org/10.1097/SLA.0b013e318279560b.
16. Brett-Fleegler M, Rudolph J, Eppich W, et al. Debriefing assessment for simulation in healthcare: development and psychometric properties. Simul Healthc. 2012;7(5):288–94. https://doi.org/10.1097/SIH.0b013e3182620228.

Simulation-Based Training for Assessment of Competency, Certification, and Maintenance of Certification

15

Scott C. Watkins

Introduction

Simulation-based training (SBT) is an education technique that enables clinician learners to practice and hone skills in an environment that replicates clinical practice without posing injury or harm to patients [1, 2]. Interprofessional education (IPE) has been defined by the World Health Organization as an education activity when "*students from 2 or more professions learn about, from, and with each other to enable effective collaboration and improve health (page 7)*" [3]. Interprofessional SBT embeds the learner in a realistic clinical team in a simulated clinical environment. The objective of interprofessional education (IPE) is to permit different professions to learn in a setting that is representative of their current or future practice [4]. Simulation-Based Training offers clinicians the opportunity to practice and evaluate the competency, proficiency and efficacy of their technical and non-technical skills [2, 5]. Simulation-Based Training IPE has been used extensively in undergraduate medical (UME) and nursing education and is now beginning to spread into graduate medical education (GME), continuing medical education (CME), continuing professional development (CPD) and maintenance of certification (MOC) [6, 7].

Evolution of Healthcare Education and Training

Traditionally, clinicians have been taught in discipline and specialty specific silos limiting the ability to learn from interactions with other clinicians and limiting the ability to learn to practice in an increasingly team-based healthcare system [4, 8–10]. Modern healthcare systems are intrinsically team-based, yet the skills needed

S. C. Watkins (✉)
Vanderbilt University Medical Center, Department of Anesthesiology, Nashville, TN, USA
e-mail: scott.c.watkins.md@gmail.co

J. T. Paige et al. (eds.), *Comprehensive Healthcare Simulation: InterProfessional Team Training and Simulation*, Comprehensive Healthcare Simulation,
https://doi.org/10.1007/978-3-030-28845-7_15

to function in such systems are not traditionally taught nor are they inherent to novice or even seasoned clinicians [4]. Today's clinician must possess the ability to foster development of shared mental models, participate in shared decision-making, and care for patients with varying degrees of self-engagement from the medically illiterate to the fully engaged, technologically savvy healthcare consumer. The transition from training in silos to training as teams has been driven in part by the recognition that failures in clinical practice are often related to failures in team-based and non-technical skills (NTS) of providers. The landmark patient safety report *To Err Is Human: Building a Safer Health System* identified breakdowns in communication, teamwork and other acts of human error as some of the leading contributors to errors in healthcare [11]. The recognition that breakdowns in healthcare teams contribute to patient harm has been substantiated by other organizations and investigators since the publication of *To Err is Human* [11–15]. The Joint Commission identified "communication" as the root cause in 60% of reported sentinel events from 2011 to 2013 [12]. Kohn and colleagues suggested that many adverse events in healthcare could be avoided with improved teamwork and that interprofessional miscommunication is one of the primary barriers to effective teamwork in healthcare [11–15]. Simulation-based training IPE is particularly useful for helping clinicians improve non-technical (NTS) and team-based practice skills. Nearly two decades after Kohn and colleagues called for team training to improve patient safety, the use of SBT and IPE SBT are slowly integrating into all levels of clinical training. Simulation-based training and IPE have reached a tipping point in undergraduate clinical training, and are now rapidly expanding into post-graduate training, continuing professional development, primary certification and maintenance of certification (MOC) [16].

Evolution from Time-Based to Competency-Based Healthcare Education

Traditionally, clinicians including physicians, nurses and other healthcare professionals have obtained degrees, certification and/or licensure through completion of a period of training followed by a knowledge based assessment [17]. This method has been very effective in producing clinicians that "know" and "know how" but does nothing to ensure that these clinicians are competent to practice, i.e. "shows how" and "does" [18]. A number of changes associated with the modern healthcare system have led to calls for outcome-based education and competency-based certification/licensure [19–21]. Outcome or competency-based education requires that a clinician demonstrate competence before being allowed to treat patients or perform specific procedures. The requirement that competence be demonstrated prior to engaging in patient care opens the door for simulation, which can assess competence in a setting that approximates clinical care [19]. This has led to widespread calls for a shift from "time-based" education to "competency-based" education for clinicians. The call for competency-based education has come from many fronts including clinicians, healthcare employers, patients, insurance companies, healthcare accreditation agencies and the public, and is driven by expectations for higher quality and safer care [2, 22–24]. As a result, a number of organizations and certifying bodies have incorporated simulation-based education and assessment modalities to ensure competence including the Medical Council of Canada (Canada - physicians), General Medical Council (United Kingdom - physicians), National Board of Osteopathic Medical Examiners (America - osteopathic physicians) and the United States Medical Licensing Examination (America - allopathic physicians) [25–27]. In addition to the above agencies, numerous other credentialing, specialty, government, and educational agencies, have recognized the value of SBT for training and assessment of clinicians [26, 28, 29]. Building on the World Health Organization's report on interprofessional education, a group of health professional educators representing American schools of nursing, medicine, dentistry, pharmacy and public health convened an expert panel in 2011 to develop a list of core competencies for interprofessional collaborative (IPC) practice [3, 30, 31]. The panel identified the following core competencies for interprofessional collaborative practice; *Values/Ethics for IP Practice, Roles/Responsibilities, IP Communication and Teams and Teamwork* [31]. The purpose of the core competencies is to help health professional schools better prepare clinicians for future collaborative practice.

Applying IPE and SBT to Competency-Based Education

The prevailing model of competency in medical education and training is that of Miller [18]. Miller described the acquisition of competence as a progression through four levels of competence and depicted them as *Miller's Pyramid* [18]. The four levels of competence in ascending degrees of expertise are *knows, knows how, shows how,* and *does* [18]. (See Fig. 15.1) Traditional methods of assessing clinician competence have relied on standard cognitive examinations or the acquisition of continuing medical education credit [25]. These methods are not suitable for assessing advanced levels of competence observed in the upper levels of Miller's pyramid or the degree of expertise expected of experienced clinicians. The lower levels of Miller's pyramid (*knows* and *knows how*) are easily taught and assessed using standard cognitive examinations, e.g. multiply choice exams, while the upper levels are difficult to teach and even more difficult to assess. [18, 32, 33] It has long been assumed that *shows how* and *does* are best learned through clinical experience and

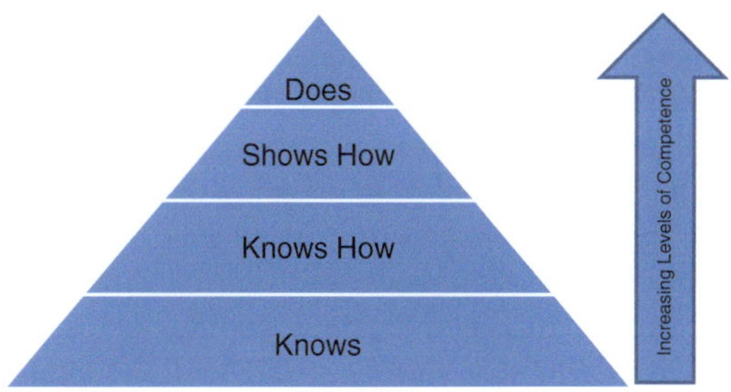

Fig. 15.1 Miller's Pyramid of Clinical Competence. (Adapted from Miller [18])

assessed through direct clinical observation, but these levels may lend themselves to experiential learning models such as SBT and IPE [18, 32–34]. Simulation-based training is evolving from primarily an educational technique to a multidimensional technique for teaching, learning and assessing varying levels of competency from novice to expert [25].

What makes SBT and team-based IPE an effective educational modality for clinicians can be explained in part by adult learning theory and by our understanding of the evolution of professional competence and expertise [5, 35]. As adult learners, clinicians tend to be independent, goal directed learners motivated by a desire to gain knowledge that can be integrated into daily practice [35]. Clinicians desire that the knowledge they gain be "*timely, relevant and practical*" [19]. Simulation-based training satisfies this desire by providing the ability to apply and practice new knowledge in a setting that closely resembles clinical practice, thus fulfilling the expectations of society and that of the clinician to be lifelong "practitioners" of his/her respected field [4]. Theories of adult learning in SBT are often modeled after Kolb's 4-stage experiential learning cycle [36, 37]. In Kolb's model, learning follows a cyclic path from the initial experience of a *concrete event* to *reflection* on the event followed by *thinking* about the event and finally to *practicing or performing* knowledge learned from the event [37, 38]. Concrete experiences are central to adult learning in Kolb's model [37]. Application of Kolb's model to SBT does not require a stretch of imagination. Learners participate in a clinical scenario (concrete event), debrief on the event (think and reflect) and complete the cycle by practicing or performing with new knowledge in a subsequent simulation or in clinical practice [37, 38]. The "event" replicated in SBT is largely unimportant, as it merely serves as an opportunity to think and reflect before "practicing and performing". This enables SBT to be utilized for and tailored to a diverse range of learner groups [36]. SBT permits learners to deal with crises and uncertainties, to err and make mistakes in a low stakes, yet clinically relevant environment.

Based on social learning theory, the replication of clinical scenarios using SBT offers both advantages and disadvantages to learners [39]. The opportunity to learn in a setting that is reflective of one's practice is certainly advantageous, but has certain limitations. Some have suggested that SBT fails to offer learners important communication and socialization opportunities that are critical to skill development and can only be obtained through clinical experiences [40–42]. These important interpersonal communication skills are only developed through interactions with other professions and clinicians in the work place setting [40]. While this does raise concern for a limitation of SBT that occurs in specialty specific and discipline specific silos, it brings attention to the value of interprofessional and interdisciplinary SBT. Training with IPE in the simulated clinical setting may permit the accelerated replication of interpersonal communication skills that are traditionally learned through associations with others in the clinical arena. The adult experiential learning application models of IPE and SBT fit well with the migration from time-based to competency-based education and training [17].

Simulation-Based Training permits the assessment of clinician competence in environments that closely resemble direct clinical observation with the ability to develop standardized and predictable assessments without the risk of harm to patients [25]. Governing bodies including health professional boards, professional societies, and state and federal governments have well established assessment tools and standards for assuring clinician competence. However, these agencies have not kept pace with the evolving nature of clinical education and expectations of society and have only recently begun to embrace SBT as a methodology for assuring clinician competence [25, 35, 43]. The future of SBT for assuring clinician competence appears bright and is driven by a number of factors including; society's demand for improved safety in healthcare, the establishment of core competencies for practice, the shift from time-based to competency-based certification, time limited certification, a shift away from standard, one time cognitive examinations to continuous life-long learning for recertification, the incorporation of screen based simulation techniques within computer based licensure exams and standardization and accreditation of simulation centers by organizations that oversee certification and licensure [25, 26, 35, 44].

Using SBT for High Stakes Assessment and Certification of Competence

The demands of the general public for improved patient safety and increased reliability in healthcare has created challenges for clinical learners and teachers alike. It is no longer acceptable for students and novice clinicians to learn "on the job" or practice and hone skills through direct patient care [45]. At the same time, clinicians are expected to receive standardized, reproducible, and comprehensive education [46]. The evolution of healthcare over the past few decades has created an environment that is not conducive to either learners, the assessment of learners, or learning through patient care, i.e. *see one, do one, teach one*, which is now largely considered inappropriate by clinicians, patients and society [27, 44, 45, 47]. This has opened the door and increased the demand for alternative means of training and assessing clinicians that has allowed SBT to emerge as a safe and effective means to learn and practice clinical skills [38].

Simulation-based training has been used in a diverse array of contexts and clinical settings. The new mantra of medical training is now "*see one, simulate many, demonstrate competence, do one when qualified (page 52)*" [48]. The growth of simulation in healthcare for training and assessment is driven by some of the same factors that have driven the use of simulation in industries such as nuclear power and aviation, which have better safety track records than that of healthcare [47]. The value and importance of simulation for maintaining public safety is evident by the emphasis placed on SBT by high reliability industries. The nuclear power industry devotes one out of every six weeks to simulation-based training for its workforce. [Personal communication M.B. Weinger M.D.; 5/15/2017] For decades, the aviation industry has required pilots to demonstrate competency in a flight simulator before embarking on their first flight [25, 49]. Commercial and military pilots are required to participate in simulations and team training exercises throughout their career [49]. Industries continue to rely on simulation to maintain safety despite the absence of evidence to support its continued use. The evidence for simulation is provided by the long track record of safety and high reliability demonstrated by these high risk industries [25]. Simulation was initially introduced in healthcare as an educational modality, but has evolved overtime to become a useful modality for education, research, assessment, quality improvement, quality assurance and system safety [1]. Simulation-based training and assessment has emerged as a safe and effective modality for ensuring a range of skills and competencies at all levels of healthcare [27, 46].

The utility of simulation has been explored and demonstrated in a diverse array of healthcare contexts including procedural skills, acute care skills, team training, crisis management, interprofessional communication, clinician/patient communication, evaluations of system safety, enhancement of quality improvement initiatives and emergency and disaster preparation [16, 38, 46, 50–52]. The utility for simulation in healthcare is limited only by its relative infancy in healthcare and by the imagination of its users.

Despite the recent explosion in interest for simulation for healthcare assessment, SBT has been used for assessment and certification purposes in healthcare for many decades Summative SBT in the form of standardized patients has been used for the assessment of medical student competency since the 1960's [25, 53]. In fact, most clinicians have participated in and/or been assessed by simulation at some point in their career. The bodies that provide resuscitation certification to healthcare providers, e.g. the American Heart Association, have employed simulation based education and assessment for many years [25]. Odds are that all practicing clinicians have at some point in their career participated in one of these courses that are often required for maintenance of clinical privileges for anyone engaged in patient care. One of the earliest simulation mannequins was Resusci-Anne, which was introduced in the 1960's and is still widely employed today, largely unchanged in design [46]. The use of simulation for resuscitation certification employs the full range of simulation modalities and technologies from low fidelity to high fidelity. Currently, all American Heart Association (AHA) basic and advanced resuscitation courses involve the use of SBT including; part-task trainers (chest compression and airway skills), medium fidelity mannequins (chest compression and ventilation skills), high-fidelity mannequins (application of algorithms to simulated codes and code team skills) and screen-based and web-based simulation modules for assessment and self-guided study [25]. In addition, most resuscitation courses consist of an interprofessional group of learners, thus much of the SBT that occurs in these courses is interprofessional in nature. Recent work suggests that using SBT to augment the stress of learners during simulated resuscitations actually improves skill retention for up to 6 months, long a weakness of biennial resuscitation programs [54].

Feedback is an inherent component of any effective SBT and plays a crucial role in the acquisition of knowledge from SBT. It is often suggested that simulation exercises are simply excuses to debrief [1]. Until recently, much of this feedback was in the form of "formative" feedback intended to help learners identify gaps in knowledge or performance. Formative feedback is a form of "low stakes" assessment. Formative feedback or assessment is not intended for high stakes decisions such as those used for competence, certification or licensure. In order for SBT to evolve from a formative assessment modality to a modality for high stakes assessment several considerations must be addressed. Summative assessments must demonstrate more robust psychometrics than that of formative assessments [55, 56]. Simulation-based training is a relatively expensive educational and assessment methodology; requiring a larger investment of time, human resources, specialized expertise and capital infrastructure than a pen and paper exam [5]. This expense is compounded when SBT is used for summative assessment with the added costs of developing psychometrically sound assessments, standardization of assessments and accreditation of simulation facilities and faculty [55, 56]. This cost is offset by the increasing demands of both clinicians and the general public for competency-based training and assessment to insure the highest quality and safety of patient care, which cannot be provided by traditional assessment modalities but may be provided by SBT [5]. The primary benefit of psychometrically sound summative assessments is the ability to make high stakes decisions regarding competency at the upper levels of Miller's pyramid [35, 56]. Simulation has the ability to assess knowledge, higher cognitive functions (critical thinking and clinical decision making), leadership/teamwork skills, and technical proficiency, in a performance based and standardized setting that poses minimal harm to patients [2]. Simulation has been widely adopted across healthcare disciplines and specialties as an educational modality, but its adoption as a modality for high-stakes assessment, licensure, certification, and maintenance of certification has lagged [46].

Anesthesiology as a Model for Simulation for Competency-Based Education

It should come as no surprise that the specialty of anesthesiology has been one of the early adopters of high stakes simulation-based assessment, as it was one of the first specialties to adapt simulation from aviation and incorporate SBT into the training process [57]. The following sections will use the specialty of anesthesiology and the journey from undergraduate medical education to maintenance of certification in the United States (US) system to illustrate how the use of simulation for training and assessment can be employed in competency-based medical education.

The Role of Simulation in Undergraduate Medical Education and Licensure

Future physicians are exposed to SBT at a majority of medical schools in the US, and all medical students in the US are assessed using simulation prior to graduation and licensure [6, 16]. In the US, medical students must complete three examinations (Steps) composing the United States Medical Licensing Examination (USMLE) administered by the National Board of Medical Examiners (NBME). The first part of the USMLE examination (Step 1) is completed after the second of 4 years of medical school. This examination is largely knowledge based and composed of multiple-choice questions, but with the recent transition to computer-based examinations the USMLE began to incorporate screen based clinical scenarios into the exam.

Prior to graduation from medical school, allopathic medical students in the US must complete USMLE Step 2. This examination incorporates simulations in the form of patient scenarios in which students are tasked with applying knowledge to make appropriate clinical decisions [25, 58]. In 2004, the NMBE added a second part to Step 2, known as Step CS (clinical skills). This entirely simulation-based examination consists of a series of twelve standardized patient (SP) examinations in which the examinee has 15 minutes to interact with the SP followed by 10 minutes to complete a written note including history and physical examination, differential diagnosis, assessment and plan. Step 2 CS was introduced to address increasing evidence that poor interpersonal and clinical skills were attributing to decreased patient satisfaction, decreased patient safety, increased medical errors and increased malpractice claims [25, 59, 60]. Step 2 CS is able to assess unique competencies that are not possible to measure on multiple-choice examinations including interpersonal communication skills, proficiency in written and spoken English, professionalism and clinical skills (e.g. physical diagnosis and examination) [25]. The use of SPs for assessment of undergraduate medical education has been in use since the 1960's and is one of the most studied and validated simulation based methods for high stakes assessment of healthcare trainees [25, 60, 61]. An extensive body of evidence exists to support the use of SPs for high stakes assessment for both medical and nursing trainees [25, 60, 61].

Following graduation from medical school and completion of 1 year of postgraduate training, US physicians are eligible to complete Step 3 of the USMLE. Step 3 is composed entirely of complex, interactive screen based clinical scenarios [25, 62]. Clinical management skills of examinees are assessed as they manage a series of screen-based simulated patients. The examinee must assess and manage the simulated patient beginning with the chief complaint. The performance of examinees is compared to those of experienced clinicians through a thoroughly validated algorithm [25, 63–65]. The computer based Step 3 examination is able to assess levels of Miller's pyramid that are not easily assessed on standard cognitive examinations [25, 64, 65]. Although, these examinations are expensive to develop, validate and administer, the ability to assess higher levels of competence and unique skills justifies the added cost [25].

Licensure for physicians in the United States is governed at the state level with each state having unique, although similar, requirements for licensure and renewal of licensure. Physician licensure is typically renewed every 2–3 years and does not require any demonstration of clinical knowledge or competence beyond the documentation of a predetermined number of CME credits [25]. This process does little to ensure maintenance of clinical standards or competence of clinicians. The responsibilities for insuring physicians achieve and maintain clinical competence falls on the specialty boards.

The Role of Simulation in Graduate Medical Education and Primary Certification

The Accreditation Council for Graduate Medical Education (ACGME) governs medical residency training in the US. In 1999, the ACGME in collaboration with the American Board of Medical Specialties (ABMS) identified six core competencies that define competency for all medical residents, thus providing a framework for post-graduate medical training programs. The six competencies are *patient care, medical knowledge, practice-based learning and improvement, interpersonal and communication skills, professionalism,* and *system-based practice* [66]. The six core competencies are described in Table 15.1. Recently, the ACGME identified specialty specific steps called *Milestones* to mark trainees' progress towards achieving competence [66]. Residency training programs now monitor and evaluate trainees based on their progression from novice to expert level performance [66]. Under the Milestones system, trainees are expected to demonstrate competence in the knowledge and skills associated with each progressive milestone before progressing in his or her training. Training programs may employ a range of assessment tools to measure trainees' progress along the Milestones pathway including written and oral exams, direct clinical observation, objective structured clinical examinations (OSCEs), simulation-based assessments or a combination of methods [34]. Programs are expected to evaluate trainees' performance on and progress toward Milestones competencies using Miller's stages of competency [66].

Table 15.1 ACGME Six Core Competencies

Practice-based Learning and Improvement	Show an ability to investigate and evaluate patient care practices, appraise and assimilate scientific evidence, and improve the practice of medicine.
Patient Care and Procedural Skills	Provide care that is compassionate, appropriate, and effective treatment for health problems and to promote health.
Systems-based Practice	Demonstrate awareness of and responsibility to the larger context and systems of health care. Be able to call on system resources to provide optimal care (e.g. coordinating care across sites or serving as the primary case manager when care involves multiple specialties, professions or sites).
Medical Knowledge	Demonstrate knowledge about established and evolving biomedical, clinical, and cognate sciences and their application in patient care.
Interpersonal and Communication Skills	Demonstrate skills that result in effective information exchange and teaming with patients, their families and professional associates (e.g. fostering a therapeutic relationship that is ethically sound, uses effective listening skills with non-verbal and verbal communication; working as both a team member and at times as a leader).
Professionalism	Demonstrate a commitment to carrying out professional responsibilities, adherence to ethical principles and sensitivity to diverse patient populations.

Adapted from – http://www.abms.org/board-certification/a-trusted-credential/based-on-core-competencies/

ACGME Accreditation Council for Graduate Medical Education

In 2011, the American Board of Anesthesiology (ABA) required that all residents in anesthesiology participate in at least one simulated clinical case each year [46]. The ABA cited evidence from a multi-institutional study demonstrating the validity of SBT for assessing residents [67]. Soon the American Board of Anesthesiology (ABA) will introduce an OSCE into the examination process for primary certification in anesthesiology. This OSCE will likely include a range of SBT including standardized patients, partial task trainers, computer-based and mannequin-based simulations [34]. OSCEs have been used for certification in anesthesiology since the Royal College of Anaesthetists [RCOA) of the United Kingdom included it in their examination in the 1990's and it continues to be a part of their two-part examination process [34, 68, 69]. The RCOA OSCE assesses a range of clinical, technical and non-technical skills including resuscitation, anesthesia equipment, history and physical examination and interpretation of statistics and data [34, 68]. The Israeli National Board Examination in Anesthesiology incorporated objective structured clinical evaluation (OSCE) into the Israeli board examination in 2003 [43]. The OSCE consists of five stations, which evaluate the management of trauma, resuscitation, operating room crises, mechanical ventilation and regional anesthesia. The technical skills and non-technical skills of examinees is assessed using a checklist and global rating scale respectively [43]. The Royal College of Physicians and Surgeons of Canada (RCPSC) added screen-based simulations to its oral examination for anesthesiology in 2010 and in 2015 launched an initiative to transform GME in Canada into competency-based medical education, called "Competence by Design [34, 70].

Graduate medical education is slowly but steadily moving towards competency-based training, although US residency programs currently remain time-based [19, 34]. At present, two subspecialty boards, anesthesiology and general surgery, have incorporated SBT as a requirement for primary certification. Research within the field of anesthesiology has shown that SBT can be an effective tool for training and assessment in non-technical skills, e.g. communication, teamwork and professionalism and the ACGME core competencies, e.g. systems-based and practice-based learning that can be inherently difficult to teach and assess using traditional knowledge based or direct observation methods [26, 67, 71, 72].

Simulation for Maintenance of Certification in Anesthesiology

In 2005, all 24 specialty boards governed by the ABMS transitioned to "time-limited" certification, thus requiring physicians to demonstrate ongoing learning and competence every 5–10 years to remain specialty board certified [25]. The ABMS is responsible for certifying physicians in 145 specialties and subspecialties [25]. Prior to 2005, physicians were certified for life. This change came in part due to ongoing expectations from the public that physicians maintain knowledge and skills throughout their practice career [19]. This was further driven by the recognition that traditional continuing medical education (CME) programs have failed to demonstrate any tangible change in physicians' practice and the knowledge gained from CME programs is seldom translated into practice [19, 73, 74]. The new time-limited certification process, known as ABMS Maintenance of Certification (MOC) consists of four parts common to all specialties. The four parts provide a framework for measuring the ACGME six core competencies and are intended to ensure physicians develop lifelong learning skills and requires demonstration of the six core competencies on an ongoing basis [25, 75]. The four parts are - professionalism and professional standing (I), lifelong learning and self-assessment (II), assessment of knowledge, judgment, and skills (III), and improvement in medical practice (IV) [75]. The MOC provides a standardized framework for the component specialty boards to follow, but each board is responsible for determining the specific elements to satisfy the core competencies. Given the need to demonstrate a diverse array of competencies including communication, teamwork and professionalism, it was determined that traditional methods of continuing education and assessment were inadequate. This has led to increased interest in simulation for continuing education and MOC, and the use of SBT has been endorsed by both the ACGME and ABMS [19, 25, 46].

In 2010, the American Society of Anesthesiology (ASA) in collaboration with the American Board of Anesthesiology (ABA) began offering a high-fidelity simulation-based course to satisfy part IV of MOC. The ASA has endorsed a network of simulation centers to provide the courses to practicing anesthesiologists. The content of the course is developed by each center using a framework of required material supplied by the ASA. The courses are specifically designed to satisfy the Practice Performance Assessment and Improvement (PPAI) element of the ABMS requirements for MOC [19, 76]. Simulation was chosen as a PPAI activity for its ability to stimulate reflection and practice improvement. Participants are able to experience a crisis or high acuity event in a setting that elicits an appropriate sense of urgency and permits time for reflection following the event [19]. The use of challenging clinical scenarios *"deliberately incorporates an experiential strategy to activate the learners to reflect on ways to improve their practice (page 111)"* [19]. The course specifically targets clinical situations associated with mortality and morbidity, such as cardiovascular collapse and hypoxemia and those that require active crisis management skills [19]. This opportunity to engage in a crisis and reflect following the crisis on one's performance is believed to foster a greater willingness to change one's clinical practice [19]. Following the simulation course, participants are required to submit three opportunities for improving his/her practice that were identified during the course and provide a follow up report to the ASA at 3 months on the status of his/her identified practice improvements. Participants in the first few years of the MOC simulation course reported a higher rate of implementation of practice improvement and changes than historically reported following traditional CME programs [19]. In an analysis of practice improvement plans submitted during the first 2 years of the course, 94% of participants reported successfully implementing at least one practice improvement and 79% implemented three or more practice improvements within 3 months of completing the simulation course [19, 76]. Interestingly, those participants who targeted or included interprofessional colleagues in their plans had a much higher likelihood of reaching their improvement goals [19].

With the addition of the MOC simulation course, the ASA has been able to support the ABMS mission to promote life-long learning and self-assessment [19, 77]. Currently, anesthesiology is the only specialty offering specialty board endorsed simulation-based training to fulfill portions of MOC. Other specialty boards permit clinicians to use SBT training to satisfy MOC, but do not develop the material or courses [25, 26]. Participation in the simulation course was initially required for all anesthesiologist seeking MOC. In 2016, despite the overwhelming favorable response from those that had completed the course, the ASA made participation in the simulation course voluntary due in part to backlash from members over the costs and time required to participate in the simulation course [19, 76, 78]. In 2016, the ASA announced a new series of screen-based simulation experiences, called *Anesthesia SimSTAT* [79]. The screen-based simulation modules focus on management of emergencies and enable anesthesiologists to access the education material anytime from anywhere, thus addressing the complaints regarding costs and time associated with participation in live simulation courses.

The ASA was not the first certifying body to offer simulation for certification or MOC. The Australian and New Zealand College of Anesthetists have developed a simulation-based course for their specialists and trainees. The course titled *Effective Management of Anesthetic Crises (EMAC)* was started in 2002 and is a requirement of anesthesiology training and recommended for Maintenance of Professional Standards (MOPS) [80]. The two and a half day course is designed to promote practice improvement, and a majority of participants surveyed have reported making changes to their practice following the course [80, 81]. In addition to certifying and licensing bodies, other organizations have realized the value of SBT for insuring the competence and safe practice of clinicians. The Controlled Risk Insurance Company (CRICO) provides medical professional liability, claims and risk management for the Harvard University system of hospitals, clinicians and providers [82]. CRICO has incentivized participation in annual simulation based crisis training for the clinicians of the Harvard medical system by providing discounts and rebates on liability coverage premiums. This is driven by a belief that simulation based training leads to reduced medico legal claims and improved patient safety [46, 82–84].

SBT for MOC is still in its infancy with opportunities for practicing clinicians to engage in such activities remaining limited. Fortunately, the interest in SBT for MOC is growing and SBT activities are appearing on the agenda of CME conferences and meetings of professional societies with increasing frequency.

Simulation for Certification in Other Medical Specialties

The other specialty that has employed SBT for certification of its clinicians is general surgery. In 2008, the American Board of Surgery (ABS) made simulation a requirement for primary certification [25, 26]. Residents in general surgery are required to complete two simulation based educational modules: the Fundamentals of Laparoscopic Surgery (FLS) and Advanced Trauma Life Support (ATLS) [25, 26, 85]. The FLS program assesses both cognitive and technical skills using a hybrid examination that includes a computer-based multiple-choice exam and hands-on examination using a laparoscopic task trainer *(FLS Laparoscopic Trainer Box)* [25, 26, 85]. Both ATLS and FLS use a combination of simulation modalities including screen-based, standardized patients and mannequin-based simulations.

Technical, procedure-based fields, e.g. minimally invasive surgery and gastroenterology, seem well suited for training and assessment using high fidelity simulations. Many commercially produced task trainers are available for procedural training and assessment including gastrointestinal endoscopy, bronchoscopy, endovascular procedures, ultrasonography and echocardiography [25]. The American Board of Internal Medicine (ABIM) introduced simulation training as an option for satisfying MOC for interventional cardiologists in 2004 [26]. The United States Food and Drug Administration has mandated that physicians performing endovascular carotid artery stent procedures undergo extensive training that includes a simulation component prior to being credentialed to perform the procedure [86, 87]. The training program has proven highly effective with novice clinicians able to perform the procedure with comparable skills as those with clinical experience [86, 87]. The rapid rise in availability and interest in robot assisted surgery has generated interest in simulation based and virtual reality (VR) augmented training platforms to train and certify surgeons in the use of this rapidly evolving technology [88]. The unique interface between surgeon and surgical robot control would suggest virtual and augmented reality simulation training modalities would be the ideal method for training robotic surgeons [88]. The learning curve for new procedures is known to be steep and associated with an increased patient risk even for experienced clinicians, thus it seems likely that simulation-based training will become the standard for initial training and competency assessment for new invasive procedures and products [88].

Role of Simulation in Nursing and Allied Health Professional Development

Simulation has a well-established role in the education and training of health professionals at the undergraduate level. So it comes as no surprise that simulation is playing an expanding role at the graduate and continuing professional development level. The opportunities for simulation-based training are unlimited. New health professional graduates are entering the workforce having been trained using simulation and are expecting that simulation will continue to be a part of their ongoing training and professional development [89]. The expectation for ongoing training opportunities that support clinician competence and contribute to reduced patient harm has been echoed by a number of professional nursing organizations including the National League for Nursing, American Nurses Association, and the American Association of Critical Care Nurses [90]. Many new nurses are exposed to simulation based training as early as orientation to their first clinical position. Medical facilities are using simulation to expose and assess new graduates in standardized clinical scenarios to ensure new nurses are on boarded with the necessary clinical skills without compromising patient safety [7]. These simulation-enhanced orientations have proven to be beneficial with reports of reduced orientation time, reduced staff turnover and improved staff retention [90–92].

New nurses often find the transition from theory based education to the demands of clinical practice challenging, and many will experience increased work related stress associated with this transition period [93]. New nurses often report feeling unprepared for the day-to-day demands of clinical practice and/or lack proficiency in basic skills expected of a nurse graduates [93]. The stress associated with transition to practice and perceived lack of competence for clinical practice may contribute to the attrition rate for new nurses and nurses returning to practice [94, 95]. Simulation based training has proven efficacy in undergraduate nursing education, so SBT seems a logical choice for helping ease the difficulties encountered by new nurses transitioning to practice [96, 97].

The demand for advanced practice registered nurses (APRN) in the United States (US) is rapidly outpacing the existing workforce of APRNs and the ability of the current education system to produce new APRN graduates [98]. A shortage of APRNs in the US has been forecasted unless innovative changes are made to the existing APRN education and training system [99]. Simulation based training offers a number of opportunities to evolve the existing APRN education model and help scale up the number of APRN graduates. In the modern healthcare system, APRNs must possess the skills to practice in and lead interprofessional and multidisciplinary teams. The development of interprofessional collaborative skills has been highlighted in the Core Competencies for Interprofessional Collaborative Practice [31]. Interprofessional practice skills require practice and training to develop, but opportunities to develop these skills can be limited, especially in traditional siloed education systems [99]. Simulation affords an opportunity for APRN students to engage with other health professional students in clinical IPE simulations to hone interprofessional skills and prepare for future practice. Time spent in simulated clinical experiences has been recognized as equivalent to time spent in clinical training for preparing undergraduate nursing students and will likely prove true for the training of advanced practice nurses and other health professionals [40, 100]. Incorporating simulation into innovative curricula offers an opportunity to scale up existing education and training of health professionals to meet increasing patient demands.

Clinicians must look for innovative ways to maintain existing skills and develop new skills to keep pace with the increasing complexity of our modern healthcare system and the patients we serve. Simulation based training continues to play an increasing role in meeting the demands for innovative education and training. Simulation offers clinicians an opportunity to develop specialized skills for care of complex patients and complex patient encounters where traditional training methods pose unacceptable risk to patients and/or clinicians. Examples of such training include the use of simulation for training nurses and respiratory therapists to manage critically ill patients on extracorporeal membranous oxygenation (ECMO) or IPE simulations for training healthcare teams to improve emergency preparedness and the management of high risk situations, e.g. natural disasters, mass casualties, active shooter scenarios and chemical spills [101–104].

Many organizations are turning to simulation to assess the ongoing competencies of health care providers to maintain quality assurance, patient safety and to satisfy regulatory bodies. Regulatory agencies in the US healthcare system such as the Joint Commission require healthcare organizations to regularly assess specific competencies of nurses caring for patients in their accredited facilities [7]. The Joint Commission does not provide assessment methods for healthcare organizations to use; yet expect the assessments to be more vigorous than self-assessments or simple check offs. Simulation based training and assessment affords organizations a modality for helping staff develop new skills, maintain existing skills and fulfill regulatory agency requirements [105].

Simulation-Based Training for Remediation

As healthcare moves from a time-based certification system to a competency-based system, it will be necessary to develop systems for assessing and remediating clinicians with lapsed competency or who fail to demonstrate adequate competence. Simulation is a logical choice for assessing the competence of clinicians, who have been out of practice, experienced lapses in skills or have failed to maintain competence. Simulation-based training will not only provide a means to evaluate these clinicians but will provide an opportunity for these clinicians to retrain in a setting that is standardized and safe. Existing systems for evaluating clinicians with lapsed competence are based on cognitive examinations and possess the inherent limitations of such assessments, i.e. they can assess *knows* and *knows how* but are unable to assess *shows how* and *does*. Rosenbatt and colleagues developed a SBT program to assess and retrain anesthesiologists with lapsed skills, which has been successful in remediating clinicians and returning clinicians to practice following lengthy absences [106]. This method of assessing and remediating clinicians with lapsed skills is likely to become more common as SBT plays an increasing role in primary certification, recertification, and maintenance of certification. Simulation based assessments developed for primary certification such as the Fundamentals of Laparoscopic surgery are now being explored for assessing practicing clinicians for recertification and/or for remediation when indicated [85, 107].

Limitations of Using Simulation for Competency Certification

Although simulation-based training is being embraced by even the smallest of medical facilities, SBT opportunities for clinicians practicing away from major academic medical centers remain limited. The options for participants seeking SBT for high stakes assessment is further limited to a small but growing number of accredited simulation-training centers. At present, three organizations offer accreditation of simulation centers; the American College of Surgeons, the American Society of Anesthesiologists (ASA), and the Society for Simulation in Healthcare [25]. The widespread use of SBT is limited by a number of factors including the cost associated with the technology and expertise heavy educational modality, the availability of skilled SBT educators and facilitators, the additional time and logistics of conducting SBT especially IPE SBT for both the trainer and trainee and a resistance to change that seems to plague healthcare [108]. True interprofessional simulation based training is even scarcer. The financial, time and logistical resources and constraints associated with SBT are amplified in IPE [4]. In addition, the expertise required to develop successful IPE SBT modules exceeds that required for single specialty learning experiences. It is imperative that the IPE exercise be inclusive of all learners and learning objectives and goals be relevant to all learners [4]. As a result, many IPE learning opportunities focus on the non-technical aspects of interprofessional practice such as communication, coordination, leadership, teamwork and shared decision making [4, 109]. Finally, despite a growing appeal and a growing body of simulation based literature and research, the evidence to support a direct patient care benefit of SBT or IPE SBT has not emerged [1, 110].

Future Directions

The costs, logistics and expertise required for simulating the clinical environment with standardized patients, computer driven mannequins and low/high tech task trainers has limited the spread of SBT. In order for SBT to expand to meet the demands and training needs of the healthcare workforce, alternative means of delivering SBT must be explored. The field of anesthesiology has been a leader in the healthcare simulation movement with its introduction of screen-based, virtual reality simulations for MOC [79]. The force behind the development of these educational modules was driven by the need to scale up the availability of SBT and to provide standardized education programs to a large number of practicing clinicians across a large geographic area. It is likely that other healthcare fields will follow suit and expand the availability of screen-based and virtual reality (VR) simulations. Screen-based and VR simulation may soon become the predominant simulation technology for health professional education as the costs of developing VR and screen based simulations decrease and access to VR platforms becomes as widespread as the nearest smartphone.

Conclusion

The use of simulation-based training and interprofessional SBT for high stakes assessment of competency is still in its relative infancy. The use of SBT for certification and recertification has been limited by the costs associated with this type of training relative to traditional educational modes, the availability and opportunities of training programs, and the need for vigorous psychometric evidence to support this assessment modality. With increasing public demands for safer care and increasing acceptance from various organizations and governing bodies, it is likely that SBT in healthcare will follow the path of other high-risk industries in which SBT is a mainstay. The future for SBT and assessment of competency is extremely bright and one can expect to see increasing demands and options for SBT in assessing certification, licensure, CPD, CME and MOC.

References

1. Gaba DM. The future vision of simulation in health care. Qual Saf Health Care. 2004;13(suppl 1):i2–i10.
2. Cates LA, Wilson D. Acquisition and maintenance of competencies through simulation for neonatal nurse practitioners: beyond the basics. Adv Neonatal Care. 2011;11(5):321–7.
3. World Health Organization. Framework for action on interprofessional education and collaborative practice (No. WHO/HRH/HPN/10.3): World Health Organization; 2010.
4. Boet S, Bould MD, Layat Burn C, Reeves S. Twelve tips for a successful interprofessional team-based high-fidelity simulation education session. Med Teach. 2014;36(10):853–7.
5. Lenburg CB. The framework, concepts and methods of the competency outcomes and performance assessment (COPA) model. Online J Issues Nurs. 1999;4(2):1–12.
6. Palaganas JC, Brunette V, Winslow B. Prelicensure simulation-enhanced interprofessional education: a critical review of the research literature. Simul Healthc. 2016;11(6):404–18.
7. Hallenbeck VJ. Use of high-fidelity simulation for staff education/development: a systematic review of the literature. J Nurses Prof Dev. 2012;28(6):260–9.
8. D'amour D, Oandasan I. Interprofessionality as the field of interprofessional practice and interprofessional education: an emerging concept. J Interprof Care. 2005;19(sup1):8–20.
9. Robertson J, Bandali K. Bridging the gap: enhancing interprofessional education using simulation. J Interprof Care. 2008;22(5):499–508.
10. Gawande A. Cowboys and pit crews. The New Yorker. 2011;26.
11. Donaldson MS, Corrigan JM, Kohn LT, editors. To err is human: building a safer health system, vol. 6: National Academies Press; 2000
12. Villemure C, Tanoubi I, Georgescu LM, Dubé J-N, Houle J. An integrative review of in situ simulation training: implications for critical care nurses. Can J Crit Care Nurs. 2016;27:22–31.
13. Leipzig RM, Hyer K, Ek K, Wallenstein S, Vezina ML, Fairchild S, et al. Attitudes toward working on interdisciplinary healthcare teams: a comparison by discipline. J Am Geriatr Soc. 2002;50(6):1141–8.
14. Meurling L, Hedman L, Sandahl C, Felländer-Tsai L, Wallin C-J. Systematic simulation-based team training in a Swedish intensive care unit: a diverse response among critical care professions. BMJ Qual Saf. 2013:bmjqs-2012-000994.
15. Reader TW, Flin R, Mearns K, Cuthbertson BH. Interdisciplinary communication in the intensive care unit. Br J Anaesth. 2007;98(3):347–52.
16. Okuda Y, Bryson EO, DeMaria S, Jacobson L, Quinones J, Shen B, et al. The utility of simulation in medical education: what is the evidence? Mt Sinai J Med. 2009;76(4):330–43.
17. Hodges BD. A tea-steeping or i-Doc model for medical education? Acad Med. 2010;85(9):S34–44.
18. Miller GE. The assessment of clinical skills/competence/performance. Acad Med. 1990;65(9):S63–7.
19. Steadman RH, Burden AR, Huang YM, Gaba DM, Cooper JB. Practice improvements based on participation in simulation for the maintenance of certification in anesthesiology program. J Am Soc Anesthesiol. 2015;122(5):1154–69.
20. Bhandari M, Montori V, Devereaux PJ, Dosanjh S, Sprague S, Guyatt GH. Challenges to the practice of evidence-based medicine during residents' surgical training: a qualitative study using grounded theory. Acad Med. 2003;78(11):1183–90.
21. Curry L, Purkis IE. Validity of self-reports of behavior changes by participants after a CME course. Acad Med. 1986;61(7):579–84.

22. ten Cate O. Competency-based postgraduate medical education: past, present and future GMS. J Med Edu. 2017;34(5).
23. Koster A, Schalekamp T, Meijerman I. Implementation of competency-based pharmacy education (CBPE). Pharmacy. 2017;5(1):10.
24. Foth T, Holmes D. Neoliberalism and the government of nursing through competency-based education. Nurs Inq. 2017;24(2).
25. Levine AI, Schwartz AD, Bryson EO, DeMaria S Jr. Role of simulation in US physician licensure and certification. Mt Sinai J Med. 2012;79(1):140–53.
26. Ross BK, Metzner J. Simulation for maintenance of certification. Surg Clin N Am. 2015;95(4):893–905.
27. Willis RE, Van Sickle KR. Current status of simulation-based training in graduate medical education. Surg Clin N Am. 2015;95(4):767–79.
28. Langsley DG. Medical competence and performance assessment: a new era. JAMA. 1991;266(7):977–80.
29. Hatala R, Kassen BO, Nishikawa J, Cole G, Issenberg SB. Incorporating simulation technology in a Canadian internal medicine specialty examination: a descriptive report. Acad Med. 2005;80(6):554–6.
30. Holtschneider ME, Park CW. Interprofessional education: implications for nursing professional development practice. J Nurses Prof Dev. 2015;31(4):242–3.
31. Panel IECE. Core competencies for interprofessional collaborative practice: report of an expert panel. Washington, D.C.: Interprofessional Education Collaborative; 2011.
32. Aronowitz T, Aronowitz S, Mardin-Small J, Kim B. Using objective structured clinical examination (OSCE) as education in advanced practice registered nursing education. J Prof Nurs. 2017;33(2):119–25.
33. Rushforth HE. Objective structured clinical examination (OSCE): review of literature and implications for nursing education. Nurse Educ Today. 2007;27(5):481–90.
34. Hastie MJ, Spellman JL, Pagano PP, Hastie J, Egan BJ. Designing and implementing the objective structured clinical examination in anesthesiology. J Am Soc Anesthesiol. 2014;120(1):196–203.
35. Ziv A, Rubin O, Sidi A, Berkenstadt H. Credentialing and certifying with simulation. Anesthesiol Clin. 2007;25(2):261–9.
36. Stocker M, Burmester M, Allen M. Optimisation of simulated team training through the application of learning theories: a debate for a conceptual framework. BMC Med Educ. 2014;14(1):69.
37. Kolb DA, Boyatzis RE, Mainemelis C. Experiential learning theory: previous research and new directions. Perspectives on thinking, learning, and cognitive styles. 2001;1(2001):227–47.
38. Brunette V, Thibodeau-Jarry N. Simulation as a tool to ensure competency and quality of care in the cardiac critical care unit. Can J Cardiol. 2017;33(1):119–27.
39. Bandura A, Walters RH. Social learning theory, vol. 1. Englewood Cliffs, NJ: Prentice-hall; 1977.
40. Larue C, Pepin J, Allard É. Simulation in preparation or substitution for clinical placement: a systematic review of the literature. J Nurs Educ Pract. 2015;5(9):p132.
41. Berragan L. Simulation: an effective pedagogical approach for nursing? Nurse Educ Today. 2011;31(7):660–3.
42. Leigh GT. High-fidelity patient simulation and nursing students' self-efficacy: a review of the literature. Int J Nurs Educ Scholarsh. 2008;5(1):1–17.
43. Berkenstadt H, Ziv A, Gafni N, Sidi A. Incorporating simulation-based objective structured clinical examination into the Israeli National Board Examination in Anesthesiology. Anesth Analg. 2006;102(3):853–8.
44. Jensen JB, Torsher LC. Simulation and continuing professional development. Int Anesthesiol Clin. 2015;53(4):60–9.
45. Ziv A, Wolpe PR, Small SD, Glick S. Simulation-based medical education: an ethical imperative. Acad Med. 2003;78(8):783–8.
46. Steadman RH, Huang YM. Simulation for quality assurance in training, credentialing and maintenance of certification. Best Pract Res Clin Anaesthesiol. 2012;26(1):3–15.

47. Ziv Stephen D Small Paul Root Wolpe A. Patient safety and simulation-based medical education. Med Teach. 2000;22(5):489–495.
48. Murphy JG, Torsher LC, Dunn WF. Simulation medicine in intensive care and coronary care education. J Crit Care. 2007;22(1):51–5.
49. Gordon S, Mendenhall P, O'Connor BB. Beyond the checklist: What else health care can learn from aviation teamwork and safety: Cornell University Press; 2012.
50. Cant RP, Cooper SJ. Use of simulation-based learning in undergraduate nurse education: an umbrella systematic review. Nurse Educ Today. 2016.
51. Wayne DB, Butter J, Siddall VJ, Fudala MJ, Linquist LA, Feinglass J, et al. Simulation-based training of internal medicine residents in advanced cardiac life support protocols: a randomized trial. Teach Learn Med. 2005;17(3):202–8.
52. Wayne DB, Didwania A, Feinglass J, Fudala MJ, Barsuk JH, McGaghie WC. Simulation-based education improves quality of care during cardiac arrest team responses at an academic teaching hospital: a case-control study. Chest J. 2008;133(1):56–61.
53. Whelan GP, McKinley DW, Boulet JR, Macrae J, Kamholz S. Validation of the doctor–patient communication component of the Educational Commission for Foreign Medical Graduates Clinical Skills Assessment. Med Educ. 2001;35(8):757–61.
54. DeMaria S Jr, Bryson EO, Mooney TJ, Silverstein JH, Reich DL, Bodian C, et al. Adding emotional stressors to training in simulated cardiopulmonary arrest enhances participant performance. Med Educ. 2010;44(10):1006–15.
55. Boulet JR. Summative assessment in medicine: the promise of simulation for high-stakes evaluation. Acad Emerg Med. 2008;15(11):1017–24.
56. Boulet JR, Swanson DB. Psychometric challenges of using simulations for high-stakes assessment. Simulations in critical care education and beyond. Des Plains: Society of Critical Care Medicine; 2004. p. 119–30.
57. Gaba DM, DeAnda A. A comprehensive anesthesia simulation environment: re-creating the operating room for research and training. Anesthesiology. 1988;69(3):387–94.
58. Dillon G, Boulet J, Hawkins R, Swanson D. Simulations in the United States medical licensing examination™(USMLE™). Qual Saf Health Care. 2004;13(suppl 1):i41–i5.
59. Vincent C, Phillips A, Young M. Why do people sue doctors? A study of patients and relatives taking legal action. Lancet. 1994;343(8913):1609–13.
60. Levine AI, Swartz MH. Standardized patients: the "other" simulation. J Crit Care. 2008;23(2):179–84.
61. Cohen DS, Colliver JA, Marcy MS, Fried ED, Swartz MH. Psychometric properties of a standardized-patient checklist and rating-scale form used to assess interpersonal and communication skills. Acad Med. 1996;71(1):S87–9.
62. Dillon GF, Clauser BE. Computer-delivered patient simulations in the United States Medical Licensing Examination (USMLE). Simul Healthc. 2009;4(1):30–4.
63. Clauser BE, Subhiyah RG, Piemme TE, Greenberg L, Clyman SG, Ripkey D, et al. Using clinician ratings to model score weights for a computer-based clinical-simulation examination. Acad Med. 1993;68(10):S64–6.
64. Clauser BE, Margolis MJ, Swanson DB. An examination of the contribution of computer-based case simulations to the USMLE step 3 examination. Acad Med. 2002;77(10):S80–S2.
65. Dillon GF, Clyman SG, Clauser BE, Margolis MJ. The introduction of computer-based case simulations into the United States Medical Licensing Examination. Acad Med. 2002;77(10):S94–S6.
66. Nasca TJ, Philibert I, Brigham T, Flynn TC. The next GME accreditation system—rationale and benefits. N Engl J Med. 2012;366(11):1051–6.
67. Schwid HA, Rooke GA, Carline J, Steadman RH, Murray WB, Olympio M, et al. Evaluation of anesthesia residents using mannequin-based simulation a multiinstitutional study. J Am Soc Anesthesiol. 2002;97(6):1434–44.
68. Bromley LM. The objective structured clinical exam-practical aspects. Curr Opin Anesthesiol. 2000;13(6):675–8.
69. McIndoe A. Modern anaesthesia training: is it good enough? Br J Anaesth. 2012;109(1):16–20.

70. Levine MF, Shorten G. Competency-based medical education: its time has arrived. Can J Anesth. 2016;63(7):802–6.
71. Buyske J. The role of simulation in certification. Surg Clin N Am. 2010;90(3):619–21.
72. Watkins SC, Roberts DA, Boulet JR, McEvoy MD, Weinger MB. Evaluation of a simpler tool to assess nontechnical skills during simulated critical events. Simul Healthc. 2017;12(2):69–75.
73. Studdert DM, Mello MM, Gawande AA, Gandhi TK, Kachalia A, Yoon C, et al. Claims, errors, and compensation payments in medical malpractice litigation. N Engl J Med. 2006;354(19):2024–33.
74. Fanning R, Gaba D. The role of debriefing in simulation-based learning. Simul Healthc. 2007;2(2):115–25.
75. SpecialtiesABoM. Steps toward initial certification and MOC [cited 2017 05/15/2017]. Available from: http://www.abms.org/board-certification/steps-toward-initial-certification-and-moc/.
76. McIvor W, Burden A, Weinger MB, Steadman R. Simulation for maintenance of certification in anesthesiology: the first two years. J Contin Educ Health Prof. 2012;32(4):236–42.
77. Iglehart JK, Baron RB. Ensuring physicians' competence—is maintenance of certification the answer? 2012. p. 2543–9.
78. Weinger MB, Burden AR, Steadman RH, Gaba DM. This is not a test! Misconceptions surrounding the maintenance of certification in anesthesiology simulation course. J Am Soc Anesthesiol. 2014;121(3):655–9.
79. Adam Levine, Arna Banerjee, Wendy Bernstein, Lawrence Chu, Samuel DeMaria, Ronald Levy, Rebecca Minehart, John Rask. Anesthesia SimSTAT: Amercian Society of Anesthesiologists and CAE Healthcare; 2017 [cited 2018 2/26/18]. Available from: http://www.asahq.org/education/simulation-education/anesthesia-simstat.
80. Weller J, Morris R, Watterson L, Garden A, Flanagan B, Robinson B, et al. Effective management of anaesthetic crises: development and evaluation of a college-accredited simulation-based course for anaesthesia education in Australia and New Zealand. Simul Healthc. 2006;1(4):209–14.
81. Weller J, Wilson L, Robinson B. Survey of change in practice following simulation-based training in crisis management. Anaesthesia. 2003;58(5):471–3.
82. Arriaga AF, Gawande AA, Raemer DB, Jones DB, Smink DS, Weinstock P, et al. Pilot testing of a model for insurer-driven, large-scale multicenter simulation training for operating room teams. Ann Surg. 2014;259(3):403–10.
83. Hamman WR, Beaudin-Seiler BM, Beaubien JM, Gullickson AM, Orizondo-Korotko K, Gross AC, et al. Using simulation to identify and resolve threats to patient safety. Am J Manag Care. 2010;16(6):e145–50.
84. Riley W, Meredith LW, Price R, Miller KK, Begun JW, McCullough M, et al. Decreasing malpractice claims by reducing preventable perinatal harm. Health Serv Res. 2016;51(S3):2453–71.
85. Surgeons SoAGaE. Fundamentals of laparoscopic surgery 2018 [cited 2018 2/26/2018]. Available from: http://www.flsprogram.org/.
86. Dawson DL. Training in carotid artery stenting: do carotid simulation systems really help? Vascular. 2006;14(5):256–63.
87. Van Herzeele I, Aggarwal R, Choong A, Brightwell R, Vermassen FE, Cheshire NJ. Virtual reality simulation objectively differentiates level of carotid stent experience in experienced interventionalists. J Vasc Surg. 2007;46(5):855–63.
88. Broderick R, Langness S, Ramamoorthy S. Training and credentialing in robotics. In: Robotic colon and rectal surgery. Cham: Springer; 2017. p. 17–22.
89. Leigh G. The simulation revolution: what are the implications for nurses in staff development? J Nurses Prof Dev. 2011;27(2):54–7.
90. Cato DL, Murray M. Use of simulation training in the intensive care unit. Crit Care Nurs Q. 2010;33(1):44–51.
91. Beyea SC, Slattery MJ, von Reyn LJ. Outcomes of a simulation-based nurse residency program. Clin Simul Nurs. 2010;6(5):e169–e75.

92. Ackermann AD, Kenny G, Walker C. Simulator programs for new nurses' orientation: a retention strategy. J Nurses Prof Dev. 2007;23(3):136–9.
93. Jung D, Lee SH, Kang SJ, Kim J-H. Development and evaluation of a clinical simulation for new graduate nurses: a multi-site pilot study. Nurse Educ Today. 2017;49:84–9.
94. Bisholt BK. The learning process of recently graduated nurses in professional situations—experiences of an introduction program. Nurse Educ Today. 2012;32(3):289–93.
95. Wu T-Y, Fox DP, Stokes C, Adam C. Work-related stress and intention to quit in newly graduated nurses. Nurse Educ Today. 2012;32(6):669–74.
96. Shin S, Park J-H, Kim J-H. Effectiveness of patient simulation in nursing education: meta-analysis. Nurse Educ Today. 2015;35(1):176–82.
97. Cant RP, Cooper SJ. The value of simulation-based learning in pre-licensure nurse education: a state-of-the-art review and meta-analysis. Nurse Educ Pract. 2017;27:45–62.
98. Safriet BJ. Federal options for maximizing the value of advanced practice nurses in providing quality, cost-effective health care. The future of nursing: leading change, advancing health. Washington, DC: Institute of Medicine; 2011. p. 443–75.
99. LeFlore JL, Thomas PE. Educational changes to support advanced practice nursing education. J Perinat Neonatal Nurs. 2016;30(3):187–90.
100. Kardong-Edgren S, Willhaus J, Bennett D, Hayden J. Results of the National Council of State Boards of Nursing national simulation survey: part II. Clin Simul Nurs. 2012;8(4):e117–e23.
101. Fehr JJ, Shepard M, McBride ME, Mehegan M, Reddy K, Murray DJ, et al. Simulation-based assessment of ECMO clinical specialists. Simul Healthc. 2016;11(3):194–9.
102. Smith SJ, Farra SL. National Disaster Health Consortium: competency-based training and a report on the American nurses credentialing center disaster certification development. Nurs Clin. 2016;51(4):555–68.
103. Evans AB, Hulme JM, Nugus P, Cranmer HH, Coutu M, Johnson K. An electronic competency-based evaluation tool for assessing humanitarian competencies in a simulated exercise. Prehosp Disaster Med. 2017;32(3):253–60.
104. Kotora JG, Clancy T, Manzon L, Malik V, Louden RJ, Merlin MA. Active shooter in the emergency department: a scenario-based training approach for healthcare workers. Am J Disaster Med. 2014;9(1):39–51.
105. Kaddoura MA. New graduate nurses' perceptions of the effects of clinical simulation on their critical thinking, learning, and confidence. J Continuing Edu Nursing. 2010;41(11):506–16.
106. Rosenblatt MA, Abrams KJ. The use of a human patient simulator in the evaluation of and development of a remedial prescription for an anesthesiologist with lapsed medical skills. Anesth Analg. 2002;94(1):149–53.
107. Hafford ML, Van Sickle KR, Willis RE, Wilson TD, Gugliuzza K, Brown KM, et al. Ensuring competency: are fundamentals of laparoscopic surgery training and certification necessary for practicing surgeons and operating room personnel? Surg Endosc. 2013;27(1):118–26.
108. Sinz EH. Anesthesiology national CME program and ASA activities in simulation. Anesthesiol Clin. 2007;25(2):209–23.
109. Zwarenstein M, Goldman J, Reeves S. Interprofessional collaboration: effects of practice-based interventions on professional practice and healthcare outcomes. Cochrane Database Syst Rev. 2009;3(3).
110. Cook DA, Hatala R, Brydges R, Zendejas B, Szostek JH, Wang AT, et al. Technology-enhanced simulation for health professions education: a systematic review and meta-analysis. JAMA. 2011;306(9):978–88.

Part IV

Application of Simulation-Based Interprofessional Education in Clinical Practice

Teamwork in the Operating Room 16

Edwin Tomoya Ozawa and Sohail K. Mahboobi

Introduction

The operating room (OR) environment is a unique space within the clinical setting, bringing together many backgrounds, disciplines, beliefs, attitudes, and styles of training into a confined area where patient care is directed at a concentrated focal point. The operating room setting can be classified as a complex system, where multiple steps must be followed in order to accomplish single tasks, and where an overwhelming amount of equipment, supplies, and infrastructure intersect in a high stakes environment. Complex systems and high stakes environments in which team training is of great importance include aviation and nuclear power, which are industries that share similar properties with healthcare in terms of the complexity of technology interfacing with human performance [1–3].

The history of simulation in healthcare is closely tied with the perioperative domain. David Gaba and colleagues at Stanford University were instrumental in developing teamwork training in the OR setting of anesthesia care, by studying teamwork and Crew Resource Management (CRM) principles developed by the commercial aviation industry. In a landmark paper, Gaba et al. discussed initial attitudes and perceptions of trainees undergoing simulation training in one of the original ACRM (Anesthesia Crisis Resource Management) protocols [4]. Hence, the tradition of interprofessional team training had its roots in the operating room. Early studies were primarily focused solely on anesthesia personnel; however, more complex scenarios require active participation from a broad spectrum of specialties and professions. Hence, Crew Resources Management became known as Crisis

E. T. Ozawa (✉) · S. K. Mahboobi
Tufts University School of Medicine, Lahey Hospital & Medical Center, Department of Anesthesiology, Burlington, MA, USA

J. T. Paige et al. (eds.), *Comprehensive Healthcare Simulation: InterProfessional Team Training and Simulation*, Comprehensive Healthcare Simulation,
https://doi.org/10.1007/978-3-030-28845-7_16

Resource Management in the perioperative domain and was initially developed within the anesthesia specialty, then spread to other members of the operating room, including nursing and technical staff and other members who may not have experienced simulation as part of their professional training. Crisis resource management encompasses ordinary and critical clinical scenarios to provide participants an opportunity to improve assessment of situation, critical decision making, team management and utilization of available resources to improve outcomes [5].

Ideally, interprofessional education (IPE) should be reinforced while professionals are in the early stages of their training or practice to introduce the culture of joint interdependence and to break down existing silos. For instance, at our institution, a successful team-training course bringing together nursing and medical students was created based on the TeamSTEPPS® training program. A longitudinal study was constructed to study the effect of a teamwork training intervention on observed behaviors and self-reported attitudes. The study found that self-reported attitudes about teamwork did not change as a result of training, but observed team performance did improve, although not to statistical significance. Such training brings together two professional groups that would normally not intersect during their routine educational experiences [6].

Interprofessional education also has great intrinsic value for existing teams where some degree of familiarity exists between members. Surgeons, anesthesiologists, certified registered nurse anesthetists (CRNAs), operating room nurses, surgical technicians, perfusionists, and other support staff may work in the same area and interact on a both a social and professional level on a daily basis. However, involving these same individuals in regular training exercises can provide insight into team dynamics, and reinforce the benefits of effective teamwork during challenging or stressful situations. Antedotes of poorly managed crisis situations are ubiquitous, and the root cause of the majority of these are often attributable to poor communication and teamwork [7]. The remainder of this chapter will discuss strategies to combat these impediments (using simulation, team training, and CRM), as well as the considerations and challenges that must be addressed in order to successfully implement effective team training.

Motivations for Team Exercises and Training

Simulation in the perioperative domain can have two different, but mutually exclusive objectives. One objective is to provide training on a particular topic. Another objective is to examine the hospital system for processes or flaws that could jeopardize patient safety. If the objective is purely educational, then the goals of the training are to ensure that members understand certain principles and have the opportunity to practice these in a safe environment. This is followed by a debriefing session for participants to reflect on the experience and develop new insights and ways of thinking that will carry over to real life practice.

There are established curriculums such as TeamSTEPPS®, which are gaining widespread acceptance, are tailor-made for the simulation environment [8].

TeamSTEPPS®, in particular, provides a construct for how a team should respond effectively during a challenging and high stakes situation. The lessons, especially with regards to leadership, are applicable to non-crisis situations as well, such as managing a unit or a department [9]. In one particular well-cited study, Weaver et al. discussed the effects of the training curriculum in the OR service line, versus controls [10]. The study examined trainee reactions, learning, and behaviors in the OR environment, as well as the use of established questionnaires (the Hospital Survey on Patient Safety Culture (HSOPS) and the Operating Room Management Attitudes Questionnaire (ORMAQ). This study revealed that individuals from the trained groups showed significant increases in the quantity and quality of pre-surgical procedure briefings, as well as the use of quality teamwork behaviors during actual cases.

In a similar study, Armour Forse et al. found that implementing a TeamSTEPPS® training program at the Creighton University School of Medicine improved teamwork and communication as measured by self-assessment surveys completed by team members, in both the OR and the post-anesthesia care unit (PACU) [11]. Stakeholder groups included anesthesiologists, CRNAs, surgeons, residents, nurses, and scrub technicians. The study also found improvements in surgical outcomes as measured by Surgical Quality Improvement Program (SQIP) parameters (such as antibiotic administered within one hour of incision, and DVT prophylaxis administration), and lower complications as measured by National Surgical Quality Improvement Program (NSQIP) for surgical morbidity and mortality (decreased mortality immediately after training). Of note, the authors measured improvements in OR staff team skills, staff communications, OR efficacy in case starts and room turnover, and patient evaluations.

As mentioned previously, a second use for team-based training is to "stress test" the hospital system for performance gaps that could cause patient harm. At our institution, the concept of "gap analysis" through simulation was introduced by the simulation center as a quality and safety tool. This is a term often used in management circles and is the comparison of actual performance with desired performance. The term "gap analysis" as used in our institution refers to a "gap" or a difference between expected performance and reality. It could also pertain to the difference between what is considered optimum performance, versus what is the predicted actual performance.

The use of simulation-based training provides a systematic way of investigating the system for latent threats. An initial threat assessments or "gap" comes from the voiced concerns of staff members who feel that suboptimal performance is likely under specific conditions. With OR mock "codes" (e.g., cardiopulmonary arrest), these specific conditions can be duplicated and performance can be monitored and recorded. Novel and locally authored checklists can be used as assessment tools to determine the degree to which "gaps," if they exist, contributed to sub-optimal performance as well as the degree of failure in performance. Following the mock code, once objective data are collected, an after-action report can be generated to provide recommendations for improvements in order to close the gaps. This process needs to be iterative. Once improvements or adjustments to the system are made based on the after-action reports, the scenarios should be repeated to demonstrate gap closure. This process will serve to validate the use of the proposed assessment tools and methodology.

The process of proactively assessing and planning responses to crises, and thereby closing performance gaps, is closely related to the concept of *organizational mindfulness*. This is an emerging principle in healthcare which encourages not only individuals or teams, but the institution as whole to understand how they will respond, especially in an unanticipated and stressful situation. For instance, during a mass casualty incident, or an active shooter incident, simulation can be used to plan for such an event and identify *gaps* far in advance of an actual situation, where additional resources need to be brought to bear. This response can occur at many levels. Planning may take place on an individual, departmental, institutional, or even a community level. Weick and Sutcliffe are social psychologists who developed some of the initial groundwork, laying the foundation of the concept [12]. They define mindful organizing as the "collective capability to detect and correct errors and unexpected events," and they describe five dimensions of organizational mindfulness: preoccupation with failure, reluctance to simplify interpretations, sensitivity to operations, commitment to resilience, and deference to expertise [13]. Mindful organizing is a trait of high reliability organizations, exemplified by groups such as the United States Navy SEALs and aircraft carrier deck crews.

Cognitive Aids

Cognitive aids and checklists are a relatively new concept in the field of healthcare, although their use has been accepted for quite some time in the aviation industry. The Stanford Cognitive Aids Group defines cognitive aids (used interchangeably with "checklists") as "structured pieces of information designed to enhance cognition and adherence to medical best practices." [14] One should note that the implementation of checklists is only effective if it is tested in the clinical environment it is designed for, and team members who use the checklist(s) practice using it regularly. Institutions should invest time and resources in adapting or developing their own checklists to address a wide variety of rare but high-stakes adverse events.

To illustrate, a checklist development methodology was presented by a group from several Harvard Medical School-affiliated institutions. In an article published by Ziewacz et al., ten critical OR events were selected for checklist development. The methodology began with an extensive literature review to identify the most common life-threatening OR crises and whether there were any tested principles or protocols to manage the events. After identification of the events, an expert group from within the organization met to develop drafts of the checklist for 12 events using best evidence-based practice from literature, and then tested them iteratively in a simulated environment to create a final product. The end-user utility of the checklists was tested by two surgical teams in a simulated environment, and the research group found that the teams were more likely to adhere to critical steps in the management of crises when the checklist was made available, with statistical significance ($p = 0.007$) [15]. Unfortunately it is much more difficult to test the impact of the checklists on actual clinical care, and the authors certainly indicate that future research should attempt to establish the link between the use of cognitive aids and patient outcomes.

Stakeholders

The OR brings together many individuals from varied professions. The list may include physicians of multiple specialties, certified registered nurse anesthetists, OR nurses, scrub technicians, anesthesia technicians, equipment representatives or technicians, students, and support staff. It is important to understand what each stakeholder brings to IPE and the team. Interprofessional teamwork requires the collaboration of several stakeholders, all of whom harbor unique skills, competencies, and activities that must be well understood to successfully understand and model simulations targeted at improving team performance.

It is worthy to note that simulation-based team training is especially important for *contingency teams*, who may not work regularly together. Just like a group of people coming together for a pick-up basketball game on a Sunday afternoon, individual team members should understand the rules of game and what positions they need to play (such as point guard, forward, or center), in order to achieve a common goal. Simulation based training may allow individuals to learn these ground rules and skills needed to participate, even though as a team they may not know or have worked with other individuals.

The role that physicians and nurses play in crisis management and patient care is obvious, however other groups and skill sets are crucial for the functioning of the OR team. For example, in our institution, our support staff plays a vital role in the management of crises by assisting in the management of non-clinical tasks such as moving beds and equipment, bringing supplies, etc. Anesthesia technicians are familiar with all equipment and supplies and are able to bring needed supplies and/or equipment to an OR on short notice. Anesthesia technicians are also able to set up, operate, and troubleshoot equipment such as invasive monitors (arterial lines, pulmonary artery catheters), blood scavenging systems and rapid transfuser systems.

It is interesting to note that perceptions of teamwork in the OR setting can differ based on specialties. For instance, a study performed by Makary et al. found that physicians tend to view their teamwork skills as better than it is perceived by nurses [16]. In this study, the group developed a novel Safety Attitudes Questionnaire, based on a refinement of the existing Intensive Care Unit Management Attitudes Questionnaire, in an attempt to create a standardized measurement tool for OR teamwork quality. The authors tested for differences in ratings of communication and collaboration that surgeons, anesthesiologists, surgical technicians, CRNAs, and OR nurses gave to each other. The results indicated that teamwork ratings for each OR caregiver differed considerably by caregiver type, and that physicians tended to view teamwork as high across all disciplines, whereas non-physicians tended to rate teamwork among physicians as lower. It is interesting to note that the authors felt that the lack of perceived teamwork by surgeons among nurses may be contributing to the low job satisfaction that seems to be pervasive in the nursing profession.

Another stakeholder group that utilizes simulation for training in the OR are perfusionists. The use of simulation-based training for this group is emphasized, especially for rare but critical events. Sistino et al. described the use of a commercially available computer-driven simulator (the Orpheus Perfusion Simulator) to develop both basic skills, as well as advanced emergency skills for cardiopulmonary perfusionists [17]. In this study, the authors developed recorded simulation scenarios to promote teamwork, communication, and patient awareness during cardiac surgery requiring cardiopulmonary bypass. In the simulation, the cardiopulmonary perfusionist faculty members played the multidisciplinary roles including a cardiac surgeon, an anesthesiologist, OR nurses, and a perfusionist in two separate sets of four simulation-based training scenarios. The first set of simulations were scripted for poor teamwork and communication, and the second set for effective teamwork and communication. The scenarios were viewed by a focus group consisting of cardiopulmonary perfusion students who were able to accurately rate the quality of teamwork and communication by listing keywords from an established peer evaluation tool. It can be assumed that the students gained insight and knowledge from the observation of, rather than direct participation in, simulation scenarios, although this effect was not directly measured by the study.

Operating room technicians may not have exposure to simulation training as part of their professional training, however, they can benefit greatly from team training. Simulation for manual and technical skill are available for surgical technicians, but generally, interprofessional education is not a core component. Perkins et al. described a pilot curriculum for surgical (scrub) technicians and OR nurses based on the American College of Surgeons Advanced Trauma Operative Management (ATOM) course [18]. Combined teams of surgical technicians and OR nurses were enrolled in a daylong eight-hour training session consisting of didactic presentations for the first half, and simulation-based training with a surgeon in ATOM for the second half. The study demonstrated that the knowledge base of both nurses and surgical technicians displayed significant improvement in didactic knowledge (the primary measure) with statistical significance ($p = 0.0008$), while rating the course quality as very high.

It is often the case that teams have a need for simulation training, but their organizations may not have the resources to provide it. Paige et al. developed a Mobile Mock OR to provide interprofessional team training at the point of care for institutions that may lack resources or expertise to provide such training [19]. Equipment included a computer-controlled manikin and an inanimate cholecystectomy model. The standardized training scenario involved four participants per session including a surgeon, scrub technician, nurse anesthetist, and a circulating nurse, performing a mock cholecystectomy in which an intraoperative crisis occurs. Team members were asked to self-rate performance before and after a training intervention with respect to team competencies of role clarity, anticipatory response, cross-monitoring, and overall team cohesion and interaction. Analysis of the ratings based on a 6-point Likert scale demonstrated an improvement in perceived teamwork skills with statistical significance in 4 of 15 items measured after the training intervention. The four items included role clarity ($p = .02$), anticipatory response ($p = .01$), cross monitoring ($p < .01$), and team cohesion and interaction ($p < .01$). This study suggested that OR teams, the majority of which have poor teamwork skills at baseline, may benefit from point of care simulation training.

Case Study: Power Failure in the Operating Room

Often times an interprofessional team of leaders that manage the OR may identify gaps in performance or resources that need to be addressed. This may come about because of a sentinel event, or because of issues found during a hospital inspection by agencies such as the Joint Commission, both scenarios of which have occurred at our institution. Policies can be written in an attempt to overcome these gaps. However, it may not be enough for a task force or a committee to brainstorm about best practices, or to investigate best practices at other institutions and incorporate them unaltered into their own environment which may possess a different culture or workflow. This case study contains all of the elements described above in this chapter, and highlights the successful use of simulation to address an institutional problem involving multiple stakeholders.

In our institution, leadership had perceived a gap regarding how a power failure in the OR setting would be managed. During a Joint Commission (JC) inspection, reviewers noted that the existing power failure policy was inadequate and did not address perioperative patient safety concerns. The existing policy only made provisions for loss of power affecting such functions as suction, plumbing, and lighting but contained no information regarding the management of power failure during a surgical procedure. To address the issue, a planning cycle consisting of the drafting of a power failure checklist and the testing of the checklist in a simulated clinical environment was created. Furthermore, it was discovered that there was no specific policy regarding a "threat assessment" with respect to exactly what equipment in the OR was at risk during total power loss. It was understood that the majority of critical OR devices would still be operable because of backup battery power, however, a comprehensive list of what equipment would fail immediately had not been generated. Furthermore, there were uncertainties regarding how long certain battery-powered devices would be able to run without power.

Although the threat of power failure is a low probability, in a high stakes environment the consequences of power loss are potentially life-threatening and the management uncertain. Despite reassurances from institutional leaders in engineering and the physical plant that such an event was unlikely, a real-life close call and the subsequent inspection of the arrangement of power distribution to the OR revealed a weak point. It was determined that failure due to fire in one particular compartment could have potentially led to the loss of power to a sizeable number of operating rooms, independent of the presence of backup generators and the emergency power grid.

A novel method for policy development utilizing simulation was proposed to address the management and performance gap identified by the JC inspection. The existing policy was revised to direct the maintenance of a complete inventory of equipment that could be affected by power loss, and also to create a single page checklist to be placed in the binder of important OR documents located at the circulating nurses' computer station. Prior to the policy revision, a thorough literature search regarding the topic of power failure in the OR was conducted. The literature search revealed the processes that other institutions had put in place due to experiencing a catastrophic power loss, such as from a hurricane.

Following the review of the literature, a protocol development team was assembled with representatives from anesthesiology, surgery, nursing, and OR technical staff and facilities support to draft a preliminary protocol. By combining information gathered from literature and voiced experiences and concerns of team members, an initial protocol and checklist was created. A simulation scenario was then created to test the protocol. A laparoscopic gastric bypass scenario was selected because it is a case that is routinely performed at our institution and this case involves a laparoscopic bowel anastomosis. Due to the complexity of this surgical procedure, a total power failure would pose significant challenges for the entire OR team A hybrid manikin was assembled using available elements from the simulation lab to make the simulation more real.

The simulation training scenario was executed in our simulation center with our standard mock OR setup including an anesthesia machine, monitors, and laparoscopic video equipment. All critical electrical equipment was connected to a single electrical cable which could be disrupted at will. The participants included an attending general surgeon, surgery resident, two anesthesia attending physicians, a scrub tech, and a circulator nurse. Participants were oriented to the power failure scenario and protocol in advance. The starting point of the scenario was midpoint during a routine laparoscopic gastric bypass surgery where the surgeons were performing the gastrojejunostomy anastomosis. Following the exercise, a debriefing session was performed with all participants, including our institution Safety Officer. Participants were asked individually to critique the scenario using the plus delta evaluation technique (first reflecting on what went well, and then discussing what could be done better). The exercise was also video recorded and was reviewed collectively by the group during the debriefing process.

The exercise was repeated at a later date in-situ with the participation of an engineer from the physical plant who was able to disrupt power to an actual OR. The participants were expanded from the first iteration to include general surgery attending and resident, anesthesia attending physicians, CRNA, scrub tech, anesthesia tech, and a circulator nurse. The previous scenario in the simulation lab included blackout conditions necessitating battery powered light sources. In the actual OR environment, participants benefited from automatic battery powered backup lighting (Bodine Ballast emergency lighting) which enabled individuals to continue their management of the situation, although to complete the open anastomosis battery powered light sources were still required.

The exercise helped to uncover deficiencies in the proposed protocol, most notably the need to designate the circulating nurse as the team leader. In addition, the importance of determining the exact extent of power failure, the need to illuminate instrument tables, and the need for backup light sources in multiple operating rooms were noted. Our policy and checklist were then modified to address these concerns prior to approval by the OR Policy Committee and rollout to our staff during an annual all-hands training event. See Fig. 16.1 for the sample OR Power Failure checklist. From our experience with this process, we concluded that our methodology is a powerful tool that can be used to assist in the development of hospital policies and protocols, especially for rare critical events. The need for a group of people sharing a work unit to come together to resolve an issue through a creative process helps to foster the spirit of cooperation. Individuals from different disciplines can collaborate in a safe environment and help to brainstorm as a team solutions that then can be codified into a document or checklist. In this way, all members feel that they have contributed to the project, creating more of a sense of teamwork and collaboration that may not routinely exist.

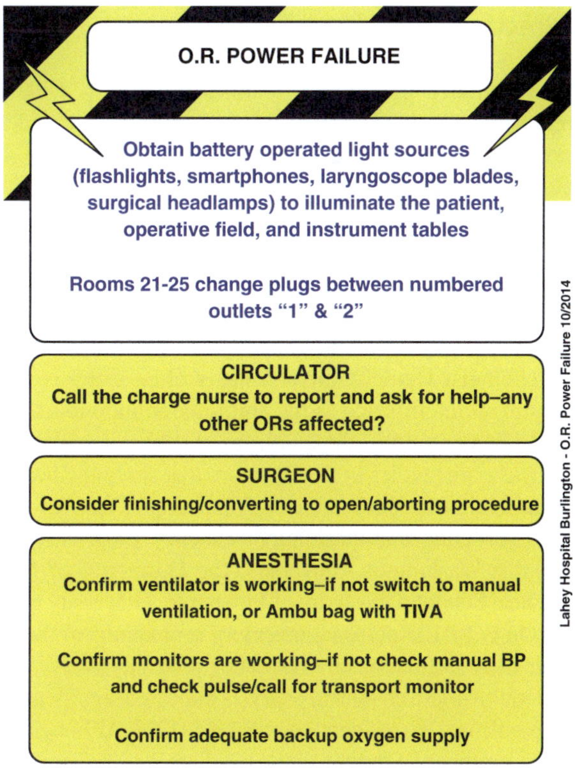

Fig. 16.1 Sample OR Power Failure checklist

Challenges to Implementation of IPE in the Perioperative Domain

Time, resources, and coordination of schedules are all significant factors that need to be considered when planning simulation-based team exercises. Support from leadership is crucial for maximizing the engagement of participants and hence increasing the chances for success. At our institution, one component of operating room team training is to identify high-value sentinel events and a restricted number of personnel who can participate in the simulations. In reality, it is very difficult to find the time and resources to allow all member to participate directly in a simulation training scenario. One solution to overcome the difficulties of involving everyone directly in a training exercise is to create a shared experience. Utilizing our existing video learning management system, we have been able to run a limited number of training exercises which are then broadcasted to the auditorium so that all members of the operating room staff are able to view and participate in a discussion. In this manner, through an all-hands meeting of operating room staff, the issues related to the specific scenarios can be brought to everyone's attention and lessons can be learned by all who participate in this exercise.

Directions for Future Research

As mentioned previously, TeamSTEPPS® is a widely used instructional tool in many domains, and its principles are widely accepted at institutions and in simulation labs. Some of the major concepts addressed within TeamSTEPPS® include closed-loop communication, giving feedback, transfer of care communications, situational awareness, and cross monitoring. Although instructors may embrace these concepts, in reality, there is not an established method for directly training these principles. Investigations into team psychology and attention are warranted. For instance, in the business literature, much attention is given to emotional intelligence as a way to enhance communication, leadership, and teamwork [20, 21]. The psychologist Daniel Goleman has written extensively on the subject, and defines emotional intelligence as the ability of an individual to identify, assess, and control one's own emotions, the emotions of others, and that of groups [22].

There are studies in the literature that study the benefits of Emotional Intelligence in the healthcare environment. For example, Talarico et al. performed a study of five U.S. academic anesthesiology residency programs, which included 339 residents (George Washington University, the University of Miami, UMDNJ - New Jersey Medical School, University of Pittsburgh, University of Texas Health Science Center). BarOn EQ-i:125 personal inventory evaluations of the residents were compared with their daily evaluations by residency program faculty. Univariate correlation analysis and multivariate canonical analysis indicated significant correlation with, and likely to be predictors of, resident performance [23]. Although results from this paper appear to be promising, further work needs to be performed to determine how emotional intelligence training can impact teamwork in the OR or healthcare environment.

Closely related to the subject of emotional intelligence is mindfulness, which is a topic that has gained much attention in recent years. The Merriam-Webster dictionary defines mindfulness as the practice of maintaining a nonjudgmental state of heightened or complete awareness of one's thoughts, emotions, or experiences on a moment-to-moment basis [24]. A review article in the management literature by Good et al. suggested that contemplative studies and techniques to increase mindful attention to emotional cues may improve teamwork skills [25]. The authors provided a model in which the practice of mindfulness can lead to a range of benefits by strengthening the ability to pay attention. This in turn leads to augmented personal skills in the domains of cognition, emotion, behavior, and physiology. As with emotional intelligence, the improved personal skills lead to workplace benefits in the domains of job performance, relationships with colleagues, and personal well-being. Further studies need to be conducted to determine what impact mindfulness has on teamwork, leadership, communication, conflict management, and relationships in the clinical setting.

Conclusion

Simulation-based, multidisciplinary team training first evolved from the Operating Room environment and became the standard for other training in other areas of the hospital environment. The OR is one of the most complex working environments in any hospital, and the stakes are extremely high. Checklists, team training with TeamSTEPPS®, and gap analysis are important applications of simulation in OR team training. Interprofessional simulation can be used to teach and reinforce practices, and also to foster a proactive culture to ferret out latent threats and address them.

It is important to be cognizant of the fact that not only nurses and physicians, but many other people with other jobs also have a role to play, and contribute to the OR team at large. These individuals from diverse backgrounds should be included in the planning and execution of interprofessional simulation and training. There are of course significant challenges in bringing all groups together to participate in training simultaneously, but creative solutions can be generated to overcome some of these obstacles, for example through the use of media or technology.

Future research should look at the role of empathy, compassion, mindfulness, and emotional intelligence training on team performance in the OR. The augmentation of non-technical skills through contemplative practices in synergy with simulation-based training may be of great benefit to the healthcare industry that values compassion and empathy as some of its core values.

References

1. Cooper GE, White MD, Lauber JK, editors. Resource management on the flightdeck: proceedings of a NASA/industry workshop (NASA CP-2120). Moffett Field: NASA-Ames Research Center; 1980.
2. Harrington D, Kello J. Systematic evaluation of nuclear operator team skills training. Paper presented at the American Nuclear Society, San Francisco, 1991.

3. Kim SK, Park JY, Byun SN. Crew resource management training for improving team performance of operators in Korean advanced nuclear power plant. 2009 IEEE International Conference on Industrial Engineering and Engineering Management, Hong Kong, 2009, pp. 2055–59.
4. Gaba D, Howard S, Fish K, Smith B, Sowb Y. Simulation-based training in anaesthesia crisis resource management(ACRM): a decade of experience. Simul Gaming. 2001;32(2):19.
5. Gaba DM. Crisis resource management and teamwork training in anaesthesia. Br J Anaesth. 2010;105(1):3–6.
6. Bourgeois D, Nepomnayshy D, Frontiero L, Frederick A. Optimizing Simulation-Based Interdisciplinary Teamwork Training for Medical and Nursing Students and Evaluating Its Long-term Effects. Burlington: Lahey Center for Professional Development and Simulation.
7. Leonard M, Graham S, Bonacum D. The human factor: the critical importance of effective teamwork and communication in providing safe care. Qual Saf Health Care. 2004;13(Suppl 1):i85–90.
8. About TeamSTEPPS. Content last reviewed June 2019. Agency for Healthcare Research and Quality, Rockville, MD. [Online] Available from: https://www.ahrq.gov/teamstepps/about-teamstepps/index.html [Accessed 2nd December 2019].
9. TeamSTEPPS® 2.0 for Long Term Care. Content last reviewed May 2019. Agency for Healthcare Research and Quality, Rockville, MD. [Online] Available from: https://www.ahrq.gov/teamstepps/longtermcare/index.html [Accessed 2nd December 2019].
10. Weaver SJ, Rosen MA, DiazGranados D, et al. Does teamwork improve performance in the operating room? A multilevel evaluation. Jt Comm J Qual Patient Saf. 2010;36(3):133–42.
11. Armour Forse R, Bramble JD, McQuillan R. Team training can improve operating room performance. Surgery. 2011;150(4):771–8.
12. Weick KE, Sutcliffe KM. Managing the unexpected: resilient performance in an age of uncertainty. 2nd ed. San Francisco: Jossey-Bass; 2007.
13. Weick CE, Sutcliffe KM, Obstfeld D. Organizing for high reliability: processes of collective mindfulness. Vol 1. Stanford: JAI Press; 1999.
14. Cognitive Aids in Medicine. [Online] Available from: http://med.stanford.edu/cogaids.html [Accessed 2nd December 2019].
15. Ziewacz JE, Arriaga AF, Bader AM, et al. Crisis checklists for the operating room: development and pilot testing. J Am Coll Surg. 2011;213(2):212–17.e10. https://doi.org/10.1016/j.jamcollsurg.2011.04.031.
16. Makary MA, Sexton JB, Freischlag JA, et al. Operating room teamwork among physicians and nurses: teamwork in the eye of the beholder. J Am Coll Surg. 2006;202(5):746–52.
17. Sistino JJ, Michaud NM, Sievert AN, Shackelford AG. Incorporating high fidelity simulation into perfusion education. Perfusion. 2011;26(5):390–4.
18. Perkins RS, Lehner KA, Armstrong R, et al. Model for team training using the advanced trauma operative management course: pilot study analysis. J Surg Educ. 2015;72(6):1200–8.
19. Paige JT, Kozmenko V, Yang T, et al. High-fidelity, simulation-based, interdisciplinary operating room team training at the point of care. Surgery. 2009;145(2):138–46.
20. George JM. Emotions and leadership: the role of emotional intelligence. Hum Relat. 2000;53(8):1027–55.
21. Farh CICC, Seo M-G, Tesluk PE. Emotional intelligence, teamwork effectiveness, and job performance: the moderating role of job context. J Appl Psychol. 2012;97(4):890–900.
22. Goleman D. Emotional intelligence. Bantam 10th anniversary hardcover ed. New York: Bantam Books; 2006.
23. Talarico JF, Varon AJ, Banks SE, et al. Emotional intelligence and the relationship to resident performance: a multi-institutional study. J Clin Anesth. 2013;25(3):181–7.
24. Merrian-Webster Incorporated. [Online] Available from: https://www.merriam-webster.com/dictionary/mindfulness [Accessed 2nd December 2019].
25. Good D, Lyddy C, Glomb T. Contemplating mindfulness at work: an integrative review. J Manag. 2016;42(1):114–42.

Applications of Simulation-Based Interprofessional Education in Labor and Delivery

17

Colleen A. Lee, Dena Goffman, Peter S. Bernstein, David L. Feldman, and Komal Bajaj

Introduction

Two decades after the birth of the quality and patient safety movement, medical errors remain a vexing problem in hospitals with some estimating upward of 250,000 deaths per year occurring as a result of preventable harm [1]. Daunting as the task to address this issue may seem, significant strides in advancing healthcare safety have been made. The improvements can be attributed, in part, to the proliferation of simulation-based medical education (SBME). The applications and benefits of simulation-based education have been demonstrated in: (a) teaching and emphasizing

The original version of this chapter was revised. The correction to this chapter can be found at https://doi.org/10.1007/978-3-030-28845-7_20

C. A. Lee (✉)
Weill Cornell Medicine, Physician Organization-Quality and Patient Safety, New York, NY, USA
e-mail: cal9115@med.cornell.edu

D. Goffman
Department of Quality and Patient Safety, New York-Presbyterian Hospital, New York, NY, USA

Department of Obstetrics and Gynecology, Columbia University Medical Center, New York, NY, USA

P. S. Bernstein
Department of Obstetrics & Gynecology and Women's Health, Albert Einstein College of Medicine/Montefiore Medical Center, Bronx, NY, USA

D. L. Feldman
Healthcare Risk Advisors, The Doctors Company, New York, NY, USA

K. Bajaj
Department of Obstetrics & Gynecology and Women's Health, Albert Einstein College of Medicine/Montefiore Medical Center, Bronx, NY, USA

Department of Obstetrics and Gynecology, Jacobi Medical Center, NYC Health + Hospitals, Bronx, NY, USA

J. T. Paige et al. (eds.), *Comprehensive Healthcare Simulation: InterProfessional Team Training and Simulation*, Comprehensive Healthcare Simulation,
https://doi.org/10.1007/978-3-030-28845-7_17

teamwork behaviors, particularly in high-risk fields like obstetrics; (b) simplifying, standardizing and practicing effective communication strategies; (c) implementing evidence based guidelines and recommendations; and (d) recognizing and practicing all these skills in interprofessional teams for high risk situations [2].

In this chapter, unique opportunities for simulation-based interprofessional education within obstetrics will be outlined. A novel program for supporting simulation-based interprofessional education for Labor and Delivery staff by a professional liability insurer (PLI) will be described and lessons learned will be shared. Finally, a review of the utility of interprofessional simulation to introduce, improve and implement obstetric emergency checklists will be presented.

Key Learning Points

- Simulation-based interprofessional team training has contributed to advances in healthcare safety.
- Professional liability insurers (PLI) may play a unique role in supporting simulation-based interprofessional team training in high-risk fields such as obstetrics.
- Obstetrics poses some unique challenges to effective team performance and communication due to the vast number of disciplines that interact during any given emergent event.
- With numerous high-stakes, low frequency, rapidly evolving emergent events requiring astute clinical judgment and expert technical skill to optimize outcomes, simulation has proven to be an invaluable tool in the field of obstetrics.
- The best venue for conducting interprofessional simulation may depend on local circumstances and the goals for the simulation program; research has shown both in-situ and off-site simulation training offer benefits to teams.
- The success of the program described in this chapter depended on both interprofessional leadership engagement and the offering of incentives to attendees in the form of continuing education credits.
- Interprofessional simulation-based team training offers opportunities to explore medico-legal topics in medicine.
- Use of emergency checklists is a new endeavor in obstetrics; and interprofessional simulation offers an opportunity to introduce, improve and implement these checklists.

A Novel Approach to Supporting Interprofessional Simulation-Based Team Training in Obstetrics: The Role of a Professional Liability Insurer

Professional liability insurers (PLI) function similarly to most traditional insurance companies, by collecting premiums and providing coverage for losses. In the world of medicine, malpractice insurance often represents a significant portion of the expense in providing care, both for hospitals and individual providers. For PLIs, lowering premiums and reducing payouts benefits the company and the insured.

There are a number of ways to accomplish this goal. Chief among these strategies can be encouraging practices that reduce the incidence of adverse outcomes.

Healthcare Risk Advisors (HRA) provides risk management and claims services to a number of major academic medical centers (AMC) in a large metropolitan area. In this case, the mission of HRA (a subsidiary of The Doctors Company Group) and those of the AMCs are aligned, as both are working to promote high quality care, foster superb communication, and encourage appropriate documentation. All of these may reduce the number of adverse events and potential lawsuits, and limit liability when there is a lawsuit. To this end, HRA have supported and facilitated its hospitals and their providers in their pursuit of initiatives which aim to reduce adverse events and improve communication and documentation. The longest standing initiative is in Obstetrics where the clinical leadership has developed and sustained a best practices program [3].

A critical aspect of this program has been a team training initiative that not only includes the teaching of crew resource management with TeamSTEPPS®, but also utilizes simulated drills that give providers a chance to practice these skills in a safe environment. While these drills have been helpful in improving teamwork and communication, they have also had an impact on adverse events and likely on malpractice incidence. Most recently, HRA worked with its hospitals and clinicians to develop a technical skills simulation program focused on specific high-risk deliveries – shoulder dystocia and vacuum deliveries. In all of these programs, the hospitals worked together as a collaborative to both develop standards for training, and ensure all members of the obstetrics staff participated, especially attending physicians. HRA facilitated these programs by providing a common meeting space and also by collecting de-identified data. In addition, it provided incentives and penalties to ensure compliance with the standards developed by the expert clinicians in the hospitals' obstetrics and gynecology departments. As a result of this and other initiatives, HRA's partner insurance carrier has been able to offer individual physician malpractice premiums that are significantly lower than policies offered by other carriers in New York. Clinicians have found the collaborative to be both informative and helpful as they carry out their duties to provide optimal care with minimal risk to patients.

Support of hospitals and individual providers is not unique, as similar programs exist throughout the country. A number of lessons have been learned as a result of this program and others like it that HRA have supported in other high-risk areas, such as the Emergency Department and Surgery. For any such program to be successful, clinical leaders, especially department chairs, must be supportive from the outset. Without such support it is difficult to ensure that clinicians will follow best practices. Administrative support from hospital executives is also critical, especially financial officers who must be willing to invest in these initiatives using limited resources. While this company has provided much of the resources necessary for these initiatives, the hospitals are ultimately providing the funding and so must be assured that these limited resources are wisely spent. Using malpractice data to demonstrate deficiencies in the delivery of care is a useful way of demonstrating this need, since malpractice cases generate significant expense to the institutions. Like any quality initiative, these programs require leaders, typically innovators and early adopters from each of the hospitals who are willing to give of their time and expertise to develop and implement programs. These clinicians typically spend a few hours per week devoted to these programs, and while there is usually overlap with their other hospital responsibilities, this is not always the case. Finally, it is important to have data that support simulation programs to reduce risk. As with many safety initiatives, this cannot always be in the form of outcome data. Ideally, one should be able to show a reduction in the number of malpractice claims after an initiative is begun. However, this is often quite difficult to do, since laws change, and the nature of what kind of case gets brought is constantly changing. HRA have used a combination of de-identified outcomes data, along with process measures, and survey data to demonstrate that over time, the supported simulation programs have at least played a part in reducing adverse events, and subsequent malpractice claims.

Interprofessional Simulation-Based Team Training for Obstetrics

Supporting Evidence

According to a 2004 study of cases involving perinatal death or permanent injury, the leading root cause of errors in 75% of cases were communication and systems issues that resulted in barriers to effective team performance [4]. Recognizing the need to address such significant gaps in obstetrical teams' performance, several professional organizations, including American College of Obstetrics and Gynecology (ACOG), Association of Women's Health, Obstetric and Neonatal Nurses (AWHONN), American Academy of Pediatrics (AAP), and Society for Maternal-Fetal Medicine (SMFM) among others, published a call to action in 2011 outlining steps to improve team performance within obstetrics, including the use of drills and simulations [5]. These groups also urged training in the principles of crew resource management and adoption of standardized communication tools, such as Situation-Background-Assessment-Recommendation (SBAR), as effective strategies to improve team performance [5], both of which are highly amenable to simulation-based practice.

Obstetrics poses some unique challenges to effective team performance and communication. In any given patient encounter on a labor and delivery unit, there are often multiple health care professionals involved. The obstetrical team is complex and may include attending obstetricians (MD), resident physicians, certified nurse midwives (CNM), physician's assistants (PA) or nurse practitioners (NP), registered nurses (RN) and other support staff. This core team frequently interacts with other specialties, including maternal-fetal medicine specialists, anesthesia personnel, and neonatologists. When emergencies arise, a host of other disciplines may become involved, including gynecologic oncology surgeons, interventional radiologists, and critical care physicians. The sheer numbers and variety of staff necessitates that interprofessional teamwork training become an integral part of the culture of highly reliable obstetrical units [6]. With numerous high-stakes, low frequency, and rapidly evolving emergent events that require astute clinical judgment and expert technical skill to optimize patient outcomes, simulation has proven to be an invaluable tool in the field of obstetrics. Although evidence of obstetrical simulation improving clinical practice or reducing adverse events is limited [7], several studies have shown promising results. In a 2006 study in the United Kingdom (UK), Draycott et al. demonstrated a significant reduction in 5 minute Apgar scores below 6 and hypoxic ischemic encephalopathy (HIE) after implementation of an interprofessional obstetrics emergency training course [8]. In 2008, this same group showed a significant decrease in birth injury rates despite similar rates of shoulder dystocia after requiring all staff to attend an annual, one-day course involving emergency drills and fetal heart rate (FHR) tracing interpretation [9]. In an interrupted time-series study in the UK, Crofts et al. demonstrated that the introduction of an obstetric emergency training program for management of shoulder dystocia resulted in both improved management and clinical outcomes, specifically, a reduction in the incidence of brachial plexus injuries [10]. In the United States, Inglis et al. achieved similar results when they studied the frequency of brachial plexus injury over 9 years during which a simulated shoulder dystocia protocol was initiated at their institution [11]. A pilot study out of the Netherlands published in 2015 showed increased patient satisfaction scores after implementation of an interprofessional team training program in an obstetrical collaborative [12].

In order to achieve improvements in outcomes, as outlined above, teams must be prepared to work optimally together, particularly in the event of unexpected emergencies.

In-Situ Versus Off-Site: Pros and Cons

The best venue for conducting interprofessional simulation may depend on local circumstances and the goals for the simulation program. An off-site simulation center provides a distraction-free environment where teams can focus on the learning objectives of the program. Alternatively, performing simulations in-situ may provide additional benefits such as uncovering latent systems risks. Off-site simulation is more resource-intensive with regard to space, ancillary personnel, faculty time and ability to back-fill staff pulled from the unit to attend an off-site course. In-situ training may be accomplished within the unit, utilizing available staff and low-technology simulators. One randomized controlled trial comparing the effectiveness of eclampsia training in local hospitals versus a simulation center noted improvement in management of eclampsia irrespective of the location of training [13]. Two studies from Denmark in 2015 that directly compared in-situ and off-site simulation, found that the setting had no effect on knowledge, attitudes, stress or evaluation of the simulation; although those who participated in the in-situ simulations felt more authenticity in the experience and also discovered more latent risks needing to be addressed at the systems level [14, 15]. Another study from an academic hospital's operating room found significantly improved staff perception of both safety and teamwork 6–12 months after implementing an in-situ interprofessional simulation program [16]. Others have found similar results with regard to improved skill, confidence and attitudes after in-situ simulation; and also found that in-situ is less resource-intensive [17].

Given that both team and individual outcomes appear to be similar in either venue, the choice between executing in-situ versus off-site simulations depends on the desired outcome and available resources. In fact, some may choose to do both.

Lessons Learned from a Comprehensive Interprofessional Simulation Program

In July 2010, one large, multi-campus academic medical center in New York City implemented a comprehensive interprofessional obstetrical simulation course supported by its PLI as described earlier. All obstetrical personnel (MD, PA, RN, and CNM) were expected to attend a half-day, off-site course on a yearly basis. Given the availability of an off-site simulation center and a busy inner city labor floor that afforded limited opportunities for in-situ simulation, an off-site venue was thought to be best to accomplish the goals of the program. Courses were offered approximately ten times per academic year and consisted of stations where interprofessional teams rotated through various obstetrical emergencies. Different scenarios were presented each year, including postpartum hemorrhage, shoulder dystocia, operative vaginal delivery, cord prolapse, emergent cesarean delivery and eclampsia, with content chosen based on need as determined by Quality Assurance case review. Team training principles were embedded into each simulation scenario to allow teams to practice these important tools, while also working on clinical knowledge and technical skill. The course included an interactive medico-legal component presented by an attorney from the PLI. Participants completed pre- and post-course surveys, which included demographic information, confidence and attitude questions. Post-course feedback from these evaluations was utilized to shape the simulation curriculum. The course was generally well received by participants and had full support from departmental leadership, which contributed to sustainability and expansion of the program. Some valuable lessons were learned over the first 6 years of this program and are highlighted in Table 17.1.

This course demonstrated several key strategies for success from a programmatic perspective. First, it was truly interprofessional in nature. Course faculty felt strongly about ensuring that teams participating in simulations mirrored, as closely as possible, the team structure on the clinical units; therefore, courses were held only when representation from each discipline could be assured. In order to accomplish this, the course had to be considered a priority with evident interprofessional leadership engagement. Support from the PLI was helpful in gaining buy-in, but enlisting input from all departments in the planning of the course was also critical. For example, after presenting a full-day, multi-station course in the first year, and receiving feedback from both participants and their leaders about the difficulties involved in scheduling and staffing, the course was pared down to a half-day, two station format that was easier for both providers and nurses to attend. Finally, another valuable lesson learned was the offering of incentives to participants in the form of continuing education (CE) credits. The fact that participants received CE credits for attendance validated the importance of the program and provided incentive to rearrange schedules, and/or work overtime, in order to attend the course.

Table 17.1 Progression of Curriculum Revisions to Comprehensive Obstetrical Simulation Course

	Year 1	Year 2	Year 3 and Beyond
Schedule	Full day, 5 stations	Change: Half-day, 3 stations Rationale: less resource intensive; ability to focus on specific skills with less stations	Change: 2 megasims Rationale: increased focus on specific skills; lengthy debriefing for participants to acquire debriefing skills for clinical practice
Clinical Content	PPH, Operative vaginal delivery, eclampsia, shoulder dystocia, medico-legal	Change: Cord prolapse, emergent Cesarean delivery, shoulder dystocia (w/ breaking bad news component) Rationale: based on participant feedback from previous year; new focus by department on disclosure after adverse events	Change: 2 OB emergencies (including, but not limited to previously covered scenarios) Rationale: based on participant feedback from previous year as well as needs assessment from department QI program
Teamwork Content	Communication skills: SBAR Closed-loop Call-out/check back Directed communication	Change: briefs, debriefs, huddles, plus all previously learned communication skills Rationale: continued rollout of team training program	Change: all previously learned team training skills plus escalation skills (CUS*, 2-challenge) Rationale: continued rollout of team training program
Participants	OB personnel: MFM Attendings OB/GYN Attendings Fellows Residents PA RN CNM	Change: addition of Neonatology and Pediatrics providers Rationale: Often involved in disclosure of adverse events (particularly infant injuries after shoulder dystocia)	Change: addition of Anesthesiology providers Rationale: Anesthesia personnel are part of daily team in L&D
Incentives	None	Change: provided CME and CEU credits Rationale: to recognize provider's commitment to attending course	Same

Abbreviations: *OB* obstetric, *PPH* postpartum hemorrhage, *QI* quality improvement, *SBAR* Situation-Background-Assessment-Recommendation, *CUS* TeamSTEPPS® tool for expressing "I'm **concerned**. I'm **uncomfortable**. This is a **safety issue**.", *MFM* Maternal-Fetal Medicine, *OB/GYN* Obstetrician/Gynecologist, *PA* physician's assistant, *RN* registered nurse, *CNM* certified nurse midwife, *L&D* labor and delivery, *CME* continuing medical education, *CEU* continuing education unit (Nursing-specific)

This interprofessional obstetrical simulation-based team training course had other unique aspects, including a medico-legal component, and an opportunity to introduce obstetric emergency checklists. The role of simulation to explore medico-legal topics in medicine has been sparsely covered in the literature. In 2008, Goffman et al. found that provider documentation significantly improved after shoulder dystocia simulations with a documentation component [18]. Building on these findings, the planning committee for the interprofessional simulation-based obstetrical team training course decided to incorporate a simulated deposition after the shoulder dystocia scenario. A predetermined physician-nurse pair agreed to participate in a mock deposition in front of their peers on the notes they had written immediately after their simulated shoulder dystocia delivery. An attorney from the PLI agreed to attend each course to perform the deposition. Due to the abbreviated form the course took after its first year, the deposition portion was modified to an interactive session lead by the same attorney given at each course. Topics covered in these talks ranged from documentation strategies to debriefing with the interprofessional team after an event to the importance of disclosure of adverse events and how to approach these conversations with patients. Although not formally studied, feedback from attendees about this portion of the experience was consistently positive in course evaluations.

Another newer, novel focus for IPE is the exploration of tools (algorithms and checklists) to help facilitate seamless teamwork, standardize management and optimize team function [19]. The introduction of emergency checklists into clinical practice is a relatively new endeavor in medicine, in general, but particularly in obstetrics. In 2014, ACOG District II introduced the Safe Motherhood Initiative (SMI) - a set of bundles focused on the leading causes of maternal morbidity and mortality- obstetric hemorrhage, hypertensive emergencies and venous thromboembolism in pregnancy [20]. These bundles contain recommendations and guidelines for effective management of these particular emergencies, including emergency checklists for hemorrhage and eclampsia. The checklists were piloted in the interprofessional simulation-based team training course in order to obtain feedback for implementation in the clinical setting. Faculty realized quickly that broader-scale testing of these obstetrical emergency checklists was necessary in order to improve the tools and ascertain effective strategies for implementation into clinical practice, as had been achieved for operating room emergency checklists [19]. Collaboration with a neighboring institution allowed broader testing of these novel checklists using interprofessional simulation-based training with a group previously unexposed to these tools.

Introducing, Improving and Implementing Obstetrical Emergency Checklists through Simulation

Obstetrics, as noted earlier, is a high stakes environment where relatively rare, acute events have the potential for catastrophic maternal and neonatal outcomes. It seems logical that these events should be amenable to similar improvement strategies such as those explored for operating room emergencies [19]. Given the paucity of literature on the feasibility of crisis checklists in obstetrics, Bajaj et al. decided to pilot and validate the checklists developed for obstetrical emergencies as part of the American College of Obstetricians and Gynecologists (ACOG) District II Safe Motherhood Initiative (SMI) [21]. The goal was to understand and learn from groups about the usability and utility of the SMI obstetric emergency checklists in improving obstetric team performance during simulated clinical events, as well as inform checklist revision and implementation [21].

Interprofessional obstetric healthcare teams undergoing regularly scheduled training at a simulation center were recruited to participate in the randomized-controlled trial. In both the eclampsia and obstetric hemorrhage scenarios, 80% of the teams utilized the checklist when it was available to them. There was no significant improvement in percentage of overall completion of all critical actions when teams had the checklist available in either scenario. Despite this, the checklists were well received by participants, with the majority reporting that if they themselves were a patient experiencing an emergency, they would want a checklist to be utilized. The interprofessional teams provided substantial feedback regarding the checklist content, design, and application, which resulted in significant revision of the checklists. This feedback highlights the importance of input by frontline staff in the design and implementation process. The majority of participants expressed the need for additional training and offered strategies for implementation of the checklists within their clinical environment. For example, the participants suggested specific locations to keep the checklists and stressed the importance of practice through in-situ simulation.

Piloting checklists in simulated settings provides an opportunity to hone checklists based on participant feedback while sharpening their skills at utilizing them and managing critical scenarios. Extending practice into the clinical environment allows for thoughtful implementation and practice.

Conclusion

Multiple studies have shown that checklists can improve outcomes and those that have not highlight the need for a renewed focus on checklist implementation and coaching. Simulation provides a useful environment for achieving these goals. In this environment where real patients are not at risk, providers can focus on checklist design, piloting their use with modifications based on feedback. This will allow for implementation planning and effective hands-on training and may ultimately translate into interprofessional teams taking better care of their patients.

Interprofessional simulation-based medical education has been successfully deployed within obstetrics with a variety of aims including reduction of patient harms, risk mitigation, and the validation of crisis checklists [21]. The applications of simulation will continue to expand for the ever-evolving care of patients in Labor and Delivery.

References

1. Makary MA, Daniel M. Medical error- the third leading cause of death in the US. BMJ. 2016;353:i2139.
2. Gaba DM. The future vision of simulation in health care. Qual Saf Health Care. 2004;13(Suppl 1):i2–i10.

3. Goffman D, Brodman M, Friedman AJ, Minkoff H, Merkatz IR. Improved obstetric safety through programmatic collaboration. J Healthc Risk Manag. 2014;33:14–22.
4. The Joint Commission. Sentinel Event Alert: Preventing Infant Death and Injury during Delivery. Joint Commission Perspectives, Volume 24, Number 9, September 2004, pp. 14–15(2).
5. AAFP, AAP, ACNM, ACOG, ACOOG, AWHONN, SMFM. Quality patient care in labor and delivery: a call to action. Joint Statement. Dec 2011. Accessed from acog.org.
6. Goffman D, Lee C, Bernstein P. Simulation in maternal-fetal medicine: making a case for the need. Semin Perinatol. 2013;37(3):140–2.
7. D'Alton ME, Bonanno CA, Berkowitz RL, et al. Putting the "M" back in maternal-fetal medicine. Am J Obstet Gynecol. 2013;208(6):442–8.
8. Draycott T, Sibanda T, Owen L, Akande V, Winter C, Reading S, Whitelaw A. Does training in obstetric emergencies improve neonatal outcome? BJOG. 2006;113(2):177–82.
9. Draycott TJ, Crofts JF, Ash JP, Wilson LV, Yard E, Sibanda T, Whitelaw A. Improving neonatal outcome through practical shoulder dystocia training. Obstet Gynecol. 2008;112(1):14–20.
10. Crofts JF, et al. Prevention of brachial plexus injury—12 years of shoulder dystocia training: an interrupted time-series study. BJOG Int J Obstet Gynaecol. 2016;123(1):111–8.
11. Inglis SR, Feier N, Chetiyaar JB, Naylor MH, Sumersille M, Cervellione KL, Predanic M. Effects of shoulder dystocia training on the incidence of brachial plexus injury. Am J Obstet Gynecol. 2011;204(4):322.e1–6.
12. Truijens SE, Banga FR, Fransen AF, Pop VJ, van Runnard Heimel PJ, Oei SG. The effect of multiprofessional simulation-based obstetric team training on patient-reported quality of care: a pilot study. Simul Healthc. 2015 Aug;10(4):210–6.
13. Ellis D, Crofts JF, Hunt LP, Read M, Fox R, James M. Hospital, simulation center, and teamwork training for eclampsia management: a randomized controlled trial. Obstet Gynecol. 2008;111(3):723–31.
14. Sørensen JL, van der Vleuten C, Rosthøj S, Østergaard D, LeBlanc V, Johansen M, Ekelund K, Starkopf L, Lindschou J, Gluud C, Weikop P, Ottesen B. 'In situ simulation' versus 'off site simulation' in obstetric emergencies and their effect on knowledge, safety attitudes, team performance, stress, and motivation: study protocol for a randomized controlled trial. Trials. 2013;14:220.
15. Sørensen JL, Navne LE, Martin HM, Ottesen B, Albrecthsen CK, Pedersen BW, Kjærgaard H, van der Vleuten C. Clarifying the learning experiences of healthcare professionals with in situ and off-site simulation-based medical education: a qualitative study. BMJ Open. 2015;5(10):e008345.
16. Hinde T, Gale T, Anderson I, Roberts M, Sice P. A study to assess the influence of interprofessional point of care simulation training on safety culture in the operating theatre environment of a university teaching hospital. J Interprof Care. 2016;30:251–3.
17. van Schaik SM, Plant J, Diane S, Tsang L, O'Sullivan P. Interprofessional team training in pediatric resuscitation: a low-cost, in situ simulation program that enhances self-efficacy among participants. Clin Pediatr (Phila). 2011;50(9):807–15.
18. Goffman D, Heo H, Chazotte C, Merkatz IR, Bernstein PS. Using simulation training to improve shoulder dystocia documentation. Obstet Gynecol. 2008;112(6):1284–7.
19. Arriaga AF, Bader AM, Wong JM, et al. Simulation-based trial of surgical-crisis checklists. N Engl J Med. 2013;368:246–53.
20. Safe Motherhood Initiative. American College of Obstetricians and Gynecologists. Available at: http://www.acog.org/About-ACOG/ACOG-Districts/District-II/SMI.
21. Bajaj K, Rivera-Chiauzzi EY, Lee C, Shepard C, Bernstein PS, Moore-Murray T, Smith H, Nathan L, Walker K, Chazotte C, Goffman D. Validating obstetric emergency checklists using simulation: a randomized controlled trial. Am J Perinatol. 2016;33(12):1182–90.

Applications of Simulation-Based Interprofessional Education in Critical Care Settings and Situations: Emergency Room, Trauma, Critical Care, Rapid Response, and Disasters

18

John T. Paige, Laura S. Bonanno, and Deborah D. Garbee

Introduction

Although effective interprofessional teamwork is an integral component of providing safe, quality care to patients throughout the healthcare system, its importance is particularly essential in the critical care setting [1–3]. In this setting, patients are often at their most vulnerable point, and lifesaving interventions are time sensitive and occur in highly dynamic conditions [4]. With advances in care, such situations are becoming more common as increasingly sicker patients are successfully treated and nurtured back to health. In response to this trend, specialized interprofessional teams have arisen within acute care hospitals to assist with the timely identification and treatment of clinically deteriorating patients: rapid response, code, trauma, burn, and stroke [5–7]. In addition, interprofessional care has taken on a more prominent role in the emergency department and the critical care units [1, 3]. Part and parcel of this emphasis on critical care is the recognized need for effective and efficient management of mass casualties resulting from a disaster [8]. Clearly, effective team interaction is desirable in the critical care setting to ensure that the right intervention occurs at the right time [9, 10].

J. T. Paige (✉)
Department of Surgery, Louisiana State University (LSU) Health New Orleans School of Medicine, New Orleans, LA, USA
e-mail: jpaige@lsuhsc.edu

L. S. Bonanno
Nurse Anesthesia Program Director, Louisiana State University (LSU) Health School of Nursing, New Orleans, LA, USA

D. D. Garbee
Associate Dean for Professional Practice, Community Service and Advanced Nursing Practice, Professor of Clinical Nursing, LSUHSC School of Nursing, New Orleans, LA, USA

J. T. Paige et al. (eds.), *Comprehensive Healthcare Simulation: InterProfessional Team Training and Simulation*, Comprehensive Healthcare Simulation,
https://doi.org/10.1007/978-3-030-28845-7_18

Simulation-based training (SBT) is an ideal modality for addressing such a need. Its ability to mimic low frequency and/or high risk clinical situations such as acute cardiac arrest, anaphylactic shock, major trauma, and respiratory failure allows interprofessional teams to practice treatment algorithms and team coordination without risk to a patient. As a result, team members have the opportunity to internalize and refine care interventions to help them become automatic in a real clinical setting.

This chapter will examine the role of interprofessional SBT in preparing healthcare providers to better treat critically ill patients and address mass casualty situations. First, it will briefly discuss a framework for viewing modern healthcare teams and the key interprofessional competencies needed to help them treat patients effectively. Next, it will review current applications of interprofessional SBT to better treat critically ill patients. Finally, it will discuss potential obstacles to conducting such training and strategies to overcome them.

The Healthcare Industry as a Complex Adaptive System and the Role of Interprofessional Compentencies

From an organizational psychology point of view, interprofessional healthcare teams demonstrate characteristics that are present in a complex adaptive system (CAS). Such a system has multiple independent components whose combined functions result in an outcome or behavior that is more than the sum of these individual parts. In this type of framework, team members are autonomous and act according to internalized basic rules of behavior. The autonomous behavior affects the entire team, and can result in non-linear influences. A small action by one member might have a profound impact on the team function. For example, failure of one member to speak up regarding a change in patient status could result in the care team pursuing an improper treatment plan. This situation can produce both unpredictable and entirely new team behaviors. Furthermore, the team itself reacts and responds to the changing conditions based on its "remembered" past actions as well as the environment in which it functions. Nonetheless, teams often move toward a certain behavior or interaction based on attractors "leading" them to that action [11].

Conceptualizing interprofessional teams within a CAS framework emphasizes the importance that communication, collaboration, and interaction among members have on the quality and safety of the treatment provided to the patient in a critical care setting. An interprofessional healthcare team, therefore, is more than the sum of its individual members. How a team communicates and interacts involves more than the particular skills each person brings to the team. In other words, teams enhance the complicated delivery of care to critically ill patients by enhancing the abilities of individual members through their working together. Thus, the training of healthcare personnel who care for the critically ill should be *within* a team structure. Such interprofessional team training has a positive impact on team behaviors as well as patient process and outcome measures in a variety of healthcare settings and situations [12–14]. Key to its effectiveness is an understanding of the organizational culture and context within which it occurs, each learner's background and experience, and the underlining principles of effective teamwork [15]. Equally important is the use of sound educational concepts in the design and implementation of the particular training curriculum needed and its pragmatic integration into the overall educational structure [16]. Finally, effective faculty development to train the trainers is essential, and should include a focus on interprofessional core principles as well as consensus-building and group facilitation skills [17].

The care of critically ill patients requires training in certain knowledge, skills, and abilities (KSAs) for clinicians treating them. Such KSAs involve cognitive, technical, and interpersonal components. Important cognitive elements include the treatment algorithms for respiratory and cardiac arrest. Technical aspects include endotracheal intubation, intravenous access, and cardiopulmonary resuscitation. Interpersonal features focus on decision-making, assertiveness, situation awareness, and communication. In addition to teaching these cognitive, technical, and interpersonal KSAs, training programs should also address the interprofessional component of teamwork and the recognized competencies and capabilities related to it. Although the particular interprofessional domains identified vary somewhat internationally, much overlap exists (Fig. 18.1) [18]. Most importantly, all frameworks include teamwork as a core interprofessional competency. In the United States, the domains initially identified by the Interprofessional Education Collaborative (IPEC) are now competencies subsumed within an overall interprofessional collaboration domain [19]. Such consolidation is now more common in approaches to teaching and training interprofessional KSAs. For example, the Center for Interprofessional Studies and Innovation at the Massachusetts General Hospital Institute of Health Professions recently adopted an integrated model of interprofessional education in

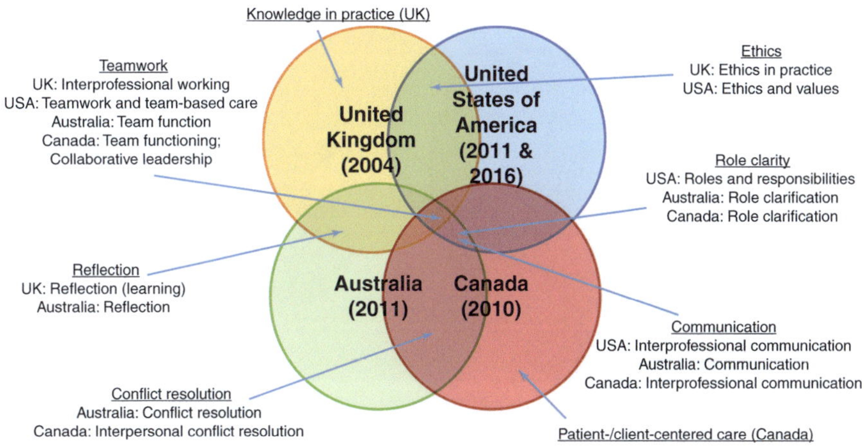

Fig. 18.1 Interprofessional Competencies and Capabilities. Although interprofessional competencies and capabilities can vary somewhat in different countries, many of them overlap. The teamwork competency is universal. The communication and role clarity capabilities are widely recognized as well

which professional competence, in this case related to interprofessional collaboration, is treated as a way of being and not just necessary KSAs that must be learned [20]. Thus, learning occurs within multiple contexts, uses various modalities, and remains patient-centered, resulting in a team member who is "competent in any context" [20].

Simulation-based techniques and modalities are well suited to help instill interprofessional competencies in learners. In fact, the use of high fidelity simulation is desirable in the acute care setting, given its ability to provide immersive, authentic training opportunities for team members to practice technical and nontechnical skills [15]. Such high fidelity SBT experiences afford ample material for discussion and reflection in the after-action debriefings that follow them. Also, simulation-based modalities can address a wide range of needs and gaps in the critical care setting, as explored in the next section.

Current Applications of Simulation-Based Modalities in the Critical Care Setting

The benefit of employing interprofessional SBT to improve the care of critically ill patients is the flexibility with which it can address multiple levels and a variety of issues within the acute care environment (Fig. 18.2). It can focus on the team unit, a clinical microsystem, an institution and its organization, or an entire geographic locale. It can address team coordination and communication, microsystem

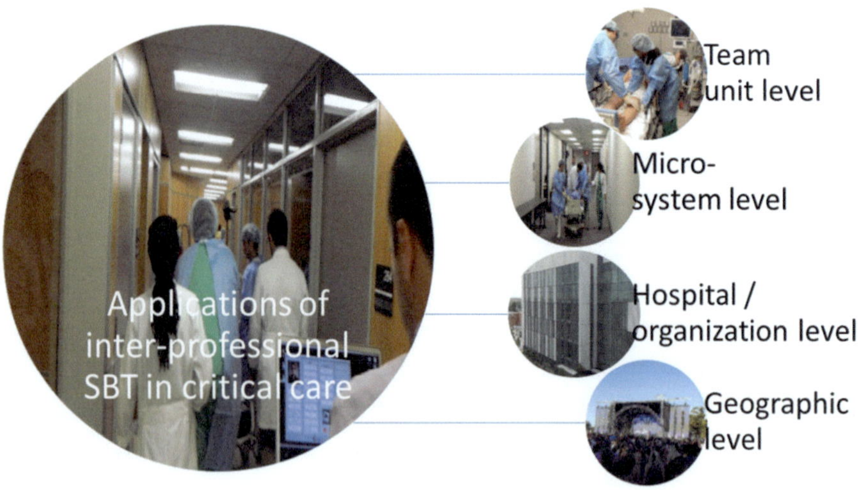

Fig. 18.2 Applications of simulation-based training in critical care. One of the advantages of simulation-based training in the acute care setting is its ability to address issues related to care and collaboration on multiple levels, including the team itself, the clinical microsystem in which the teams operate, the hospital/organizational environment, and the overall regional/geographic setting

resiliency, organizational structure, or disaster preparedness. Combined, such a diversity of applications enhances SBT's utility, since it creates the possibility to address multiple levels of a healthcare entity simultaneously. This fact is especially apparent when SBT occurs in situ rather than when it happens outside the actual clinical environment ex cura [21].

Certainly, interprofessional SBT often targets training and education at the team unit level when addressing critical care issues (Table 18.1) [22–29]. Such training typically occurs in situ, and focuses on physicians and nurses. Kirkpatrick's framework of training effectiveness is useful for evaluating its impact [30]. Such analysis demonstrates positive participant reaction to training (Level 1) as well as the acquisition of KSAs through the training (Level 2). On occasion, change in participant

Table 18.1 Recent examples of the effectiveness of simulation-based training of interprofessional teams caring for critically ill patients

Team Unit Author	Participants	Intervention	Assessment	Outcomes (Kirkpatrick level)
Emergency Department				
Paltved et al. (2017) [22]	Physicians and nurses	In situ medical scenarios (urosepsis, chronic obstructive pulmonary disease exacerbation, acute pancreatitis)	1. Trainee Reactions Score (self-report) 2. Safety Attitudes Questionnaire (self-report)	1. Positive reaction to training (Level 1) 2. Increase in safety climate and teamwork climate scores (Level 2)
Truta et al. (2018) [23]	Physicians, residents, and nurses	Single day didactic and in situ simulation-based training sessions involving medicine and trauma scenarios	1. Nontechnical skills for emergency medicine tool (observer)	1. Increase in all domains of tool for all professions (Level 2)
Intensive care				
George and Quatrara (2018) [24]	SICU physicians and nurses	In situ simulation-based scenario (increased intracranial pressure in traumatic brain injury patient)	1. Knowledge test 2. Teamwork Skills Scale (self-report)	1. Increase in scores with one month retention (Level 2) 2. Increase in TSS scores with one month retention (Level 2)
Emani et al. (2018) [25]	Pediatric CCU physicians and nurses	Five day didactic and in situ simulation-based training sessions	1. Simulation experience questions 2. Team dynamics and performance tool (self-report) 3. Time measurements and frequency counts (observer)	1. Positive reaction to sessions (Level 1) 2. Increase in team dynamic and performance scores (Level 2) 3. Increase in frequency of closed loop communication (Level 2)

(continued)

Table 18.1 (continued)

Team Unit Author	Participants	Intervention	Assessment	Outcomes (Kirkpatrick level)
Rapid Response/Code				
Theilen et al. (2017) [26]	Pediatric Medical Emergency Team physicians and nurses	Weekly in situ simulation-based training of deteriorating medical and surgical pediatric patients	1. Response time to deteriorating patient over 3 years 2. PICU admissions and bed days over 3 years 3. Mortality	1. Decrease in time in recognition of patient deterioration, response by staff, and escalation to PICU (Level 3) 2. Decrease in PICU admissions and bed days with cost savings (Level 4) 3. Overall hospital decrease (Level 4)
Gilfoyle et al. (2017) [27]	Pediatric resuscitation team resident physicians, nurse practitioners, nurses, and respiratory therapists	Single day session involving didactic components and simulation-based training scenarios (cardiogenic shock, unstable ventricular tachycardia, asystole)	1. Clinical Performance Tool (observer) 2. Time to treatment (observer) 3. Clinical Teamwork Scale (observer)	1. Increase in scores (Level 2) 2. Decrease in time to initiation of chest compressions and defibrillation (Level 2) 3. Increase in scores (Level 2)
Trauma				
Sadideen et al. (2016) [28]	Burn resuscitation team physicians, residents, and nurses	Ex cura simulation-based training scenario (pediatric burn)	1. Post training survey (self-report)	1. Realistic and useful for training (Level 1)
Sullivan et al. (2017) [29]	Trauma teams physician residents and nurses	Ex cura simulation-based training sessions using sharp and blunt trauma scenarios	1. T-NOTECHS (observer)	1. Improvement in communication and interaction skills (Level 2)

behavior in the clinical environment (Level 3) as well as improvement in patient outcomes (Level 4) result from such training [21]. Targeted teams include those in specific hospital settings such as the emergency department (ED) and intensive care units (ICUs) as well as those with specific designations such as rapid response teams, code teams, and trauma teams. SBT scenarios usually address actual crises and patient conditions that the particular team will encounter, and sessions tend to focus on both technical and nontechnical skills acquisition. Assessment of technical skills include use of clinical checklists and time to treatment, whereas nontechnical skills are typically evaluated using established instruments designed to assess some of the aforementioned team-based competencies (e.g. leadership, mutual support, communication, etc.). This diversity of applications and its associated encouraging results reveal the widespread use in today's healthcare environment of high fidelity

SBT of interprofessional teams to improve communication and collaboration in acute care settings [22–29].

In addition to addressing needs and gaps at the team unit level, interprofessional SBT can help promote improvements at higher organizational levels. In fact, SBT is very well suited for this purpose. For example, its ability to reproduce rare, uncommon, but potentially catastrophic, situations or events allows for "stress tests" of a department or line of service to identify unrecognized conditions that may exacerbate rather than mitigate threats [31]. Additionally, it can help improve an institution's care processes through prospective analysis in order to find the right balance of patient safety, clinical outcomes, and efficiency [32]. As useful, its retrospective application in recreating the conditions associated with an adverse clinical event can lead to solutions and insights beyond those found through traditional root cause analysis [32, 33]. Finally, simulation modelling and SBT can be combined to study patient throughput and flow to design care environments and processes to improve quality [32, 34].

This focus on quality improvement and safety at a systems-based level is particularly attractive in the dynamic, time sensitive environment of critical care in which any adverse event could lead to dire consequences for the patient. Not surprisingly, several examples of such an application involving interprofessional teams exist [35–38]. In certain situations, they address improving team function *and* systems-level care, particularly those activities targeting specific, disruptive, uncommon events in order to ensure that both the care team and system are prepared. Interprofessional SBT of personnel to de-escalate or handle violent behavior in the ED is illustrative. This training typically encompasses a very broad range of staff in addition to healthcare providers, including security staff, social services staff, guest services personnel, unit coordinators, and patient access specialists. These scenarios help members learn and practice protocols related to these situations, and they can identify physical plant and/or process issues that may hinder and/or improve response.

The reproducibility of interprofessional SBT scenarios also allows for institutional-wide applications. For example, the Durham Veterans Administration (VA) Medical Center [39] conducted unannounced in situ cardiac arrest interprofessional SBT exercises at varying times throughout its facility as part of a quality improvement project using the Systems Engineering Initiative for Patient Safety (SEIPS) model. In the process, it was able to identify and mitigate system related hazards in the care environment, policies, and culture of its institution. In New York City, the Patient Safety Institute at Northwell Health [40] joined forces with Lenox Hill Hospital to create an interprofessional SBT curriculum to prospectively prepare and test a new freestanding emergency department, known as Lennox Hill-Greenwich Village. This systems integration project included orienting new and experienced staff to the facility and in situ "stress tests" of the physical location prior to its opening. This approach helped uncover several latent safety threats within the facility as well as issues related to patient intake and flow.

Such institutional level interprofessional SBT can facilitate health system-wide applications through scalability. For example, collaborations within the International Network for Simulation-based Pediatric Innovation, Research and Education (INSPIRE) enabled multi-institutional work investigating pediatric resuscitation techniques in EDs. For one of these explorations, in situ SBT scenarios aided in demonstrating that adherence to pediatric cardiac arrest guidelines was not associated with ED pediatric volume [41]. In other similar projects, the in situ SBT scenarios revealed disparities in the management of pediatric hypoglycemia and sepsis between general and pediatric EDs [42, 43]. Clearly, the ability to identify gaps in performance and knowledge on such a scale provides opportunities for developing interprofessional SBT curricula targeting them.

Finally, interprofessional SBT's flexibility, reproducibility, and scalability enables the implementation of curricula and programs to address challenges to health systems within defined geographic regions. For example, in Eastern North Carolina, a Level 1 trauma center developed an in situ SBT curriculum for targeted rural EDs related to management of pediatric trauma [44]. Disaster and mass casualty preparation are other examples. These interprofessional SBT activities include annual "Disaster Day" exercises conducted at a single institution, simulated mass casualty traumas, and response exercises to pandemics [45–48]. Computer modelling simulations can assist with planning and preparation by determining surge capacities at affected healthcare entities [49].

Barriers to Interprofessional Simulation-Based Training in the Critical Care Setting and Potential Solutions

The multiple benefits of interprofessional SBT make it a very attractive modality for addressing gaps across a wide scale of settings. Barriers, however, can interfere with its implementation, and they can relate to the simulation-based nature of the training, its interprofessional quality, and even the character of the critical care environment (Fig. 18.3) [50–55]. Overlap does exist. For example, the work culture in healthcare is typically not familiar with conducting training exercises to improve team performance and systems function, be it related to the use of simulation, the interprofessional education, or the critical care component. In addition, having time to train and access to equipment or space to train are two other common challenges. Finally, curricular integration of the training is a common obstacle. Other barriers are unique to the particular character of the component of training. Salient examples include the technological challenges of simulation-based high fidelity training with its associated cost, the logistical obstacles of scheduling learners from multiple professions, and the limited space and care requirements of a critical care setting.

Developing solutions to these barriers is essential in order to unleash interprofessional SBT's full potential in the critical care environment. One important approach is to demonstrate a return on investment related to the interprofessional SBT in order to justify the perceived high cost of high fidelity simulation [56]. Using sound curricular design principles will help ensure choosing the appropriate simulation with adequate technological capability to address the objectives of the training [57]. In this manner, costly high technology simulators may be replaced with less expensive, low technology models or even table-top exercises. Applying an established

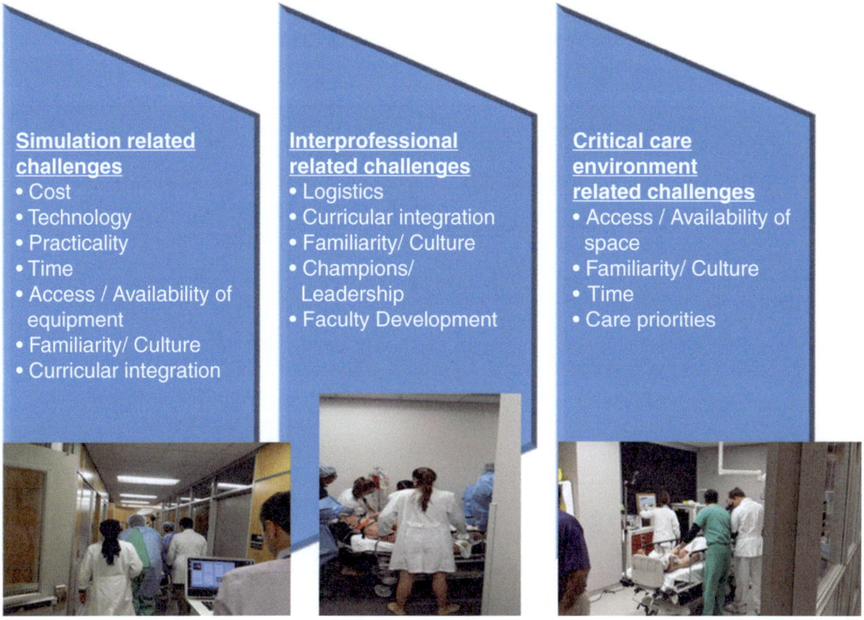

Fig. 18.3 Challenges of simulation-based training in critical care. Challenges related to implementation of simulation-based training in critical care settings can arise from issues related to the use of simulation itself, problems arising from bringing together interprofessional teams, and matters developing from the critical care environment in which the training occurs

curricular framework to the development and implementation of an interprofessional SBT program can also help address issues related to its implementation and streamlining within established educational opportunities [53, 57]. Administrative backing and the identification of a local champion within the critical care setting can assist in overcoming the logistical challenges and space requirements encountered [58]. Such leadership and support can also help overcome the cultural reticence to engage in interprofessional SBT training.

Clearly, challenges are inevitable in organizing these complex, sophisticated training exercises involving a wide range of professionals with varying degrees of background KSAs and experiences. The use of a systematic, consistent approach to developing and implementing these programs can ease the difficulties encountered. At LSU Health New Orleans, we have utilized one such structure to assist with implementation of SBT activities within the Health Sciences Center to create an interprofessional curriculum (Table 18.2). This framework known as the "5P" approach [58] divides potential barriers into task buckets of decreasing importance: (1) Finding a PATRON; (2) Developing a PLAN; (3) Locating a PLACE; (4) Assembling your PEOPLE; and (5) Choosing your PRODUCTS. Each task has strategic and tactical aspects to help identify and address potential pitfalls. Other frameworks for implementation of training programs are available in the literature related to training in domains outside of healthcare [59, 60]. The particular one

Table 18.2 Application of the 5P Approach in Establishing an Interprofessional Team Training Curriculum at the LSU Health New Orleans Health Sciences Center

Finding a PATRON		
Strategic issues	Institutional support for protected time, funding, cultural acceptance	Health Sciences backing for HRSA grant application and award to implement IPE curriculum
Tactical issues	Local champions to drive implementation	Identification of faculty champions in the Schools of Medicine, Nursing, and Allied Health to drive implementation
Developing a PLAN		
Strategic issues	Robust curriculum developed according to sound educational principles	Team training curriculum developed to address gap, teach teamwork KSAs; program evaluated on multiple Kirkpatrick levels
Tactical issues	Logistics of scheduling, implementation, assessment	Integration of training within established curricular program in School of Medicine; development of web based assessment
Locating a PLACE		
Strategic issues	Locale for training to match curricular needs	Ex cura training at School of Medicine Learning Center
Tactical issues	Securing actual space, location	Time secured to use simulation rooms monthly on Wednesday mornings
Assembling your PEOPLE		
Strategic issues	Team of expert faculty to conduct training; targeted learners for training	Faculty experienced in SBT of interprofessional teams to conduct sessions; senior students targeted in each of the Schools
Tactical issues	Faculty development for trainers; actual composition of training teams	Annual faculty development for new faculty and local champions; team composition based on scenario and scheduled accordingly
Choosing your PRODUCTS		
Strategic issues	Simulators, debriefing techniques, and assessment tools to match curricular needs	High fidelity simulation scenarios using computer-based manikins, structured debriefing, team-based assessment tool
Tactical issues	Smooth integration of simulators, debriefing, assessment tools into scenarios and sessions	Scenario creation, immediate after-action debriefing in room, electronic tablet-based completion of assessment tool

chosen is not as essential as developing a systematic approach to implementation and evaluation of an interprofessional SBT program in critical care.

Conclusion

The highly dynamic, high-risk setting of caring for the critically ill make it an ideal target area for interprofessional SBT of teams providing care. Conceptualizing such teams as a CAS emphasizes the importance of communication, collaboration, and interaction among the individual members, and the non-linear impact one individual's action can have on team function and patient well-being as a whole. A particular strength of interprofessional SBT in the critical care setting is its reproducibility and scalability, enabling training and improvement in the quality of care at the team, clinical microsystem, institutional, and regional levels. Current applications of interprofessional SBT in critical care settings reveal evidence of training effectiveness, most often at the first two levels of Kirkpatrick's framework. These training activities are complex, sophisticated, and involve a wide range of learners with diverse backgrounds. As such, challenges to successful implementation will occur. Overcoming them requires a systematic approach to address aspects including logistics, curriculum, and support. Future work in SBT in critical care domains will focus on improving patient outcomes.

References

1. Donovan AL, Aldrich JM, Gross AK, Barchas DM, Thornton KC, Schell-Chaple HM, Gropper MA, AKM L, University of California, San Francisco Critical Care Innovations Group. Interprofessional care and teamwork in the ICU. Crit Care Med. 2018;46(6):980–90.
2. Ford K, Menchine M, Burner E, Arora S, Inaba K, Demetriades D, Yersin B. Leadership and teamwork in trauma and resuscitation. West J Emerg Med. 2016;17(5):549–56.
3. Bleetman A, Sanusi S, Dale T, Brace S. Human factors and error prevention in emergency medicine. Emerg Med J. 2012;29(5):389–93.
4. Alarhayem AQ, Myers JG, Dent D, Liao L, Muir M, Mueller D, Nicholson S, Cestero R, Johnson MC, Stewart R, O'Keefe G, Eastridge BJ. Time is the enemy: mortality in trauma patients with hemorrhage from torso injury occurs long before the "golden hour". Am J Surg. 2016;212(6):1101–5.
5. Maharaj R, Raffaele I, Wendon J. Rapid response systems: a systematic review and meta-analysis. Crit Care. 2015;19:254.
6. Al-Mousawi AM, Mecott-Rivera GA, Jeschke MG, Herndon DN. Burn teams and burn centers: the importance of a comprehensive team approach to burn care. Clin Plast Surg. 2009;36(4):547–54.
7. Wang H, Thevathasan A, Dowling R, Bush S, Mitchell P, Yan B. Streamlining workflow for endovascular mechanical thrombectomy: lessons learned from a comprehensive stroke center. J Stroke Cerebrovasc Dis. 2017;26(8):1655–62.
8. National Academies of Sciences, Engineering, and Medicine, Health and Medicine Division, Board on Health Sciences Policy, Forum on Medical and Public Health Preparedness for Disasters and Emergencies. Engaging the private-sector health care system in building capacity to respond to threats to the public's health and national security: proceedings of a workshop. Washington, D.C.: National Academies Press (US); 2018.
9. Weller J, Boyd M, Cumin D. Teams, tribes, and patient safety: overcoming barriers to effective teamwork in healthcare. Postgrad Med J. 2014;90(1061):149–54.
10. Richardson J, West MA, Cuthbertson BH. Team working in intensive care: current evidence and future endeavors. Curr Opin Crit Care. 2010;16(6):643–8.
11. Pype P, Mertens F, Helewaut F, Krystallidou D. Healthcare teams as complex adaptive systems: understanding team behavior through team members' perception of interpersonal interaction. BMC Health Ser Res. 2018;18(1):570.
12. Doumouras AG, Hamidi M, Lung K, Tarola CL, Tsao MW, Scott JW, Smink DS, Yule S. Non-technical skills of surgeons and anaesthetists in simulated operating theatre crises. Br J Surg. 2017;104(8):1028–36.
13. Varpio L, Bader KS, Meyer HS, Durning SJ, Artino AR, Hamwey MK. Interprofessional healthcare teams in the military: a scoping review. Mil Med. 2018;183(11-12):e448–54.
14. Paige JT, Garbee DD, Brown KM, Rojas JD. Using simulation in interprofessional education. Surg Clin North Am. 2015;95:751–66.
15. Eddy K, Jordan Z, Stephenson M. Health professionals' experience of teamwork education in acute hospital settings: a systemic review of qualitative literature. JBI Database System Rev Implement Rep. 2016;14(4):96–137.

16. Prast J, Herlache-Pretzer E, Frederick A, Gafni-Lachter L. Practical strategies for integrating interprofessional education and collaboration into the curriculum. Occup Ther Health Care. 2016;30(2):166–74.
17. Ratka A, Zorek JA, Meyer SM. Overview of faculty development programs for interprofessional education. Am J Pharm Educ. 2017;81(5):96.
18. Thisthlethwaite JE, Forman D, Matthews LR, Rogers GD, Steketee C, Yassine T. Competencies and frameworks in interprofessional education: a comparative analysis. Acad Med. 2014;89(6):869–75.
19. Interprofessional Education Collaborative. Core competencies for interprofessional collaborative practice: 2016 update. Washington, D.C.: Interprofessional Education Collaborative; 2016.
20. Cahn PS, Tuck I, Knab MS, Doherty RF, Portney LG, Johnson AF. Competent in any context: an integrated model of interprofessional education. J Interprof Care. 2018:1–4. Epub 24 jul.
21. Armenia S, Thangamethesvaran L, Caine AD, King N, Kunac A, Merchant AM. The role of high-fidelity team-based simulation in acute care settings: a systematic review. Surg J (NY). 2018 Aug 13;4(3):e136–51.
22. Paltved C, Bjerregaard AT, Krogh K, Pedersen JJ, Musaeus P. Designing in situ simulation in the emergency department: evaluating safety attitudes amongst physicians and nurses. Adv Simul (Lond). 2017;2:4. https://doi.org/10.1186/s41077-017-0037-2. eCollection 2017.
23. Truta TS, Boeriu CM, Copotoiu SM, Petrisor M, Turucz E, Vatau D, Lazarovici M. Improving nontechnical skills of an interprofessional emergency medical team through a one day crisis resource management training. Medicine (Baltimore). 2018;97(32):e11828.
24. George KL, Quatrara B. Interprofessional simulations promote knowledge retention and enhance perceptions of teamwork skills in a surgical-trauma-burn intensive care unit setting. Dimens Crit Care Nurs. 2018;37(3):144–55.
25. Emani SS, Allan CK, Forster T, Fisk AC, Lagrasta C, Zheleva B, Weinstock P, Thiagarajan RR. Simulation training improves team dynamics and performance in a low-resource cardiac intensive care unit. Ann Pediatr Cardiol. 2018;11(2):130–6.
26. Theilen U, Fraser L, Jones P, Leonard P, Simpson D. Regular in-situ simulation training of paediatric medical emergency team leads to sustained improvements in hospital response to deteriorating patients, improved outcomes in intensive care and financial savings. Resuscitation. 2017;115:61–7.
27. Gilfoyle E, Koot DA, Annear JC, Bhanji F, Cheng A, Duff JP, Grant VJ, St George-Hyslop CE, Delaloye NJ, Kotsakis A, McCoy CD, Ramsay CE, Weiss MJ, Gottesman RD, Teams4Kids Investigators and the Canadian Critical Care Trials Group. Improved clinical performance and teamwork of pediatric Interprofessional resuscitation teams with a simulation-based educational intervention. Pediatr Crit Care Med. 2017;18(2):e62–9.
28. Sadideen H, Wilson D, Moiemen N, Kneebone R. Using "the burns suite" as a novel high fidelity simulation tool for interprofessional and teamwork training. J Burn Care Res. 2016;37(4):235–42.
29. Sullivan S, Campbell K, Ross JC, Thompson R, Underwood A, LeGare A, Osman I, Agarwal SK, Jung HS. Identifying nontechnical skill deficits in trainees through interdisciplinary trauma simulation. J Surg Educ. 2018;75(4):978–83.
30. Kirkpatrick DI. Evaluating training programs: the four levels. 2nd ed. San Francisco: Berrett-Koehler; 1998.
31. Deutsch ES, Dong Y, Halamek LP, Rosen MA, Taekman JM, Rice J. Leveraging health care simulation technology for human factors research: closing the gap between lab and bedside. Hum Factors. 2016;58(7):1082–95.
32. Paige JT, Fairbanks FJT, Gaba DM. Priorities related to improving healthcare safety through simulation. Simul Healthc. 2018;13:S41–250.
33. Slakey DP, Simms ER, Rennie KV, Garstka ME, Korndorffer JR Jr. Using simulation to improve root cause analysis of adverse surgical outcomes. Int J Qual Health Care. 2014;26(2):144–50.
34. Lundberg P, Kordorffer JR Jr. Using simulation to improve systems. Surg Clin North Am. 2015;95:885–92.

35. Krull W, Gusenius TM, Germain D, Schnepper L. Staff perception of interprofessional simulation for verbal de-escalation and restraint application to mitigate violent patient behaviors in the emergency department. J Emerg Nurs. 2018. pii: S0099–1767(18)30031-X.
36. Sanchez L, Young VB, Baker M. Active shooter training in the emergency department: a safety initiative. J Emerg Nurs. 2018;44(6):598–604.
37. Wong AH, Wing L, Weiss B, Gang M. Coordinating a team response to behavioral emergencies in the emergency department: a simulation-enhanced Interprofessional curriculum. West J Emerg Med. 2015;16(6):859–65.
38. Wong AH, Auerbach MA, Ruppel H, Crispino LJ, Rosenberg A, Iennaco JD, Vaca FE. Addressing dual patient and staff safety through a team-based standardized patient simulation for agitation management in the emergency department. Simul Healthc. 2018;13(3):154–62.
39. Barbeito A, Bonifacio A, Holtschneider M, Segall N, Schroeder R, Mark J, Durham Veterans Affairs Medical Center Patient Safety Center of Inquiry. In situ simulated cardiac arrest exercises to detect system vulnerabilities. Simul Healthc. 2015;10(3):154–62.
40. Kerner RL Jr, Gallo K, Cassara M, D'Angelo J, Egan A, Simmons JG. Simulation for operational readiness in a new freestanding emergency department: strategy and tactics. Simul Healthc. 2016;11(5):345–56.
41. Auerbach M, Brown L, Whitfill T, Baird J, Abulebda K, Bhatnagar A, Lutfi R, Gawel M, Walsh B, Tay KY, Lavoie M, Nadkarni V, Dudas R, Kessler D, Katznelson J, Ganghadaran S, Hamilton MF. Adherence to pediatric cardiac arrest guidelines across a spectrum of fifty emergency departments: a prospective, in situ, simulation-based study. Acad Emerg Med. 2018;25(12):1396–408.
42. Walsh BM, Gangadharan S, Whitfill T, Gawel M, Kessler D, Dudas RA, Katznelson J, Lavoie M, Tay KY, Hamilton M, Brown LL, Nadkarni V, Auerbach M, INSPIRE ImPACT investigators. Safety threats during the care of infants with hypoglycemic seizures in the emergency department: a multicenter, simulation-based prospective cohort study. J Emerg Med. 2017;53(4):467–474.e7.
43. Kessler DO, Walsh B, Whitfill T, Dudas RA, Gangadharan S, Gawel M, Brown L, Auerbach M, INSPIRE ImPACTS investigators. Disparities in adherence to pediatric sepsis guidelines across a spectrum of emergency departments: a multicenter, cross-sectional observational in situ simulation study. J Emerg Med. 2016;50(3):403–15.e1–3.
44. Bayouth L, Ashley S, Brady J, Lake B, Keeter M, Schiller D, Robey WC 3rd, Charles S, Beasley KM, Toschlog EA, Longshore SW. An in-situ simulation-based educational outreach project for pediatric trauma care in a rural trauma system. J Pediatr Surg. 2018;53(2):367–71.
45. Livingston LL, West CA, Livingston JL, Landry KA, Watzak BC, Graham LL. Simulated disaster day: benefit from lessons learned through years of transformation from silos to interprofessional education. Simul Healthc. 2016;11(4):293–8.
46. Saber DA, Strout K, Caruso LS, Ingwell-Spolan C, Koplovsky A. An interprofessional approach to continuing education with mass casualty simulation: planning and execution. J Contin Educ Nurs. 2017;48(10):447–53.
47. Kilianski A, O'Rourke AT, Carlson CL, Parikh SM, Shipman-Amuwo F. The planning, execution, and evaluation of a mass prophylaxis full-scale exercise in Cook County, IL. Biosecur Bioterror. 2014;12(2):106–16.
48. Biddell EA, Vandersall BL, Bailes SA, Estephan SA, Ferrara LA, Nagy KM, O'Connell JL, Patterson MD. Use of simulation to gauge preparedness for Ebola at a free-standing children's hospital. Simul Healthc. 2016;11(2):94–9.
49. Morton MJ, DeAugustinis ML, Velasquez CA, Singh S, Kelen GD. Developments in surge research priorities: a systematic review of the literature following the academic emergency medicine consensus conference, 2007–2015. Acad Emerg Med. 2015;22(11):1235–52.
50. Hosny SG, Johnston MJ, Pucher PH, Erridge S, Darzi A. Barriers to the implementation and uptake of simulation-based training programs in general surgery: a multinational qualitative study. J Surg Res. 2017;220:419–426.e2.
51. Al-Ghareeb AZ, Cooper SJ. Barriers and enablers to the use of high-fidelity patient simulation manikins in nurse education: an integrative review. Nurse Educ Today. 2016;36:281–6.

52. Sunguya BF, Hinthong W, Jimba M, Yasuoka J. Interprofessional education for whom?— challenges and lessons learned from its implementation in developed countries and their application to developing countries: a systematic review. PLoS One. 2014;9(5):e96724.
53. West C, Graham L, Palmer RT, Miller MF, Thayer EK, Stuber ML, Awdishu L, Umoren RA, Wamsley MA, Nelson EA, Joo PA, Tysinger JW, George P, Carney PA. Implementation of interprofessional education (IPE) in 16 U.S. medical schools: common practices, barriers and facilitators. J Interprof Educ Pract. 2016;4:41–9.
54. Global Forum on Innovation in Health Professional Education; Board on Global Health; Institute of Medicine. Interprofessional Education for Collaboration: Learning how to improve health from interprofessional models across the continuum of education practice: workshop summary. Washington, D.C.: National Academies Press (US); 2013.
55. Leclair LW, Dawson M, Howe A, Hale S, Zelman E, Clouser R, Garrison G, Allen G. A longitudinal interprofessional simulation curriculum for critical care teams: exploring successes and challenges. J Interprof Care. 2018;32(3):386–90.
56. Asche CV, Kim M, Brown A, Golden A, Laack TA, Rosario J, Strother C, Totten VY, Okuda Y. Communicating value in simulation: cost benefit analysis and return on investment. Acad Emerg Med. 2018;25(2):230–7.
57. Eisold C, Poenicke C, Pfältzer A, Müller MP. Simulation in the intensive care setting. Best Pract Res Clin Anaesthesiol. 2015;29(1):51–60.
58. Paige JT. Team training at the point of care. In: Tsuda S, Scott DJ, Jones DB, editors. Textbook of simulation, surgical skills, and team training. Woodbury: Ciné-med, Inc.; 2012.
59. Proctor EK, Powell BJ, McMillen JC. Implementation strategies: recommendations for specifying and reporting. Implement Sci. 2013;8:139.
60. Kilbourne AM, Neumann MS, Pincus HA, Bauer MS, Stall R. Implementing evidence-based interventions in health care: application of the replicating effective programs framework. Implement Sci. 2007;2:42.

Pre-hospital Care: Emergency Medical Services

19

Jennifer McCarthy, Amar Pravin Patel, and Andrew E. Spain

Introduction

The lack of national uniformity in Emergency Medical Services (EMS) in the United States has fostered confusion amongst the general public, politicians, and other licensed healthcare providers regarding their role. Annually, 911 receives over 37 million calls resulting in approximately 28 million patients being transported to a healthcare facility [1, 2]. These numbers, and the visible presence of ambulances on the street, belie the fact that, unless faced with a medical emergency personally, the scope of practice, system structure, and efficiency of EMS is often invisible to others [3]. It is an environment where the providers routinely have limited patient contact time and dramatically different assessment, care, and environmental realities compared to all other healthcare settings. Such circumstances lend a uniqueness and, at times, a mystique, to the EMS profession. Additionally, this limited knowledge about EMS and its providers, creates challenges for healthcare simulationists as they try to understand the intricacies of the care given, making it difficult for them to engage EMS teams and professionals in simulation-based activities for Interprofessional Education (IPE).

J. McCarthy (✉)
Seton Hall University, School of Health and Medical Sciences, Nutley, NJ, USA
e-mail: jennifer.mccarthy@shu.edu

A. P. Patel
CAE Healthcare, Sarasota, FL, USA

A. E. Spain
Society for Simulation in Healthcare, Washington, MO, USA
e-mail: aspain@ssih.org

J. T. Paige et al. (eds.), *Comprehensive Healthcare Simulation: InterProfessional Team Training and Simulation*, Comprehensive Healthcare Simulation,
https://doi.org/10.1007/978-3-030-28845-7_19

EMS Origins in the United States and its Current Provider Structure

The current EMS system in the United States arose in the late 1960s after the National Academy of Sciences's publication in 1966 of the EMS White Paper, *Accidental Death and Disability: The Neglected Disease of Modern Society*. Using data obtained from the Federal Department of Transportation (DOT), the White Paper identified that citizens who were dying on highways after traumatic accidents could be saved if military trauma care was available in the civilian sector. The federal government initiative, resulting from the White Paper, to design an EMS system drew on public safety and healthcare influences. Additionally, the EMS structure had a strong paramilitary essence shaping education and practices, something that is still evident today. Over many decades, advanced military- and hospital-based emergency medicine patient treatments infused the EMS industry. EMS systems began to change from a fully permission-based environment where transportation was handled by a private company, a funeral home, or a hospital system to one with clear guidelines and protocols put into place to create a level of independence between the prehospital and hospital provider. As the EMS systems evolved in the early years, EMS was uniquely structured and not uniformly established throughout the U.S. Some services established in fire departments, usually in large cities with ample funding, while other services remained civilian or healthcare affiliated to offset the cost. They began to leverage relationships and as the need for prehospital care grew, EMS systems continued to transform to a more independent healthcare delivery model. Even today, there are vast differences in EMS system and even with these differences the progressive nature of EMS is readily visible.

More recently, the Institute of Medicine (IOM) completed in 2007 an in-depth report on the state of emergency medicine care in the United States entitled the *Future of Emergency Medicine: Crossroads of Emergency Medical Service Care*. This report included an analysis of EMS care as an extension of emergency medicine, and it, identified a model to highlight the complex nature of EMS structure [4]. The model depicted EMS as a mixed service that is part public health, part emergency medicine, and part public safety (Fig. 19.1). This dynamic structure created confusion about the scope, practice, and purpose of the industry.

This perplexity related to which "realm" of healthcare activity EMS belongs is not the only source of confusion for individuals unfamiliar with the EMS system. Misperceptions reign regarding the personnel working in the system and the nomenclature used for each one. The current Federal EMS design includes four tiers of providers intended to provide a comprehensive system of prehospital patient care. The most recent terminology of the four levels of care are Emergency Medical Responder (EMR), Emergency Medical Technician (EMT), Advanced Emergency Medical Technician (AEMT), and Paramedic. Previous nomenclature usually began with EMT, and then the level of provider following, for instance EMT-Basic (now EMT), and EMT-Paramedic (now Paramedic). Consequently, many outside the EMS system still refer to all EMS personnel as "EMTs" without understanding the

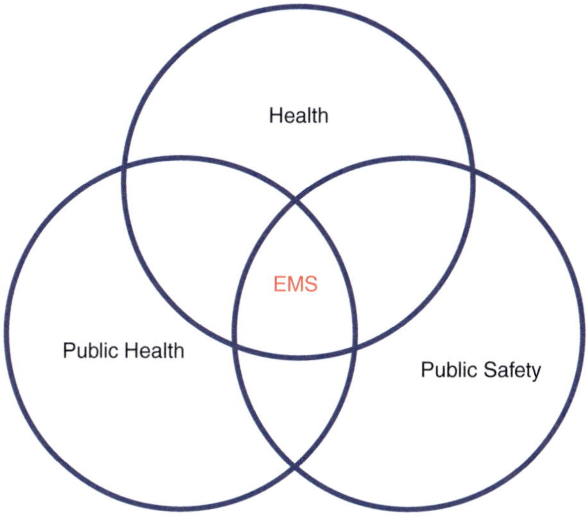

Fig. 19.1 This figure from the IOM describes the interprofessional influences evident in the current Emergency Medical Services. EMS is part health, part public safety, and part public health initiatives [4]. (Original source: NHTSA 1996)

many different levels of care each delivers. In addition, individual states do not necessarily offer all levels of the EMS licensure. Instead, each state has adopted various combinations of the four provider levels of care to meet the needs of their particular geography and demography. Furthermore, additional levels of care are included to ensure medical practices match the needs of the state.

The nationally recognized four levels of care (EMR, EMT, AEMT, and Paramedic) allow the public access to providers who are educated in current emergency medicine treatments and who meet the standards of a national credentialing body. The national curricula for each provider level promote a career ladder within the industry by building upon each prior level in depth and breadth of knowledge, skills, and abilities (KSAs) related to the accepted scope of practice. This educational system is constructed with the goal of getting the maximum lifesaving treatment to the scene of the emergency in the time required for care to be effective in improving a patient's outcome.

An EMR provider is usually the first responder arriving to an emergency before an ambulance. Many areas utilize police officers and firefighters to fill the EMR role. These providers are able to provide many of the most important lifesaving treatments that are required in the first minutes of an emergency. They include cardiopulmonary resuscitation (CPR), the use of a defibrillator, medication administration for opiate overdoses or anaphylaxis, or oxygen administration. EMT providers provide the next tier of care required to improve survivability. EMTs may bring with them automatic CPR and bleeding control devices, and they are an additional support for EMR providers. Paramedics are best described as physician extenders who are trained to provide the key components of the first 20-minutes of care to the scene of an emergency. This care is equivalent to what the patient would receive in a hospital emergency department. In some rural areas, the paramedic care providers must be able to stabilize and manage a patient for the first 40 minutes or more due to the extended transport times needed to reach a hospital.

Not universally seen within EMS systems are AEMT providers. When AEMTs are part of an EMS system, they are a resource with better patient screening and triage methodologies. Locally, their scope of practice lies between an EMT and Paramedic, and they help manage complex patients until a paramedic can arrive to the scene of an emergency. Whereas EMTs are universally first responders who compose part of an ambulance crew, paramedics may also respond in an ambulance, an intercept vehicle, or fire apparatus depending on the region. Aeromedical units bring critical care registered nurses (RNs), respiratory therapists (RTs), paramedics, and even physicians to critically ill patients at the scene of an emergency or for transfer to another facility, reducing long transport times in rural areas. Regardless of the type of vehicle in which they arrive, EMS providers have the same goal in their response to the management of patients, saving lives and expanding emergency care.

EMS Curricula

Although there are still similarities in some regions to the 1970s in how EMS manage their resources, overall the industry has significantly advanced and is far more effective and efficient. EMS have taken disaster response, management, and mitigation to a completely different level. They understand the impact and value of having competent, capable, and confident EMS providers. The need for advanced patient treatments and improved technologies drove the development of curricula of increasing length and time to allow for advancements in care outside of the hospital setting.

Today, EMS curricula utilize a competency-based structure and have stringent performance outcomes for KSAs taught [5]. The higher the level of EMS provider, the more contact hours required in completing curricula and clinical/field time. A Paramedic, therefore, has the highest KSA outcome assessments needed for completion. These assessments match the dynamic and complex scope of practice a paramedic is required to provide to any type of patient. Unfortunately, this increase in requirements in the various curricula may be contributing to a decrease in EMS volunteers nationally [6, 7]. The curricula growth is also a direct response to a number of healthcare trends resulting in ever more complex patients receiving care in an out-of-hospital setting. They include increased disease acuity, earlier hospital discharge, increased home care, a growing desire to decrease the number of individuals that visit an emergency department, and the push to manage patients at home with a referral to a specialty care or primary care physician. These trends have informed the next evolution in EMS care, the Mobile Integrated Healthcare (MIH) model discussed below in the Emerging Trends section.

EMS Regional Structure

At establishment, not every state adopted the same EMS operational structure, and forty years later, this fact continues to have a direct impact on EMS design and growth. In 1972, the first notable television series depicting paramedics was *Emergency*. This popular show depicted cutting-edge treatments, and the fire-based service model on which it was based had a huge influence on the industry. Today, each state allows different EMS services to structure their system as they feel would best serve the public. As a result, particular regions may have a mix of private-, fire-, government-, or hospital-based services that may or may not operate collaboratively. Such decisions regarding EMS structure within a community were made in the 1970's and 1980's when the current treatment models, quality assurance requirements, fiscal responsibility, and scope of practice did not exist. There is an attempt at the national level to formalize and streamline the various treatment and system models through curriculum-based instruction, federal oversight, and national accreditation. The goals of this effort are to improve patient care, patient safety, provider competence and confidence, and EMS system utilization and deployment. Nonetheless, although similar, each EMS model is unique, and a particular system is neither stronger nor more beneficial as compared to another. The implementation and utilization of a specific EMS model will always be dependent on the precise regional requirements where the care is being delivered.

Staffing Models

Just as the system structure is regionally based, so too is the staffing of a particular responding EMS unit. Some areas may utilize an EMT with a Paramedic partner while other systems utilize two paramedics. In many communities, a multi-tier response system is in place allowing for several agencies with different levels of EMS care providers to respond to a single emergency incident. Alternatively, a system may also opt to adopt a model where a variety of healthcare providers staff a single emergency response ambulance. This model can include combinations of care providers from the EMR level up to and including physicians, RNs, or other in-hospital care providers such as RTs.

In addition to the challenges in managing an EMS model and adequately staffing it, EMS agencies have also had to cope with the recent increase in the number of critical care transport vehicles in communities. These specialty transport vehicles are responsible for transporting a patient between two healthcare facilities. Their primary responsibility is to provide hospital-level, Intensive Care Unit (ICU) care in a mobile environment. As with traditional EMS units, staffing on a specialty transport vehicle is often regulated by the state office of EMS and is determined by the patient's level of disease acuity. Crew configuration may be similar to a traditional EMS vehicle, or it could include RT, RN, or even a physician. In some regions, systems opt to staff units with providers who can provide a higher level of care in order to allow the crew to take both 911 calls and critical care transport requests. These patient transfer situations have mandatory documentation and procedural criteria to ensure patient safety during transfer and transport. The documentation and procedural steps are often complex, and conflicts related to care instructions between the sending and receiving facilities are common. Today, opportunities to combat these unique situations do exist, and, by understanding current trends in the industry, we can better understand options for improving educational gaps and system processes.

Air Medical EMS

One aspect of EMS that is highly visible to the public is the air medical component. Including both rotor and fixed wing options, the growth and use of aircraft in civilian EMS arose from the sharing of trauma care methods between the military and civilian sectors. First used in 1926 in the military, the value of air medical transport and its decrease in time to definitive care was quickly recognized [8]. By the Korean War, it had evolved into the more common model of rotor wing evacuation. It was not until 1972, however, that the first civilian rotor wing service came into service based at St. Anthony's Hospital in Denver, Colorado. Rotor wing services are used for flights from emergency scenes where they meet ambulances at or near the location of a call for service, for interfacility transports between hospitals within a limited geographic range, for missions focused on search and rescue, and for the transport of organs. Fixed wing flights can transport patients thousands of miles and even between continents if needed. The staffing of air medical flights may routinely have two Paramedics or a Paramedic and Flight Nurse which is the most common for rotor-wing. Often, different personnel are either added or exchanged based on the patient needs, such as when a neonatal care team is used for the inter-facility transport of a premature infant. Today, air medical services are used for many different purposes. It is estimated that there are approximately 400,000 rotor wing and 150,000 fixed wing transports annually in the United States [9] (see Fig. 19.2).

Emerging Trends

A growing focus in prehospital medicine is the establishment and utilization of EMS providers to help patients manage all aspects of healthcare where they live. This concept presents a patient-centered focus in which healthcare resources are available in the mobile environment and brought to the patient. In this manner, EMS providers can help manage chronic diseases, provide education, or even follow-up with a patient after hospital discharge. The potential patient benefit and the increased scope of practice are significant leaps forward for EMS. Today,

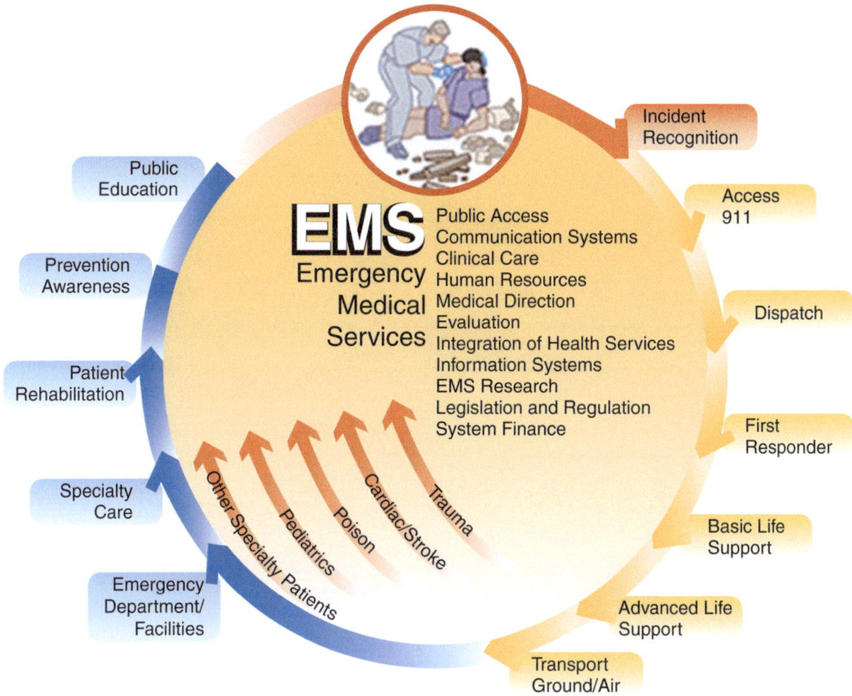

Fig. 19.2 This figure provides an overview of the aspects of the EMS system and the varied services it provides [10]

this growing trend is known as Mobile Integrated Healthcare and Community Paramedicine (MIH-CP). Figure 19.3 provides a detailed visual summary of how the Mobile Integrated Health initiate functions across a health system. Although MIH-CP has not been universally adopted, it is gaining widespread recognition, and systems are continuing to look for opportunities to address the fiscal constraints felt by the health systems to push an MIH-CP program forward. MIH-CP programs do vary based on the patient population and the needs of the area being served. Current MIH-CP initiatives are geared towards proactive patient interventions to keep individuals from being readmitted to a hospital or using the emergency department. The goal would be to triage those patients who are able to go to an urgent care, primary care, or specialty care physician setting. MIH-CP programs are integrated into the health care teams by using EMS providers with nursing, pharmacy, social services and other ancillary services to collaboratively address the needs of patients in the prehospital environment that do not fall into a 911 emergency response criteria.

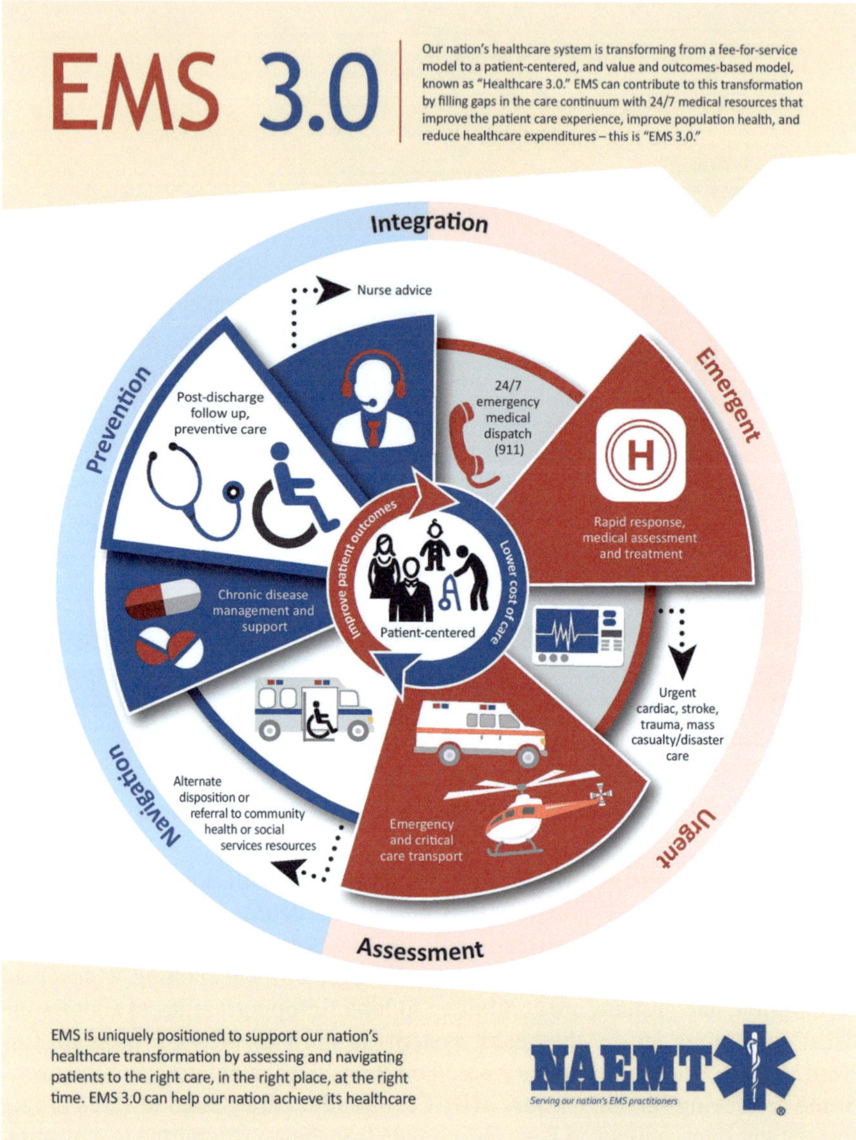

Fig. 19.3 This figure summarizes the Mobile Integrative Health initiative. Reproduced with permission from the National Association of Emergency Medical Technicians (NAEMT)

Federal agencies like The Joint Commission or the Centers for Medicare & Medicaid Services (CMS) identify and establish patient safety goals and measurable benchmarks for hospitals. Although the focus of EMS is to provide prehospital care, they directly impact many of the quality benchmarks established by these and other federal agencies. Additionally, the establishment of an MIH-CP program could bring to light the need to transition quality and patient safety goals from the hospital setting into the prehospital setting. Optimally, a collaborative approach between a healthcare system and an EMS service ensures the entire healthcare arena is meeting the needs of the patient, their family, and the community they all service. Benchmarks such as time to definitive care can easily be met when a more integrative team approach is utilized. Organizations must combat their desire to work in silos and be more collaborative, thus fostering an interprofessional relationship that allows for an entire team (EMS and hospital providers) to positively impact competence, confidence, and capability of the care team, and to meets the needs of the patient and their family members.

The Role of a Dispatch Center

To ensure consistency between call activation and emergency response, a centralized number routed through a dispatch center, is routinely utilized. While some dispatch centers are only 911 call centers, several centers primarily handle local events for critical care transport or non-emergency transport patients. Emergency Medical Dispatchers are an important part of EMS. They are responsible for information gathering, sharing, and prioritizing an emergency and non-emergency EMS response, and communicating between other agencies to ensure all members of the response team are safe. Despite their importance and impact, an Emergency Medical Dispatcher is often absent from the IPE design. Similar to the varied EMS system design between local and state agencies, dispatch centers are not structured the same. Unplanned calls for help usually follow Emergency Medical Dispatch (EMD) criteria, which select the level of response based on an evidence-based algorithm driven by the answers provided by civilians at the scene. Planned calls for non-emergency EMS assistance are typically scheduled events that require transfer of a patient to another facility for additional care or transport of the patient home after discharge. Additional circumstances do exist when an unplanned call for transport is managed in a non-emergency manner such as the activation of an MIH-CP provider. These events are handled by Emergency Medical Dispatchers who follow a strict criteria established by local, state, and federal agencies to ensure that transport is medically necessary.

Emergency Call Location and Influence

Geographic locations are routinely classified as urban, suburban, and rural. Each area has statistical and predictable emergency call types due to trends in that geographic location. Urban units tend to have the shortest response and patient contact times resulting in reduced time to complete patient care interventions [11] Suburban environments allow for both short and extended response and patient contact time dependent on the location of the hospital. As healthcare systems continue to modify their delivery model, the transport times and capability of the healthcare facilities will always be in flux. Based on their geographic location, rural areas by far have the longest response and patient contact times. This creates a unique environment where rural EMS providers must be comfortable with managing both simple and complex patients for longer periods of time resulting in a far greater number of medications and procedures to be completed. Additionally, rural EMS providers should have a greater understanding of pathophysiology, how to manage various diseases, and how to manage a critical patient for a longer period of time.

Patient Interactions

An EMS provider is trained to care for patients of all ages. No two patient interactions or presentations are alike and the EMS response can differ vastly because of a patient's own environment. EMS providers must be able to adapt to a variety of living conditions, unique family dynamics occurring at the scene, and/or specific patient religious or cultural needs. In cases where the patient or family refuses to interact with EMS providers, environmental clues must be used to facilitate interaction with the patient. The EMS provider, along with other interprofessional team members, may have to engage in detective work to ensure the care provided meets the needs of the patient.

Although the typical EMS response involves managing one patient at a time, occasionally, EMS providers may encounter two or more patients at an emergency scene. In addition, large-scale emergencies can happen and tax the EMS system. In events where the resources immediately available are less than the number of patients that need to be cared for, a mass casualty incident (MCI) is declared and the level of emergency response is increased. Regardless of the type of incident, EMS providers are prepared to handle these situations which are dynamic and often push providers outside of their comfort zone. EMS providers are trained to handle all types of illness and/or injury and to ensure that the patient and his or her family members are informed.

Interprofessional Discipline Overlap and Simulation

EMS providers almost always interact with other disciplines during a patient care response. The most probable overlap exists between dispatch, other public safety personnel, MIH-CP providers, and healthcare facilities. A variety of simulation activities/scenarios can directly improve patient outcomes focusing on this small overlap of disciplines. For example, police interacting with a simulated belligerent diabetic patient learn to recognize that this unusual behavior can also be caused by a medical condition such as hypoglycemia. Examples of simulation activities/scenarios that could benefit EMS providers could involve a patient suffering from excited delirium or managing an active shooter event with injured patients on the scene. The public call for help usually begin as an emergency call for a crime, not a medical emergency, yet the best practice approach requires an interprofessional response that includes the coordinated response of police, fire, and EMS dispatch agencies to achieve the best patient outcome [12].

If a patient is transported to a healthcare facility, it is imperative that the handoff communication involve provider-to-provider interaction to ensure there is appropriate transfer of care (e.g. report of medications administered and patient's medical history). In most cases, this hand-off would be from EMS provider to RN; however, a handoff may also occur between a RT, resident physician or attending physician. Industrial influences in the region offer unique experiences that influence EMS patient care including confined space rescue, hazardous materials decontamination, or terrain influences that require interprofessional teamwork to transfer the patient safely to a definitive treatment facility.

EMS and IPE Simulation Considerations

The key to a successful EMS response is the utilization of a team-based approach built on an understanding of the roles and capabilities of each member of the healthcare team and working together to achieve positive outcomes. An example of the success of working together is managing real world events where they occur and utilizing the individual skills of each team member to improve care. Simulating such complex care situations such as the one presented in Box 19.1 scenario is not easy but training together in a safe environment builds appropriate and positive individual and team performance characteristics to foster the learning process. Leveraging technology-based educational sessions such as simulation-based education activities allow the healthcare simulationist to design and implement realistic activities that can overcome challenges. A well-designed IPE simulation will engage human and system processes making the providers more effective and capable, the system stronger and safer, and quality of care improved.

Design Variety

The unpredictable and varied staffing, operational structure, and scope of treatment protocols make it difficult to dictate one standard for all EMS simulation

Box 19.1 Outline of How EMS Emergency Call Information May Be Provided

SCENARIO:

It is 10:00 am on a hot sunny day. A Paramedic and EMT receive a radio call:

> Medic 101, respond to 4873 Any Street for an unconscious 73-year-old female.

As they begin their response, the dispatcher advises that a home health nurse has arrived for a scheduled visit. The caller reports that the patient is breathing and has a pulse, but is not responding to verbal stimuli.

activity design. However, following best practices in healthcare simulation can ensure that organizations have an opportunity to bring structure and control in EMS education, enhance provider competency and capability, and improve system processes. It is this point in simulation-based education that healthcare simulation educators should adapt the crawl, walk, run model for simulation design. Reflection on the learning needs of an initial EMS student versus a seasoned EMS provider as well as the learning needs of other healthcare professionals makes it clear that that the design should engage, but not overwhelm the learners. An IPE simulation activity design varies based on the educational level of the learner. For a novice clinical learner, it easy to provide IPE activities focused on the expansive EMS scope of practice to raise awareness. These activities have been helpful to eliminate barriers between professionals who will ultimately be providing coordinated team-based patient care.

In 2016, the Center for Patient Safety identified ten topics to improve patient safety in EMS [13]. The following grid (Table 19.1) provides examples of how different professions can be integrated into IPE simulation activities related to the safety goals. Selection of a profession should be made by evaluating the simulation activity needs assessment, structure of EMS involved in the activity and identified learning objective(s).

Conducting a needs assessment provides guidance for planning simulation activities/scenarios (Box 19.2). Asking these types of questions (and many more) are essential in order to understand the EMS system within the larger public safety, public health, and healthcare systems. The answers to these questions are an important element in the analysis, design, develop, implementation, evaluation, and maintenance (ADDIE+M) of any simulation activity. By understanding the scope, practice, and role of the EMS providers involved in an IPE simulation activity, an educator can predict and ultimately test the flow and design of the activity. In addition, such an understanding will impact the overall time needed for the activity, the objectives, and the summative and formative assessments. These multiple factors can influence EMS's patient care; an incomplete understanding can lead to misunderstandings and create activities that are inaccurate. Obtaining as much information as possible upfront is important to support the needs assessment and design of the activity.

In designing your IPE simulation activity, it is imperative to have a communication and affective domain feedback component developed. EMS providers often overlook the importance of these two important steps in both effective patient care and impact in patient safety. Working in a less formal, uncontrolled environment also skews the providers' comparison point for "acceptable" action vs. "unacceptable" action [14, 15]. A disconnection of perspective often causes both inappropriate and hostile interprofessional interactions between EMS providers and other professions. EMS providers have higher on the job injuries, blood borne pathogen exposures, and life altering accidents than other health providers [16, 17]. It is important for healthcare team members to share experiences to foster a better understanding of the challenges faced by each clinical discipline. Designing an IPE simulation activity that allows for interaction between providers to occur in a

Table 19.1 This table provides an overview of the many professions that interact with EMS

EMS Safety Goal	Possible Team/Communication Interactions			
Airway Management	EMS and Physician (Emergency Department or Anesthesia)	EMS and Nursing	EMS and Respiratory Care	
Behavioral Emergencies	EMS and Police/Fire (As EMR)	EMS and Nursing Home Staff	EMS and Physician	EMS and Nursing (Emergency or Psychiatric)
Ambulance and Helicopter Crashes	EMS crew and Air Medical Crews	EMS and Air traffic/ Dispatch		
Device Failure	EMT and Paramedic	Paramedic and Nursing		
Medication Error	EMS and Police/Fire (pre-hospital administration of Narcan)	EMT and Paramedic	Paramedic and Paramedic	Paramedic and Nursing
Mobile Integrative Health – Community Para medicine	EMS and Nursing	EMS and Physician	EMS and Social Services	EMS and Pharmacy
Pediatric Patients	EMS and Physician	EMS and Nursing	EMS and Clergy	EMS and Suddent Infant Death Syndrome (SIDS) center
Safety Culture	EMS and Chief Quality Officer	EMS and Nursing	EMS and Physician	
Second Victim Intervention	EMS and Mental Health Professionals	EMS and Clergy		
Transition of Care ~ iPASS Illness severity Patient Summary Action List Situational awareness and planning Synthesis by reciever	Police/Fire First Responder to EMT Or Paramedic to Specialty Care Team	EMT to Paramedic Or EMS to Surgicenter	Paramedic to Nursing Or EMS to Doctor Office	Paramedic to Physician

safe environment, allows the healthcare team members to see each other's challenges. Design considerations are presented in Box 19.3. If healthcare providers can understand these challenges and responsibilities, and reflect on the impact each has towards patient safety and outcomes; the team will be in an improved position to foster a stronger team dynamic and better teamwork and communication. IPE simulation activities are an excellent way to achieve this lofty but important goal. By helping healthcare professionals collaborate and interact positively, the immediate and noticeable return any system will see is improvements in patient care and safety while also improving job satisfaction [18].

Box 19.2 Key Questions for a Needs Assessment

NEEDS ASSESSMENT:

To replicate the scenario as an IPE simulation activity, the educator will need to investigate the wide variety of issues that will be present through the various stages of this single call for EMS service. Here is a small sample of the questions that can be asked to investigate the factors involved in an IPE simulation that involves EMS.

- How is the EMS system structured?
- How does the dispatcher function and integrate with the responding crew?
- What is the scope of practice allowed for each of the EMS crew members on scene? What are the protocols in place to support this?
- Will there be an EMR on scene to assist?
- How is home health care integrated?
- In what ways will the team need to perform based on the different clinical decisions that are made throughout the transport?
- At what stage does the hospital portion of care become a part of the care process (e.g. on scene or during the transport?
- What care is delivered enroute and who might be involved if the patient is ill (extra providers in the transport)?
- When do additional resources in the hospital environment become engaged (e.g. response teams) based on the information received from the EMS unit?
- How does patient care transition from the EMS unit to the Emergency Department? Who is involved?

Box 19.3. Design Factors for EMS IPE Simulation

DESIGN CONSIDERATIONS:

While the requested or desired reasons for including EMS in an IPE activity can vary widely, there are some consistent considerations related to EMS that the educator should consider for all IPE activities where they are included:

- What are the communication concepts that must be addressed?
- What opportunities exist to break down the silos between professions and enhance the understanding and awareness of the other professions?
- How can the activity be designed to identify systems issues and challenges or to then support improving the system in the future?
- Where are the common challenges faced by each of the professions involved that can be included?
- What variations exist between the multiple EMS agencies that serve an individual area that create the need for design modifications dependent on participants?

Typical IPE EMS Activities

The most common IPE EMS simulation activities involve an overlap with other public safety departments. An EMS simulation activity may also involve a combination of public safety and hospital personnel simulating a hand-off from the prehospital to the hospital environment or hospital to a critical care transport team. Responses to doctor/dental offices or surgical centers serve as an easy conduit for transfer of care in an emergency. For example, transfer of care in an emergency department can be between EMS to RN, EMS to physician, EMS to an advanced practice provider, EMS to RT, or EMS to a specialized service such as neurology, cardiology or trauma services due to a specific code activation. A rare overlap can include transfer of care to a healthcare provider in obstetrics, burn care, or dialysis. Every EMS provider is required to complete, at a minimum, annual education competency assessments to facilitate recertification and/or re-licensure. These mandatory assessments provide opportunity to enhance the amount of EMS IPE simulation activities. Unfortunately, a significant challenge in EMS education is creating a realistic environment that mimics challenges in managing scene safety. The growing concern is being able to simulate a high-risk environment without endangering or impacting the safety of the learners. There is a balance and that balance must always weigh the importance of keeping the learners' safe regardless of the learning objective. Additionally, it is imperative that the experience involves all aspects of care to include care for the patient during movement.

An example of the value of IPE is when EMS providers are required to complete rotations with anesthesia providers in the operating room (OR) to develop clinical competence in managing an airway. Unfortunately, this training can cause the EMS provider unnecessary stress. An IPE simulation activity with anesthesia providers to provide training on airway management could improve the comfort of the EMS provider as well as prepare the EMS provider for actual hands on airway management involving an actual patient out of the hospital setting. This would allow the team to learn about each other's roles and to understand how they can work together when the EMS provider is tasked with working in the real OR environment. The key is to foster capability, confidence, and competence of the student and the other healthcare team members. Additionally, the learner begins to understand the environment, their role, their team members' roles, and the processes of that unfamiliar clinical setting. Long term, the effectiveness IPE simulation activities environment can be seen translated in the real world as the benefits to improving the quality of patient care become better known.

Most healthcare disciplines can utilize a simulation activity once as they focus solely on medical care and communication. In EMS, scenarios can be modified with environmental and fidelity factors that adjust the mandatory actions, despite the patient presentation and care requirements.

Code Activations and Patient Flow

It is important to trial an IPE simulation activity before implementation of a new policy or practice that affects patient care. Using simulation to first test a new policy allows for streamlining and improvement that otherwise would not occur before implementation. This is especially important when such policies directly impact patient care or could alter how a patient is transferred from the prehospital setting into a hospital environment. For example, a 52-year-old is experiencing chest pain and the prehospital providers determine the patient is having a heart attack. Instead of transporting the patient to the emergency department, the consulting physician advises that the patient should be taken directly to Cardiac Catheterization Lab bypassing the Emergency Department. An IPE simulation activity can also be used to improve the flow of information from the prehospital environment to the hospital. An IPE simulation activity could include a scenario where EMS and Nursing interact, and patient hand-off is required in the activity. The patient received multiple interventions before hospital arrival. There are many factors that can impede a proper patient hand off. High Emergency Department census, the high acuity patient being transferred, current patient care ratios, poor past experiences between providers; just to name a few. The simulation activity could address each of these factors and allow the providers to practice better standard patient hand off. Even less obvious simulation activities regarding the flow of information, such as EMS supply and pharmacy replenishment processes, can provide data about the time, impact, and efficiency while identifying opportunities for improvement.

Atypical IPE EMS Activities

Medical emergencies can occur in any patient care environments. Often these emergencies are rare, and the health professionals have never needed to render emergency care until the EMS arrives. Practicing medical emergencies is an easy way to implement initial IPE simulation activities between EMS and other health professions. For example, a dental hygiene medical emergency response integrates two professions that normally do not interact but may be required to because of a medical emergency during dental treatment. Facilitating patient treatments like seizure management or CPR in a dental chair can be challenging and must involve a variety of healthcare team members to ensure it is done effectively avoiding issues with unknown equipment and tight spaces. The transfer of care between the dental team and the EMS crew can be confusing because of the equipment that may have been utilized during the dental procedure. These atypical IPE with simulation activities are high risk, low yield activities that require a significant amount of preplanning to ensure it is an effective and safe teaching environment.

EMS IPE: Lessons Learned

The EMS scope of practice and the complex nature of healthcare is, unfortunately, creating a natural barrier for integrating realistic IPE simulation activities. Although cost associated with utilizing simulation-based education has continued to be a significant concern over the years, the technology is available within the industry. EMS programs have invested in the technology but have not provided educators with the foundational skills or time needed to effectively integrate IPE with simulation [19].

It is important to optimize educational opportunities both in the planning and debriefing phases with learners. By doing this early on, we hope to avoid creating a series of false assumptions which can ultimately undermine an objectively driven simulation activity. By identifying staffing levels and patterns, and their respective affiliated organization, we can further highlight the complexities related to creating an IPE simulation activity. Furthermore, this may help identify possible future IPE activities. The design of simulation scenarios should address a need, establish a competency or competencies, enhance capability, or improve a process [20].

The care provided by EMS is not just life and death decisions. EMS trauma responses account for less than 20% of the overall service activation and in some areas, the percentage is much lower [21]. It is less important to develop a situation where blood, guts, and gore are a significant part of the scenario [22]. IPE simulation activities involving EMS providers should be structured and based on data identified by evaluating the EMS services in the local region where the simulation activity will be offered. The local EMS leadership can provide a more accurate breakdown of the types of calls, amount of contact time with a patient, and the most frequently accessed destination for patient care. This information can be used to design a better simulation activity that is relevant to the learning objectives and realistic for the learners.

As you review the potential impact and implication for developing and implementing an IPE simulation activity, it is equally imperative that the value of IPE is not forgotten. The teamwork and communication needed to be successful in EMS involves the EMS team members understanding their own strengths and weaknesses. An often forgotten, but unique simulation experience involves an intraprofessional simulation focused on emergency response, care, and transport that ultimately ends with the public safety team managing a complex scene and involving the local healthcare system. Scenarios such as a mass casualty drill can create just such an intraprofessional and interprofessional simulation experience.

Scheduling EMS IPE simulation activities can be difficult. If interacting with initial learners, the curricula are packed with limited opportunity for including non-mandatory topics or activities. For experienced providers, scheduling educational opportunities around their shift rotation can be difficult. Optimally, offering a variety of opportunities to attend an IPE simulation experience ensures that all shifts can participate. By obtaining buy-in from EMS leadership, you have a greater chance of improving participation. Due to the varied EMS structures, engaging with the EMS leadership early in the process as you begin to plan your educational activity, will garner support. By showing them the value of IPE with simulation, you may find a new pivotal partner.

Conclusion

The complex varied national structure and wide-ranging level of EMS providers have resulted in a public identity problem for the EMS profession. Providers are often referred to as "ambulance drivers," yet their scope of practice allows them to perform the most advanced pharmacologic administrations and invasive procedures, in some areas without consulting a physician. EMS personnel interact with a wide range of other health professions. Including EMS in IPE simulation activities, offers a mechanism for raising awareness about EMS patient care services while also improving communication between professions that often overlap outside of the hospital. While these activities require specific questions to ensure the proper design and thus a successful activity, the EMS profession is eager to be included in IPE activities. Despite the differences in system structure, personnel staffing, or scope of practice, EMS personnel are seeking ways to improve patient safety. By involving them in an IPE simulation activity, patient safety and improved patient outcomes can become an important shared goal.

References

1. NHTSA. Review of National 911 Data Collection. July 2013. [Online] Available from: https://www.911.gov/pdf/current911datacollection-072613.pdf.
2. NASEMSO. National EMS Assessment. December 2009. [Online] Available from: https://www.nasemso.org/documents/National_EMS_Assessment_Final_Draft_12202011.pdf.
3. NHTSA. Safety in numbers. DOT HS 812 027. May 2014. [Online] Available from: https://www.ems.gov/pdf/ems-data/Provider-Resources/SafetyInNumbers_EMS_May2014.pdf.
4. Institute of Medicine. Emergency Medical services at the crossroads. Washington, D.C.: National Academies Press; 2007. Chapter 6.
5. NHTSA. National EMS Education Standards. DOT HS 811 077A. January 2009. [Online] Available from: https://www.ems.gov/pdf/education/EMS-Education-for-the-Future-A-Systems-Approach/National_EMS_Education_Standards.pdf.
6. Margolis GS, Studnek J, Fernandez AR. Will work for free. Are volunteerism rates falling? J Emerg Med Serv. 2006;31(5):48, 51.
7. Federal Interagency Committee on Emergency Medical Services. 2011 National EMS Assessment. U.S. Department of Transportation, National Highway Traffic Safety Administration, DOT HS 811 723,Washington, D.C.; 2012. [Online] Available from: www.ems.gov; page 106.
8. Martin T. Aeromedical transportation: a clinical guide. Boca Raton: Taylor & Francis Group; 2006.
9. Varon J, Wenker O, Fromm R Jr. Aeromedical transport: facts and fiction. Internet J Emerg Intensive Care Med. 2006;1(1).
10. NHTSA. What is EMS? 2007. [Online] Available from: https://www.ems.gov/whatisEMS.html.
11. Patel A, Waters N, Blanchard I, Doig C, Ghali W. A validation of ground ambulance pre-hospital times modeled using geographic information systems. Int J Health Geogr. 2012;11(1):42.
12. Roach B, Echols K, Burnett A. Excited delirium and the dual response: preventing in-custody deaths. July 2014. [Online] Available from: https://leb.fbi.gov/2014/july/excited-delirium-and-the-dual-responsepreventing-in-custody-deaths.
13. Center for Patient Safety. EMS forward: the ten patient safety topics. January 2016. [Online] Available from: http://aams.org/wp-content/uploads/2016/02/EMSFORWARD-PS-10.pdf.
14. Marx JA, Rosen P. Rosen's emergency medicine: concepts and clinical practice. 8th ed. Philadelphia: Elsevier/Saunders; 2014. p. 2507.
15. Banja J. The normalization of deviance in healthcare delivery. Business Horizons. 2010;53(2):139. [Online] Available from: https://doi.org/10.1016/j.bushor.2009.10.006.
16. Reichard A, Marsh S, Moore P. Fatal and nonfatal injuries among emergency medical technicians & paramedics. Prehosp Emerg Care. 2011;15(4):511–7.

17. Mazen ES, Kue R, McNeil C, et al. A descriptive analysis of occupational health exposures in an urban emergency medical services system: 2007–2009. Prehosp Emerg Care. 2011;15(4):506–10.
18. O'Daniel M, Rosenstein AH. Professional communication and team collaboration. In: Hughes RG, editor. Patient safety and quality: an evidence-based handbook for nurses, Advances in patient safety. Rockville: Agency for Healthcare Research and Quality (US); 2008. [Online] Available from: http://www.ncbi.nlm.nih.gov/books/NBK2637/.
19. McKenna K, Carhart E, Bercher D, Spain A, Todaro J, Freel J. Simulation use in paramedic education research (SUPER): a descriptive study. Prehosp Emerg Care J. 2015;19(3):432–40.
20. INACSL Standards Committee. INACSL standards of best practice: simulation SM Simulation design. Clin Simulat Nurs. 2016;12(S):S5–S12. [Online] Available from: https://doi.org/10.1016/j.ecns.2016.09.005; https://www.inacsl.org/INACSL/document-server/?cfp=INACSL/assets/File/public/standards/SOBPEnglishCombo.pdf.
21. MMWR: Morbidity and Mortality Weekly Report. Guidelines for field triage of injured patients. January 13, 2012. [Online] Available from: https://www.cdc.gov/mmwr/pdf/rr/rr6101.pdf.
22. Blaug G, Hochner A, Portwood J. What variables affect public perceptions for EMS meeting general community needs? J Allied Health. 2012;41(2):e39–43.

Correction to: Applications of Simulation-Based Interprofessional Education in Labor and Delivery

Colleen A. Lee, Dena Goffman, Peter S. Bernstein, David L. Feldman, and Komal Bajaj

Correction to: Chapter 17 in: J. T. Paige et al. (eds.), *Comprehensive Healthcare Simulation: InterProfessional Team Training and Simulation*, Comprehensive Healthcare Simulation, https://doi.org/10.1007/978-3-030-28845-7

The book was inadvertently published with incorrect affiliation of all the authors in Chapter 17. This has now been corrected in Chapter 17 as below:

Colleen A. Lee MS, RN[1], Dena Goffman MD[2,3], Peter S. Bernstein MD, MPH[4], David L. Feldman MD, MBA[5], Komal Bajaj MD, MS-HPEd[4,6]

[1]Weill Cornell Medicine
Physician Organization-Quality and Patient Safety
New York, NY, USA

[2]Department of Quality and Patient Safety
New York-Presbyterian Hospital
New York, NY, USA

[3]Department of Obstetrics and Gynecology
Columbia University Medical Center
New York, NY, USA

[4]Department of Obstetrics & Gynecology and Women's Health
Albert Einstein College of Medicine/Montefiore Medical Center
Bronx, NY, USA

[5]Healthcare Risk Advisors, The Doctors Company
New York, NY, USA

[6]Department of Obstetrics and Gynecology
Jacobi Medical Center, NYC Health + Hospitals
Bronx, NY, USA

The updated version of this chapter can be found at https://doi.org/10.1007/978-3-030-28845-7_17

J. T. Paige et al. (eds.), *Comprehensive Healthcare Simulation: InterProfessional Team Training and Simulation*, Comprehensive Healthcare Simulation,
https://doi.org/10.1007/978-3-030-28845-7_20

Index

J. T. Paige et al. (eds.), *Comprehensive Healthcare Simulation: InterProfessional Team Training and Simulation*, Comprehensive Healthcare Simulation,
https://doi.org/10.1007/978-3-030-28845-7

MIX
Papier aus verantwortungsvollen Quellen
Paper from responsible sources
FSC® C105338

If you have any concerns about our products,
you can contact us on
ProductSafety@springernature.com

In case Publisher is established outside the EU,
the EU authorized representative is:
Springer Nature Customer Service Center GmbH
Europaplatz 3, 69115 Heidelberg, Germany

Printed by Libri Plureos GmbH
in Hamburg, Germany